Functional Gastroenterology

Functional Gastroenterology

Assessing And Addressing The Causes Of Functional Gastrointestinal Disorders

Steven Sandberg-Lewis, ND, DHANP

Second Edition

© 2009, 2017 by Steven Sandberg-Lewis, ND

All Rights Reserved. First edition 2009 published by NCNM Press

Second edition 2017
Printed in the USA

ISBN: 978-0-692-86466-1

Illustrations by Leah Sherman, ND
Senior Editor: Kayle Sandberg-Lewis, LMT, MA, BCN Fellow

No part of this book may be reproduced or transmitted in any form or by any means, electronic or mechanical, including photocopying, recording, or by any information storage or retrieval system, without the prior written permission of the publisher, except where permitted by law.

For permission contact:
Steven Sandberg-Lewis
5331 SW Macadam Ave
Suite 380
Portland, OR 97239

e-mail: funcgastro@gmail.com

To my mother, Joyce Sandberg,
and to the memory of my father, Robert Sandberg,
for their love, support and patience.

Table Of Contents

List Of Tables And Illustrations

Tables

Illustrations

Foreword

Functional Gastroenterology*: Assessing and Addressing the Causes of Functional Gastrointestinal Disorders* by Dr. Steven Sandberg-Lewis ND, DHANP is a book that is long overdue. While many Gastroenterology texts focus on pathology, diagnosis and current drug therapy, this work views the GI tract and its function in much greater depth. In the chapters that follow, Dr. Sandberg-Lewis discusses not only the scientific aspects of gastroenterology but also the art of medicine as it pertains to the assessment of diseases and dysfunctions of the gastrointestinal tract. *Functional Gastroenterology* explores the gastrointestinal tract in terms of a living and dynamic ecosystem, its endocrinology, and its interaction with the central nervous system and the environment.

In this work, Dr. Sandberg-Lewis constructs a symphony of function, biochemistry, diet and ecosystem interactions, effects of the environment and stressors, and the gastrointestinal nervous system, which aid the practitioner in understanding how the art and science of medicine must both be used in order to achieve optimal and lasting health.

Dr. Sandberg-Lewis discusses the philosophical differences between the reductionist and holistic views of medicine noting that within the last thirty years a more biopsychosocial model of gastroenterology is emerging, but as with all changes in medicine, they are slow to be embraced by the dominant school of thought. Whereas allopathy treats the perceived gastrointestinal dysfunction with drugs and surgery to allay symptomology, the functional gastrointestinal model allows the practitioner to view the dysfunction in terms of an imbalance of the different systems that interact within the GI tract in order to maintain homeostasis. Once perceived, the practitioner will be able to provide a more specific intervention to allow the homeostatic balance to be restored rather than prescribe medications that mask symptoms of GI distress while maintaining the imbalance. Viewing the gastrointestinal dynamic in a functional and integrated manner embodies the naturopathic precepts of Tolle Causum, Tolle Totum, while following the Hierarchy of Health and the Therapeutic Order, models embraced by naturopathic medicine in order to restore optimal health.

Modern medicine, in its drive to be more efficient through managed care, often misses the opportunity to know both the patient and their disease state at the functional level. Following some routine laboratory tests, colonoscopy and perhaps a CT, it then becomes a matter of dispensing routine prescriptions to allay symptoms. Often these require additional prescriptions when the dysfunction adapts to previous ones or were incorrect to begin with. Dr. Sandberg-Lewis addresses the effects that long term drugging has upon the GI tract noting its propensity to add to the many diseases encountered there, or create new ones. In contradistinction, the functional gastroenterology model allows the practitioner to make more specific and meaningful prescriptions to stimulate the vital force, thereby allowing the healing reaction to go to completion.

With his many years of clinical experience and scholarly contributions, Dr. Steven Sandberg-Lewis has produced a work that synthesizes the integrative approach to medicine, one that naturopathic clinicians have practiced and expounded for over 100 years. To this end, Dr. Sandberg-Lewis provides the reader with diagnostic tools, laboratory evaluations and therapeutic suggestions to help the practitioner better understand the cause of the dysfunction. Understanding the many things that can lead to disease and dysfunction of the gastrointestinal tract, utilizing many time tested diagnostic and therapeutic methodologies, and melding the art and science of medicine, provides practitioners with the tools to restore and maintain health for their patients. By writing this text, Dr. Sandberg-Lewis sets a precedent and standard for other practitioners of naturopathic medicine to put down in written form the art and science of naturopathic medicine.

Thomas A. Kruzel, ND
Author of *The Homeopathic Emergency Guide*
Scottsdale, Arizona
August 2009

Acknowlegements

I wish to thank Nora Sande, who encouraged me to write and reminded me of that commitment every time we saw each other. No doubt I would not have written the first edition in just short of a year without her persistence.

Thanks to David Schleich, president of the National University of Natural Medicine (NUNM), for his vision. He created the first series of sabbaticals for NUNM professors and brought his decades of publishing experience to the creation of the NUNM Press.

Thanks to my wife, Kayle, for her tireless editing, and along with my sons Asher and Ezra for being such a supportive family.

Thanks also to copy editor, Jenny Bowlden, for graciously making repeated corrections and modifications for the first edition, and Nancy and Richard Stodart of Fourth Lloyd Productions for all their work on the second edition.

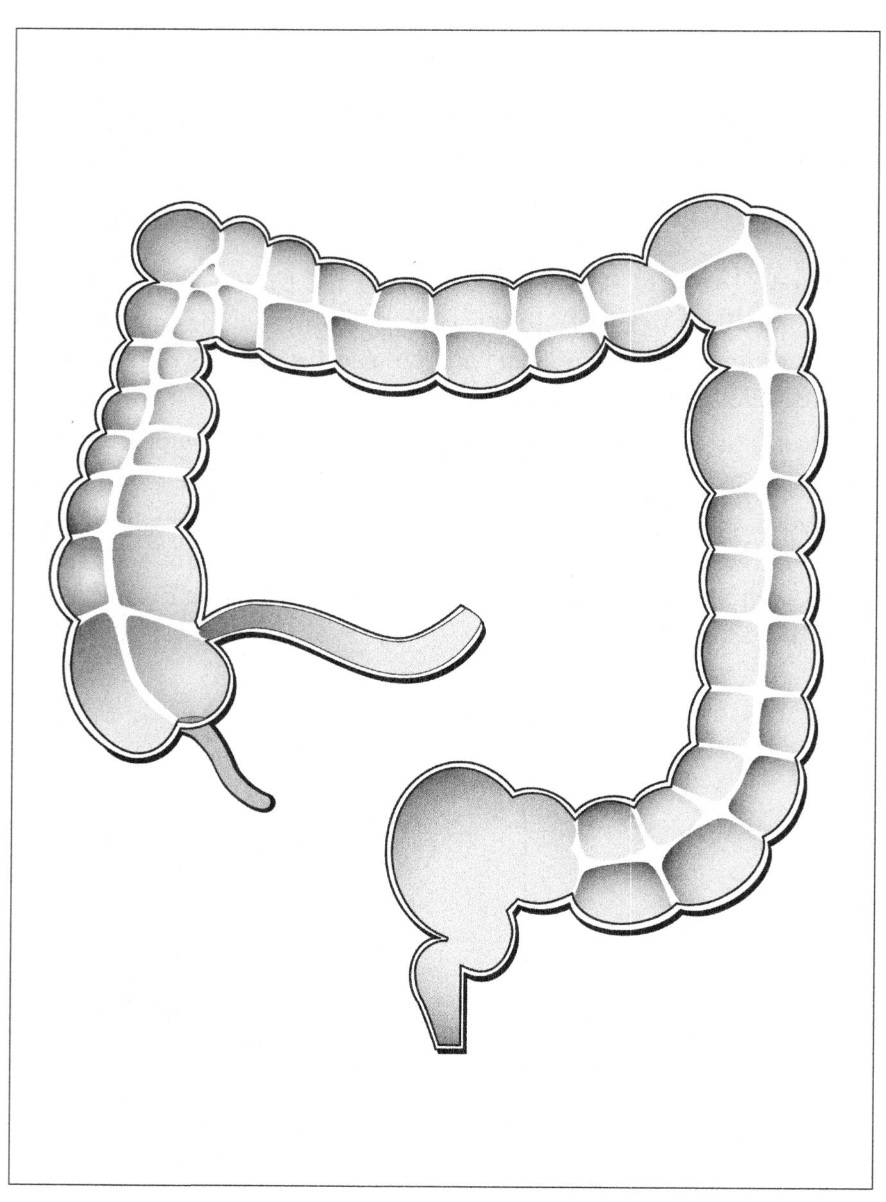

Introduction

The Medical Thought Process

Ramban, the physician (Rabbi Moshe ben Nachman– 1194-1270) is credited with first saying "you are what you eat." Someone a bit less thrifty with his words said "you are what you believe, think, feel, eat, drink, digest, absorb, tolerate or mount an immune response to, metabolize, circulate and eliminate." The latter is my approach.

This book is designed to explain the use of assessment and treatment strategies for functional conditions. The focus will be on improving normal function of the GI tract and pathologies will be discussed only as they apply to function.

How Doctors Think, by Jerome Groopman, MD (Houghton Mifflin, Boston, NY 2007) is an excellent starting point in the discussion of the thought processes of physicians. Although Groopman's work, which includes the input of psychologists Amos Tversky and Daniel Kahneman, is based on the epistemology used by allopathic physicians, it has lessons for all schools of medicine. Groopman's work motivated me to combine his findings with my own observations in the hope the reader will find this information valuable in approaching the assessment of both pathology and functional disorders.

Below are six common pitfalls in the medical thought process:

Anchoring (Groopman)

Finding a "reasonable" explanation for a patient's state should not stop further consideration of alternative diagnoses. Anchoring is the tendency to latch on to a diagnosis and stick to it. Physicians often do this because it's easy or because a particular explanation just seems "right". Being convinced too soon can lead to missing the mark and treating the patient for the wrong disorder. Perhaps the patient has more than one condition and anchoring to a single condition may prevent the consideration of a more serious co-morbidity.

Early in my career I had an office visit with a sexually active young woman complaining of vaginal itching and dyspareunia. The pelvic exam revealed a classic "strawberry cervix" and the wet prep showed

Trichomoniasis. Had I looked further, I might have noticed a mucopurulent endocervical discharge. Had I been more thorough and cultured for Neisseria gonorrhea, I would have found it (the available test in the 1970s.) I diagnosed Trichomoniasis and missed the gonorrhea. Another practitioner diagnosed it a week or two later when her dyspareunia failed to clear up.

Diagnosis Momentum (Groopman)

Related to the concept of anchoring is the concept of diagnosis momentum. It is the tendency for a diagnostic label to build belief and power to the point that it is hard to stop. A diagnosis can have weight and influence on management and treatment that defies questioning. My suggestion is to always send for the labs, films, surgical notes and biopsy reports and to not blindly accept a diagnosis handed down from another health practitioner. Make sure it makes sense to you. The patient deserves this 2nd or 3rd opinion and it will help you be a better doctor. An example is a young girl who for many years had been institutionalized for psychotic episodes. Eventually her parents were able to prevail in searching for an alternative explanation and she had the good fortune to find a doctor who re-examined the diagnosis and tested for Lyme disease. The antimicrobial treatment reversed much of her Lyme encephalitis and she no longer needed antipsychotic medication.

Confirmation Bias (Groopman)

I have frequently seen physicians find confirmation by selecting and focusing only on information that fits a diagnosis or plan of action while throwing out (or failing to recognize) information that contradicts the presumed correct path. A good example of this type of thinking is found in the homeopathic repertorization process. More obscure ("small") remedies may be ignored when going through a list of remedies. The doctor may not know the name or the abbreviation of the remedy (ie. *Arum t*) and it will be treated as if it is invisible—completely left out of the remedy selection process. Had the remedy been one familiar to the physician, it would be considered and perhaps given extra weight as a remedy choice.

Availability (From Tversky And Kahneman)

This is a tendency to jump to a conclusion about a case based on a recent experience with similar case presentations or other easily available patterns of presentation. An example was a case seen in our teaching clinic several years ago. A woman in her early fifties presented with a severe sore throat, and symptoms/signs of low grade fever and malaise. Her daughter brought her to our clinic because she had been sick for almost two weeks, was not getting well and had developed the pain in the throat. A student intern took her history and performed an ENT exam and came to the conclusion that it was a viral pharyngitis. The intern based the initial diagnosis on the fact that it was winter in Portland, Oregon and her findings seemed to fit a prolonged pharyngitis. Taking the differential a bit deeper, we re-examined the woman and found that her external throat was intensely tender to palpation over the thyroid gland and the soreness was triggered by rotating the head. The thyroid gland was palpably enlarged. This was actually a case of granulomatous thyroiditis (DeQuervain thyroiditis.) This was confirmed by an abnormally low TSH level and a sedimentation rate of 70. Certainly, this uncommon cause of painful goiter is self-limiting over a six to eight week period, but we treated her with homeopathic Spongia tosta 30C which resulted in excellent pain control.

Commision Bias (Groopman)

The rushed feeling that something must be done is something most of us will recognize. It may be more likely if the doctor has a special focus on a certain treatment approach, and more options are not immediately felt to be available. In any case, a quote from Linda Lewis, MD is apt—"Don't just do something, stand there!" Slowing down and considering what is truly appropriate is better than the mindset of action for action's sake.

Attribution Errors—Emotions In The Thought Process (Groopman)

Naturopathic students and physicians, like most health care workers, tend to develop an emotional stance toward their patients. A great quote from *How Doctors Think* is "If we feel our emotions deeply, we risk recoiling or breaking down—if we erase them we fail to care for the patient." Whether the feelings are positive or negative toward a patient does not prevent them from clouding the practitioners perspective. These are errors of attribution.

A simple example occurred in my practice. One of my patients referred his thirty year-old daughter to my practice. She had a two-year history of recurrent sinusitis. I used a procedure called "nasal specific technique" with curative effects and we were all very happy with the results. Further history and physical exam revealed that she had moderate hypertension. When we discussed taking her blood pressure at home to rule out "white coat hypertension", she said that merely the idea of having her pressure checked was daunting to her. She would not check it at home. I found myself avoiding checking her vitals as we continued to have visits around this issue. I realized during a follow-up visit that I hadn't taken a blood pressure reading in a very long time. Luckily, no health crisis had developed for her, but when I realized my avoidance of this simple test out of a desire not to stress my patient, I knew it was an error in judgment. I discussed it with her and she agreed to monitor it regularly.

Some Thoughts On Improving Medical Decision Making

Thinking Outside The Box

One of my favorite R. Crumb comics shows two men sitting in a crowded, dark space with barely enough room to move. They are discussing a small hole in the wall through which a beam of light can be seen. One suggests peeking through the hole. The other warns that that would be dangerous. The final frame shows a beautiful sunny field in a meadow where the crate sits, still holding the two men arguing about whether to peer out of the box.

Thinking and looking laterally rather than straight ahead is incredibly valuable. Looking up a differential list, researching the literature, talking to other practitioners about a case or re-reading a file from start to finish may bring up an entirely new perspective.

Pattern Recognition

Groopman describes how experienced physicians "within seconds, largely without any conscious analysis" recognize certain patterns. This process is not linear or step by step and the clues come from all directions at once.

The renowned homeopath, George Vithoulkas, explained the process of seeing the essence of homeopathic types as pattern recognition. He described how one may recognize someone from a distance not based on specific features, but on a collection of impressions—stature, posture, gait, etc. Another great homeopath, Paul Herscu, put pattern recognition in another context. He told of a trip he and his family took to Africa when they toured the plains in an open air bus. The sightseers were warned to keep their arms inside the frame of the bus. Their guides explained that lions do not recognize humans as prey when they are amalgamated into the shape of a bus, but if they can see limbs or heads as a separate outline, they may well suspect a potential meal and attack.

Alternate Anatomy

Consider variations from normal anatomy to prevent limited thinking. For example, remember that the transverse colon may be prolapsed, descending so as to compress the bladder; the cecum is in an ascending position (as far superior as the hepatic flexure) in about 6% and on the left side in about 0.5% of abdomens (Smith, G.M, "A Statistical Review of the Variations in the Anatomic Positions of the Cecum and Processus Vermiformis in the Infant," *Anat. Rec.*, 5:549, 1911.)

Strategies To Consider When The Thought Process Is Stuck

These may be used in case analysis, diagnosis, choosing a remedy, etc.

1. Ask the patient to tell the story in his or her own words again—"As if I'd never heard it before. What were your thoughts and feelings both emotionally and physically? How did it happen? … When did it happen?"
2. Consider: Is there anything that doesn't fit?
3. Could there be more than one problem/condition/disease?
4. Could the treatment have been compounded, labeled or taken incorrectly?

Here are two examples of this from my practice:

The first was a 38 year old woman on oral birth control, who complained of a brief menstrual flow occurring weekly, over the previous 3 weeks. On closer inspection, the flow always began on Sunday. It was discovered that Sunday was the only day of the week that she did not have a scheduled waking time. With no schedule, she would fail to take the daily pill, hence triggering breakthrough bleeding.

The second example relates to compounding of medications. In previous years, I prescribed a time release form of T3 (triiodothyronine) for patients with thyroid hormone conversion problems (Wilson's syndrome). At one point, I noticed that the benefits my patients had previously enjoyed from this treatment were now minimal. About a year into this phase, I received a letter from the compounding pharmacy explaining they had discovered the T3 they were using had been mislabeled by the supplier. It was actually T4. That would mean I had been prescribing miniscule amounts of T4 and no T3. Since these patients all had normal T4 levels to begin with and the capsules contained only 7.5 mcg, the treatment, although mostly harmless, was also mostly worthless.

5. Don't let finance guide you. Outline a diagnostic and treatment approach you feel is optimal for the patient. Let the patient decide whether to vary from your focus on excellence. If the case is complex, you can work with the patient to prioritize phases for your approach.
6. As discussed above under "diagnosis momentum" do not blindly accept another physician's diagnosis. Send for the biopsy, films, surgical report, etc.
7. Discuss the case with other physicians and health care practitioners. Case conferencing can open your eyes to new possibilities.

Steven Sandberg-Lewis, ND, DHANP

Chapter 1

Functional Gastroenterology

Factors Involved in the Adaptive Physiology of FGID
- *Genetics*
- *Family of origin stress and disease coping orientation*
- *Psychological factors*
- *Altered motility*
- *Altered inflammation*
- *Altered visceral sensitivity*
- *Altered intestinal permeability*
- *Food allergy and intolerance*

Rome IV Diagnostic Categories

Irritable Bowel Syndrome
- *Epidemiology of IBS*
- *Typical symptoms of IBS*
- *Subcategories of IBS diagnosis*

Biomedical Treatment of IBS
- *IBS-C specific drugs*
- *IBS-D specific drugs*
- *Treatments for IBS pain/spasm*

Naturopathic Assessment

The practice of functional gastroenterology requires the physician to

- understand normal digestive function and ecology
- assess the structure, neurology, flora, motility, secretion, detoxification and psychoneuroimmunoendocrine aspects of the patient's picture
- apply effective natural (and pharmaceutical) therapies

Reductionism as a model of the human body is still dominant in Western medicine. It is claimed that this perspective evolved from the struggle between Descarte and the Catholic church during the 17th century. Separation of mind from body—an impossible goal—was agreed upon in order to gain permission for physicians to dissect cadavers. The mind, as the seat of the soul, was to be left to the church. Physicians were to limit their study and care to the "body". This was a great step forward for the study of anatomy and pathology and a giant step backward for the understanding and treatment of functional disorders.

In the last thirty years, an integrated biopsychosocial model of disease has emerged in allopathic/biomedicine and has gone a long way to add acceptance to functional disorders. In 2016 Rome IV, the latest world conference on functional gastrointestinal disorders (FGID) expanded its discussion to include the microbiota, gut-brain axis interactions, as well as cross-cultural understanding of FGID. It is becoming closer to what is needed to understand optimal function and methods of assessment and treatment of functional GI disorders, but has yet to jump the chasm between theory and practice. This book is my attempt to fill that void.

Table 1.1 Functional GI Disorders—The Big Picture

<table>
<tr>
<td>

Early Life

- **Genetics (miasma)**
- **Prenatal Life and Birth Process**
  - Maternal stress
  - Maternal diet and medical Rx
  - Maternal alcohol/tobacco/drugs
  - Maternal environmental exposures
  - Maternal breathing patterns
  - Vaginal vs Cesarean birthing
- **Environment**
  - Air quality
  - Water quality
  - Toxic exposures
- **Psychosocial**
  - Bonding
  - Nurturing
  - Communication
  - Stressors
  - Coping/Habits
- **Nutrition**
  - Nursing or bottle feeding
  - Solid food introduction
  - Mastication
  - Hydration
- **Medical orientation**
  - Vaccination
  - Medication
  - Disease suppression
- **Rest and exercise**

</td>
<td>

Later Life

Digestive physiology

- Microflora
- Sensation
- Motility
- Inflammation

↕

GI WELLNESS vs FGID

Nutrition

Rest

Activity

Toxicity

Structural Integrity

↕

Later Life

Psychosocial function

- Nurturing
- Communication
- Life stress
- Coping/Habits
- Mindfulness

</td>
</tr>
</table>

Factors Involved In The Adaptive Physiology Of FGID

Genetics

It is believed that patients with FGID may have polymorphisms leading to altered levels of cytokines (decreases in IL-10 leading to more GI inflammation), serotonin reuptake transporters (which may raise or lower serotonin levels), G-proteins (affect CNS/enteric nervous system communication) or α-2 adrenoreceptors (change motility.) [1]

Family Of Origin Stress And Disease Coping Orientation

Children learn to relate to illness from their parents. Adults with IBS tend to have offspring with a higher risk of IBS and significantly more healthcare visits for all causes including gastrointestinal symptoms. Outpatient health care costs are also significantly higher for IBS offspring than for control children.[2] Childhood physical and emotional abuse are associated with an increased risk of adult IBS with a poor outcome.[3] An abusive history may lower the threshold at which these patients experience symptoms. Adults with IBS who do not seek healthcare treatment have a lower incidence of childhood abuse.[4] Animal studies show a significant increase in IBS following neonatal-maternal separation.[5]

Psychological Factors

In human research, psychological stress can exacerbate symptoms of IBS (and IBD), decreasing visceral pain thresholds and altering mucosal barrier function.[6] Stress also affects GI function to a lesser extent in non-IBS subjects. Psychological factors modify the experience of the disorder by the IBS patient and influence whether they seek medical care. An investigation into the psychological parameters of functional dyspepsia concluded that "symptom severity and weight loss in functional dyspepsia are determined by psychosocial factors (depression, abuse history) and somatization, and only to a lesser extent by gastric sensorimotor function."[7]

Stress often significantly increases the complaints in IBS and stress causes a shift in the host-gut microbial relationship (see Chapter 4).

Altered Motility

Both healthy subjects and patients with FGID will have increased motility in response to emotional or environmental stress. An example is that a wave of peristalsis occurs when a sudden loud noise (such as a loud clap) startles a person, but produces no perceptible symptoms. A person with a functional esophageal disorder has a stronger smooth muscle response and may experience it as pain. The greater motility responses to stress apply to the FGID generally.

In Chapter 6, as well as later in this chapter, I discuss the details of anti-CDT-B and antivinculin antibodies as an immune response to acute food poisoning or traveler's diarrhea. When above a threshold, these antibodies destroy a significant number of interstitial cells of Cajal and lead to deficient GI motility. This appears to be a major mechanism underlying the origins of irritable bowel syndrome.

Altered Inflammation

As many as 50% of IBS patients have increased activation of mucosal inflammatory cells. A 2002 immunohistology study showed various increases in intraepithelial lymphocytes, lamina propria CD3(+) cells and CD25(+) cells, neutrophils, mast cells and criteria for classic lymphocytic colitis in IBS patients compared with asymptomatic controls.[8] A second study found that 23% of patients diagnosed with irritable bowel also had lymphocytic colitis. In the control group 5% had lymphocytic colitis.[9] These details give credence to the idea that FGID may coexist with pathology and that FGID are very general categories that may be misdiagnoses of occult infections, allergic conditions, etc. The concomitance of irritable bowel syndrome (IBS) and inflammatory bowel disease has been demonstated, one more clear indication that functional and organic diseases often coexist. This becomes an extremely important concept when preventing unnecessary escalation of immunosuppressive treatments for non-responsive IBD.[47] Markers can be used to distinguish the low-grade inflammation of IBS from the gross inflammation of IBD. These include fecal calprotectin and lactoferrin.[10]

A small study from *Annals of Allergy* found that one or several foods or food additives induced the typical symptoms of IBS.[11]

Altered Visceral Sensitivity

People with functional GI disorders experience allodynia—pain in response to peristaltic smooth muscle activity. Normal enteric sensation includes distention and chemical irritation of the bowel, but there is no perception of the average peristaltic wave. In IBS research, patients also show a lower pain threshold to balloon distention of the bowel.[12] This altered sensitivity may also be induced in response to psychological stress.[13] PET scan studies suggest that visceral hypersensitivity in IBS relates to abnormal activation of brain circuits involved in emotional and cognitive modulation of sensory information. In controls, anticipation of distention leads to decreased activity in centers that down regulate pain perception (insula, anterior cingulate cortex, amygdala, and dorsal brainstem). IBS patients showed less anticipatory inactivation and therefore felt more pain,[14] as well as having increased activation of a vigilance network (dorsolateral prefrontal cortex.)[15]

Altered Intestinal Permeability

The tight junctions between enterocytes play a major role in detoxification, barrier function, water and electrolyte balance. Depending on the type of IBS, small bowel and/or colonic hyperpermeability are present.[16,17] Children with IBS have gastric, small bowel and colonic hyperpermeability.[18] The permeability may be induced by stress.[19,20] Neonatal maternal deprivation in rats induces these changes.[21] There is evidence that this altered permeability is transferable between cells. A fascinating study involved culturing healthy colonocytes with a supernatant from colonic biopsy specimens of patients with IBS.[22] Factors in the IBS supernatant induced paracellular hyperpermeability and a decreased permeability transcellularly within 48 hours! It is believed that the responsible factor is colonic lumenal serine protease.[23]

Food Allergy And Intolerance

In adults and children chronic constipation may be caused by food hypersensitivity and an elimination diet is often effective.[24,25]

Altered Intestinal Flora (See Chapter 3)

Brain-gut Axis (See Chapter 5)

Rome IV Diagnostic Categories

The six major adult categories of FGID/Disorders of Gut-brain Interaction:

1) Esophageal Disorders
2) Gastroduodenal Disorders
3) Bowel Disorders
4) Centrally Mediated Disorders of GI Pain (changed from Rome III terminology of Functional Abdominal Pain)
5) Gallbladder and Sphincter of Oddi Disorders
6) Anorectal Disorders

In addition, there are pediatric categories of FGID, detailed below.

Table 1.2 Esophageal Disorders
Functional heartburn
Functional chest pain
Functional dysphagia
Reflux hypersensitivity
Globus

Table 1.3 Gastroduodenal Disorders
Functional dyspepsia
Postprandial distress syndrome
Epigastric pain syndrome
Belching disorders
Excessive supragastric belching
(Rome III was Aerophagia)
Excessive gastric belching
Nausea and vomiting disorders
Chronic nausea/vomiting syndrome
Cannabinoid hyperemesis syndrome
Cyclic vomiting syndrome
Rumination syndrome

TABLE 1.4 BOWEL DISORDERS
Irritable bowel syndrome
Functional abdominal bloating/distension
Functional constipation
Functional diarrhea
Unspecified functional bowel disorder
Opioid-induced constipation

TABLE 1.5 CENTRALLY MEDIATED DISORDERS OF GASTROINTESTINAL PAIN
Centrally mediated abdominal pain syndrome
Narcotic bowel syndrome/Opioid-induced GI hyperalgesia

TABLE 1.6 GALLBLADDER AND SPHINCTER OF ODDI DISORDERS
Functional gallbladder disorder
Functional biliary sphincter of Oddi disorder
Functional pancreatic sphincter of Oddi disorder

TABLE 1.7 ANORECTAL DISORDERS
Functional fecal incontinence
Functional anorectal pain
Chronic proctalgia
Levator ani syndrome
Unspecified functional anorectal pain
Proctalgia fugax
Functional defecation disorders
Dysynergic defecation
Inadequate defecatory propulsion

The temporal criteria that apply to all FGID are that symptoms must have commenced at least six months before diagnosis and be active for at least three months.

TABLE 1.8 FGID: NEONATE/TODDLER
Infant regurgitation
Rumination syndrome
Cyclic vomiting syndrome
Infant colic
Functional diarrhea
Infant dyschezia
Functional constipation

TABLE 1.9 FGID: CHILD/ADOLESCENT
Functional nausea and vomiting disorders
Rumination syndrome
Cyclic vomiting syndrome
Functional nausea
Functional vomiting
Aerophagia
Functional abdominal pain disorders
Functional dyspepsia
Epigastric pain syndrome
Abdominal migraine
Postprandial distress syndrome
Irritable bowel syndrome
Functional abdominal pain—NOS
Functional defecation disorders
Functional constipation
Nonretentive fecal incontinence

A patient with FGID may also have GI pathology which must be ruled out.

Of course, a patient may have alarm symptoms, but still have FGID. Organic diseases need to be ruled out before confirmation of the diagnosis. The diagnostic work-up may include colonoscopy with colonic biopsies and tests for malabsorption/infection.

TABLE 1.10 ALARM SYMPTOMS IN FUNCTIONAL GI DISORDERS
Gastrointestinal bleeding
Onset of symptoms after age 50
Family history of colorectal cancer
Documented weight loss
Nocturnal symptoms
Predominant and severe diarrhea

In my experience, infection or overgrowth (bacterial, fungal, parasitic), allergy/intolerance, low grade inflammation, hiatal hernia syndrome and ileocecal valve syndrome must be investigated in most cases of functional GI disorders.

Functional GI disorders are no different than any condition a healthcare practitioner diagnoses, treats and manages. In a majority of cases, helping these patients requires ruling out pathology—followed by assessing and correcting:

- function of GI organs (digestive secretion, motility, elimination, detoxification)
- imbalanced flora
- nutrition and lifestyle habits
- environmental and endogenous toxicity
- stress, coping mechanisms and unresolved emotional states
- spinal and other physical circuits innervating the GI tract

Irritable Bowel Syndrome

Irritable bowel syndrome is the number one gastrointestinal diagnosis. Diagnosis of IBS—and FGID in general—is based on a combination of typical symptoms, a physical examination that is within normal limits and the absence of alarm features suggestive of an organic disease. Upper and lower gastrointestinal symptoms may overlap, and the clinical picture may match diagnostic criteria for more than one FGID. The symptoms may change over time. Patients with functional upper GI problems one year may fit the criteria for a functional lower GI condition a few years later.

Epidemiology Of IBS

For most of the world, IBS is more commonly a disorder of women although the opposite is true in India.[26] More women than men seek health care services for IBS in the United States. Women report that the phases of the menstrual cycle affect their IBS symptoms.[27] Serotonin 5-HT$_3$ receptor antagonists and 5-HT$_4$ partial agonists are reported to work more effectively for females than males. In a study of 990 adults in Jackson, Mississippi, Caucasians were 2.5 times more likely to have symptoms meeting the Rome criteria for IBS than African-Americans.[28] IBS is associated with anxiety, depression, health care visits and work loss. Anxiety and depression are more common in IBS patients than controls and anxiety increases healthcare seeking.[29,30] IBS or symptoms related to IBS (abdominal pain, diarrhea, constipation, dyspepsia) were found to be present in 54% of depressed patients and in 29% of nondepressed controls.[31] During the previous year, 24% of depressed persons visited doctors at least once because of abdominal symptoms, while only 13% of controls had done so. IBS patients not responding well to therapy rated themselves as having lower energy levels and higher degrees of memory deficits, depression, fatigue, and sleep disturbances.[32]

An article from the Mayo clinic points out that gastroesophageal reflux disease (GERD), functional dyspepsia and IBS often coexist.[33] Delayed gastric emptying may be common among them. IBS patients often have bronchial hyperresponsiveness and an association between GERD and asthma has been reported.[34]

Typical Symptoms Of IBS

At least 3 months, with onset at least 6 months previously of recurrent abdominal pain associated with 2 or more of the following:

- Improvement with defecation; *and/or*
- Onset associated with a change in frequency of stool; *and/or*
- Onset associated with a change in form (appearance) of stool

Subcategories Of IBS Diagnosis

The major subcategories of IBS are diarrhea predominant (IBS-D), constipation predominant (IBS-C), a type that is a mix of the two (IBS-M) and an unclassified type (IBS-U). A fifth is post-infectious IBS (PI-IBS) but unfortunately this important and common form is not listed in Rome IV. After an episode of bacterial gastroenteritis there may be as much as a 12-fold increased risk of developing IBS symptoms within a year. The diarrhea-predominant form is most common in this setting.[35]

A study published in the Journal of Pediatrics in 2008 found a 36% incidence of abdominal pain at six month follow-up post Salmonella, Campylobacter or Shigella associated gastroenteritis.[36] 87% of these symptomatic children (ages 3-19, of both genders) were diagnosed with IBS and 24% were diagnosed with functional dyspepsia. A 2005 study from the University of Newcastle found that smoking tobacco was associated with a 4.8 odds ratio for developing post-infectious IBS.[37] Lactose intolerance does not seem to have a higher incidence in post-infectious IBS patients versus controls,[38] but the number of IBS-D patients reporting GI symptoms following ingestion of dairy products was four-fold greater than healthy controls.[39]

Gut infection may lead to changes in the enteric nervous system which alter visceral hypersensitivity and intestinal motility. Changes in immune function are also seen in these patients. Mucosal T lymphocytes are increased and the cytokines produced are weighted toward pro-inflammatory activity. Post-infectious IBS (PI-IBS) has been shown to have an autoimmune etiology in both murine and human studies. Infectious gastroenteritis is the most significant environmental risk factor for IBS.[41] Organisms that trigger PI-IBS include Campylobacter, Salmonella, Shigella, E. coli, Giardia,[42] and viruses.[48]

Cytolethal distending toxin B (CDT-B) is produced by enteric pathogens that trigger PI-IBS. Campylobacter jejuni is the prototypical bacteria that produces CDT.[50] A partial list of other bacteria that produce CDT includes *Haemophilus ducreyi* (chancroid), *Aggregatibacter actinomycetemcomitans* (periodontitis), *Escherichia coli* (traveler's diarrhea), *Shigella dysenteriae* (dysentery), *Salmonella enterica* (typhoid fever) and *Campylobacter upsaliensis* (enterocolitis).

The interstitial cells of Cajal (ICC) are fibroblast-like cells that act as pacemakers for the migrating motor complex (MMC). A key underlying cause of small intestinal bacterial overgrowth (SIBO) is thought to be deficiency of the MMC, which moves debris and microorganisms from the stomach and small bowel down to the ileocecal valve. This motor pattern takes place during nightly fasting and between meals.[49] In a landmark study, the number of ICC were reduced in post Campylobacter jejuni gastroenteritis infected rats who eventually developed SIBO.[50] Three months after *C. jejuni* gastroenteritis, 27% of the rats had SIBO. These animals had a lower number of ICC than controls in the jejunum and ileum (0.12 ICC/villus was the threshold for developing SIBO.)

CDT-B toxin may destroy ICC by stimulating the production of autoantibodies against a cytoskeletal protein known as vinculin. The antigen-antibody complexes between anti-vinculin antibodies and cytolethal distending toxin lead to autoimmune destruction of ICC.[51]

The symptoms of IBS and SIBO are nearly identical. In a study of 202 IBS patients, 157 (78%) had SIBO based on a lactulose breath test. Of those whose overgrowth was eradicated by antibiotics (10 days of neomycin, ciprofloxacin, flagyl or doxycycline) **48% no longer met the Rome III criteria for IBS**. Patients whose treatment did not lead to eradication had no improvement in IBS symptoms.[40] Note: Bacterial stool culture does not represent small intestinal flora. A breath test is necessary for the definitive diagnosis of SIBO. A study of the recurrence of SIBO after antibiotic treatment showed an increase in treatment failure to be more common in older patients, those on chronic proton pump inhibitor therapy and status post appendectomy.[41] Appendectomy post rupture may be even more likely to lead to rapidly relapsing IBS due to adhesions secondary to chemical peritonitis. Conversely, patients with IBS undergoing appendectomy for presumed acute appendicitis have a 2.10 relative risk for having a normal appendix resected.[52]

Alterations in colonic bile acids may be common in IBS-D. Since most enteric bile is reabsorbed in the terminal ileum, the irritating effects of excess bile salts on colonic mucosa are prevented. A recent study reveals that in subjects with IBS-D the total amount and total secretion of bile acids accelerates colonic transit and increases stool volume. True bile acid malabsorption need not be present to have these effects.[53]

The standard practice treatment of post-infectious IBS is often identical to that of idiopathic IBS-D. In several of the following chapters I will outline an approach which is specific for the rational naturopathic treatment of post-infectious IBS. **In fact, I regard most cases of IBS to be related to infections or overgrowth of commensals/imbalanced flora as part of the etiology.**

Typical IBS symptoms that may accompany changes in stool frequency and consistency, including:

- straining during defecation
- stool urgency
- incomplete feeling after a bowel movement
- passing mucus
- abdominal bloating

Symptoms of upper GI dysfunction (Functional Dyspepsia) that may also be found in IBS, including:

- nausea
- epigastric pain
- uncomfortable postprandial fullness

Other extra-intestinal symptoms often associated with IBS thought to be more common than in the general population:

- lethargy
- backache
- headache
- urinary tract symptoms
- dyspareunia
- rosacea

The extraintestinal symptoms listed above may help to rule in IBS and some authors feel that when these are present a simpler work-up is warranted (note: rosacea may be more common in patients with many GI disorders including celiac, Crohn's and ulcerative colitis).[54]

Biomedical Treatment Of IBS[42]

Mild symptoms—respond well to dietary and lifestyle modifications, education, and reassurance about their disease.

Moderate to severe symptoms—anticholinergics, antispasmodics, low dose tricyclic antidepressants and/or other psychiatric medications and IBS-specific agents.

The most severe symptoms—often refractory to standard treatment. These patients will often require mental health providers, psychotropic medications, and may need frequent appointments with primary care providers to offer ongoing support throughout treatment.

IBS-C Specific Drugs

Alosetron (Lotronex): A selective 5-HT_3 receptor antagonist that was pulled from the U.S. market in 2000 due to side-effects of severe constipation, ischemic colitis, and bowel perforation.[43,44] It was re-introduced in the U.S. market in 2002 under a restricted prescribing program.

Tegaserod (Zelnorm): Tegaserod, a selective 5-HT_4 agonist, was approved for women with IBS-C and men with chronic idiopathic constipation.

In March 2007, Novartis voluntarily removed tegaserod from the U.S. and Canadian market after an FDA safety analysis of pooled data from twelve clinical trials demonstrated a statistical increase in the incidence of myocardial infarction, stroke and unstable angina. In July 2007, tegaserod was re-introduced under a restricted investigational new drug protocol, limiting its use to treatment of IBS-C and chronic idiopathic constipation in women under fifty-five years of age who meet specific guidelines. It continues to remain off market for general use.

Linaclotide (Linzess): This is a guanylate cyclase agonist

Prucolapride (Resolor, Resotran): This prokinetic agent is a 5-HT_4 agonist commonly employed by SIBO literate physicians for IBS-C. It is available from Canadian and European pharmacies. At the time of this writing, it has not yet been FDA approved in the U.S.

Methylcellulose (Citrucel): This bulking agent is safe for SIBO/IBS-C because it is non-fermentable by intestinal flora.

Psyllium (Metamucil, Konsyl and others): This natural bulking agent may be partially fermentable and therefore may or may not aggravate some SIBO/IBS-C and methane induced constipation patients. Flax and chia seeds fall into this same category.

IBS-D Specific Drugs

Loperimide (Imodium): An OTC peristalsis inhibitor which appears to have its major effects on colonic motility.

Diphenoxylate hydrochloride with atropine sulfate (Lomotil): A combination of a non-absorbable opiate plus an anticholinergic

Rifaximin (Xifaxan): A non-absorbable antibiotic which is FDA approved for IBS-D, traveler's diarrhea and hepatic encephalopathy. TARGET 1 and TARGET 2 studies found this a better treatment than placebo. In those multicenter trials, SIBO was not evaluated (they were treating IBS-D in general). Rifaximin is over 75% effective for IBS-D due to hydrogen dominant SIBO (550 mg TID for 14 days).

Rifaximin is also used by SIBO-literate physicians to treat IBS-C, SIBO with both elevated hydrogen and methane and in methane-induced constipation. In these cases it is prescribed along with either neomycin or metronidazole.

Eluxadoline (Viberzl): A mu opioid receptor agonist

Cholestyramine (Questran): A bile acid sequestrant which may be used to alter colonic bile acid levels and slow colonic transit.

Treatments For IBS Pain/Spasm

Enteric coated peppermint oil: This can be extremely effective for some patients, but as with any antispasmotic, it may aggravate GERD by relaxing the lower esophageal sphincter. It also has antimicrobial effects and therefore is an antispasmotic that does not increase the recurrence of SIBO.

Iberogast: This German herbal tincture has multiple mechanisms of action including antispasmotic, carminative and prokinetic.

Dicyclomine (Bentyl): An anticholinergic especially in IBS-D

Hyoscyamine sulfate (Levsin): An anticholinergic

Imipramine (Tofranil): A tricyclic antidepressant that reduces visceral pain and slows orocecal transit.

Amitriptyline (Elavil): As in imipramine above

Naturopathic Assessment

In addition to the Rome IV conditions we recognize the following:

- Hypochlorhydria—see Chapter 13
- Functional pancreatic insufficiency—see Chapter 14
- Ileocecal valve syndrome—see Chapter 15
- Hiatal hernia syndrome and diaphragmatic dysfunction—see Chapter 12

Assessment may include:

- Reflex point testing (Riddler's, Bennett's and Chapman's)—see Chapter 8
- Organ specific muscle testing—see Chapter 8
- Laboratory testing (stool, saliva, blood, urine, breath)—see Chapter 9

- Secretory testing (Heidelberg or gastric string test)—see Chapters 9, 13
- Transit/retention time testing—see Chapter 9
- Energetic psychology techniques

Treatment may include:

- Dietary interventions (food and clinical nutrition)
- Adequate fluid intake
- Botanical remedies
- Homeopathic remedies
- Hydrochloric acid and enzyme replacement
- Organ and tissue extracts
- Prebiotics, probiotics, lactoferrin, colostrum
- Visceral, spinal, cranial, extremity and fascial manipulation
- Therapeutic exercises, biofeedback (including neurofeedback) and breath training
- Energetic or conventional psychology interventions
- Mindfulness training
- Prescription medications

In Chapter 9 there will be an explanation of the Four R Program:

- Removal of parasites and overgrown commensals
- Replacement of digestive acid, bile and enzymes
- Re-innoculation with beneficial flora
- Repair of the mucosal lining

1 Drossman, DA *Rome III : The Functional Gastrointestinal Disorders,* McLean, VA : Degnon Associates, 2006, 3rd edition.
2 Levy, RL *Am J Gastroentero.* 2000 Feb;95(2):451-6.
3 Salmon P et al, J Behav Med 2003 Feb: 26(1):1-18
4 Guthrie, E et al *Gut.* 2003 Nov;52(11):1616-22.
5 Barreau, F et al *Pediatr Res.* 2007 Sep;62(3):240-5.
6 Gareau, MG et al *Curr Mol Med.* 2008 Jun;8(4):274-81.
7 Van Oudenhove, L et al *Gut.* 2008 Jul 14. [Epub ahead of print]
8 Chadwick, VS et al *Gastroenterology.* 2002 Jun;122(7):1778-83.
9 Tuncer, C et al *Acta Gastroenterol Belg.* 2003 Apr-Jun;66(2):133-6.
10 Petitpierre, M et al *Ann Allergy.* 1985 Jun;54(6):538-40.
11 Otten, CM et al *Clin Chem Lab Med.* 2008;46(9):1275-80.
12 Truong, TT et al *Curr Gastroenterol Rep.* 2008 Aug;10(4):369-78.
13 Gareau, MG et al *Curr Mol Med.* 2008 Jun;8(4):274-81.
14 Berman, SM et al *J Neurosci.* 2008 Jan 9;28(2):349-59.
15 Bonaz, B *J Physiol Pharmacol.* 2003 Dec;54 Suppl 4:27-42.
16 Zeng, J et al *Aliment Pharmacol Ther. 2008; 28(8):994-1002*
17 Dupont, AW *Curr Gastroenterol Rep.* 2007 Oct;9(5):378-84.
18 Shulman, RJ et al *J Pediatr.* 2008 Nov;153(5):646-50.
19 Gareau, MG et al *Curr Mol Med.* 2008 Jun;8(4):274-81.
20 Alonso, C et al *Gastroenterology.* 2008 Jul;135(1):163-172.
21 Barreau, F et al *Gut.* 2008 May;57(5):582-90.
22 Pische, T et al *Gut.* 2008 Sep 29. [Epub ahead of print]
23 Gecse, K et al *Gut.* 2008 May;57(5):591-9.
24 Carroccio A, Iacono G. Review article: Chronic constipation and food hypersensitivity: an intriguing relationship. *Aliment Pharmacol Ther.* 2006 Nov 1;24(9):1295-304.
25 Carroccio A, Di Prima L, Iacono G, Florena AM, D'Arpa F, Sciumè C, Cefalù AB, Noto D, Averna MR. Multiple food hypersensitivity as a cause of refractory chronic constipation in adults, *Scand J Gastroenterol.* 2006 Apr;41(4):498-504
26 Goshal, UC et al *Indian J Gastroenterol.* 2008 Jan-Feb;27(1):22-8.
27 Heitkemper, M et al *Biol Res Nurs.* 2003 Jul;5(1):56-65.
28 Wigington, WC et al *Clin Gastroenterol Hepatol.* 2005 Jul;3(7):647-53.
29 Mikocka-Walus, AA et al *Clin Pract Epidemol Ment Health.* 2008 May 23;4:15.
30 Hu, WH et al *Aliment Pharmacol Ther.* 2002 Dec;16(12):2081-8.
31 Hillila, MT et al *Aliment Pharmacol Ther.* 2008 Sep 1;28(5):648-54.
32 Grossi, ML et al *Int J Prosthodont.* 2008 May-Jun;21(3):201-9.
33 Talley, NJ *Drugs Today (Barc).* 2006 Jul;42 Suppl B:3-8.
34 Dickman, R et al *Curr Gastroenterol Rep.* 2006 Aug;8(4):261-5.
35 Dobronte, Z *Orv Hetil* 2006 Oct 29;147(43):2077-80.
36 Saps, M et al. *J Pediatr* 2008 Jun;152(6):812- 816.
37 Parry, SE et al. *Eur J Gastroenterol Hepatol* 2005 Oct;17(10):1071-5.
38 Parry, SE et al. *Eur J Gastroenterol Hepatol* 2002 Nov;14(11):1225-30.
39 Gupta, D et al *J Gastroenterol Hepatol* 2007 Dec;22(12):2261-5.
40 Pimentel, M et al, *Am J Gastroenterol* 2000 Dec;95(12):3503-3506.
41 Lauritano, EC et al *Am J Gastroenterol.* 2008;103(8):2031-2035.
42 Beatty JK et al, Post-infectious irritable bowel syndrome: mechanistic insights into

chronic disturbances following enteric infection. *World J Gastroenterol.* 2014 Apr 14;20(14):3976-85.

43 Chang, L et al *Am J Gastroenterol* 2006; 101: 1069-1079.

44 Horton, R *Lancet* 2001; 357: 1544-1545.

45 Kamm, MA *Aliment Pharmacol Ther* 2002; 16: 343-351.

46 Carlsson, L et al *J Pharmacol Exp The*r 1997; 282: 220-227.

47 Spiller R et al, IBD and IBS—Separate entities or on a spectrum? *Nat Rev Gastroenterol Hepatol.* 2016 Sep 26;13(10):613-21.

48 Zanini B et al, Incidence of post-infectious irritable bowel syndrome and functional intestinal disorders following a water-borne viral gastroenteritis outbreak. *AM J Gastroenterol* 2012 Jun;107(6):891-9.

49 Deloose E, Tack J, Redefining the functional roles of the gastrointestinal migrating motor complex and motilin in small bacterial overgrowth and hunger signaling. *Am J Physiol Gastrointest Liver Physiol* 2016 Feb 15;310(4):G228-33.

50 Pokkunuri V et al, Role of Cytolethal Distending Toxin in Altered Stool Form and Bowel Phenotypes in a Rat Model of Post-infectious Irritable Bowel Syndrome. *J Neurogastroenterol Motil.* 2012 Oct;18(4):434-42.

51 Pimentel M et al, Development and validation of a biomarker for diarrhea-predominant irritable bowel syndrome in human subjects. *PLoS One*. 2015 May 13;10(5):e0126438.

52 Lu CL et al, Irritable bowel syndrome and negative appendectomy: a prospective multivariable investigation. *Gut*. 2007 May;56(5):655-60.

53 Peleman C, Colonic Transit and Bile Acid Synthesis or Excretion in Patients With Irritable Bowel Syndrome-Diarrhea Without Bile Acid Malabsorption. *Clin Gastroenterol Hepatol.* 2016 Nov 14. pii: S1542-3565(16)31047-3.

54 Egeberg A et al, Rosacea and gastrointestinal disorders: a population-based cohort study. *Br J Dermato*l. 2017 Jan;176(1):100-106.

Chapter 2

The Enteric Nervous System, Gastrointestinal Hormones, And Immunity

The Enteric Nervous System (ENS)—"The Gut Brain"

The ENS is derived from the embryonic vagal and sacral neural crest cells.[1] Rich in plexi, it has as many neurons as the spinal cord. It has two types of plexi—myenteric and submucosal. The myenteric plexus is located between the longitudinal and circular muscle layers and controls motility. The submucosal plexus, located in the submucosa, responds to the contents of the lumen, regulating mucosal blood flow and epithelial cell function.

Numerous neurotransmitters are secreted by these plexi. Among these, acetylcholine is excitatory, stimulating smooth muscle contraction, increasing intestinal secretion, releasing enteric neuropeptides and increasing mucosal blood flow. In general sympathetic neurons, through release of norepinephrine, have opposing functions. Connections between the CNS and the ENS are both direct as well as mediated through the

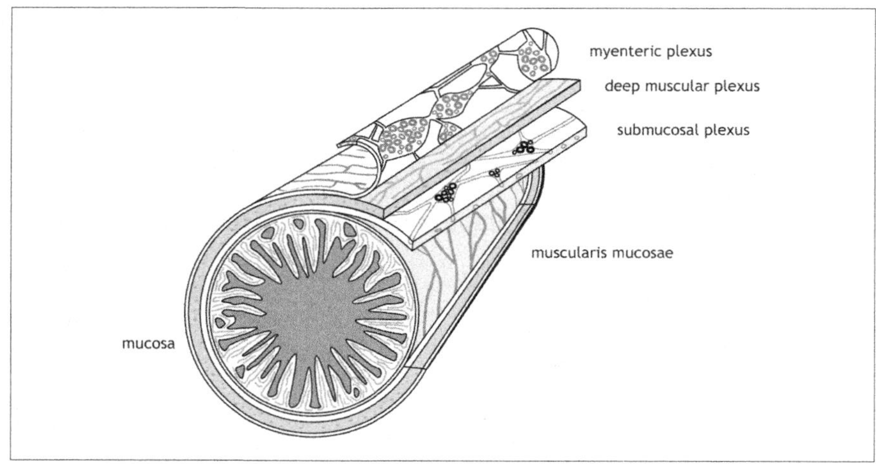

FIGURE 2.1 THE ENTERIC NERVOUS SYSTEM

autonomic system. In porcine research, cholinergic activity in the ENS triggers SIgA secretion.[2] Human enteric neurons produce chemokines and can induce chemotaxis of immunocytes during intestinal inflammation.[3] Enteric neurons appear to have the capacity to prevent the breach of the intestinal mucosa by pathogenic bacteria.[4] Immune cells in the Peyer's patches of the ileum communicate via the enteric nervous system as they sample antigens at multiple sites.[5] Commensal flora are centrally involved in the cross-talk between the CNS and ENS (see Chapter 5).

The presence of food in the intestine triggers SIgA production and parenteral nutrition compromises immunity as evidenced by a significant increase in pneumonia and intra-abdominal abscesses compared to enterally fed patients.[6] The earlier enteral feeding is established and enhanced—by the addition of glutamine and probiotics—the better the outcomes for patients with traumatic brain injury.[7,8]

GI Hormones, Paracrines And Neurocrines

Although the GI tract, including its mesenteric adipose, is the richest source of hormones, it is not organized grossly into a gland as are most endocrine organs. Instead, the enteroendocrine cells (EEC) that produce these hormones are solitary—physically isolated from each other—and scattered throughout the GI mucosa. These secretions interact with those of the pancreas to create the "soup" that regulates GI motility, secretion, blood flow and maintenance of the mucosa. G protein coupled receptors mediate the action of these GI peptides with major influence from the short chain fatty acids produced by intestinal flora. Major GI hormones/ regulating factors include:

- Cholecystokinin
- The Cholinergic-Anti-inflammatory Pathway
- Adipocytokines
- Secretin
- Somatostatin
- Motilin
- Gastrin
- Melatonin
- Serotonin

An important relationship exists between gastric acid and pancreatic function. An acid bolus entering the duodenum is a trigger for the release of secretin and cholecystokinin. These stimulate the release of bile, bicarbonate and pancreatic digestive enzymes into the duodenum. Achlorhydria or hypochlorhydria are therefore possible etiologies for functional pancreatic insufficiency.

Cholecystokinin (CCK)

Gallbladder motility and delivery of bile to the duodenum

Released from the I cells of the duodenum, CCK's major effects are to stimulate the contraction of the gallbladder and relax the sphincter of Oddi, allowing for the release of bile into the duodenum. CCK is released in the gut in response to a meal and acts via vagal afferents to induce post-meal satiety and glucose regulation. Even a moderate elevation of blood lipids may have a negative feedback mechanism on circulating CCK.[9] Hyperlipidemia is also a risk factor for pancreatic insufficiency, perhaps through this mechanism.[10,11] Along with adipocyte hormones, because of its effect on appetite, CCK may be important in maintenance of normal body weight. The combination of chronic elevation of TNF- α and CCK may induce the cachexia of anorexia nervosa and anxiety disorders. Curiously, intravenous CCK has been found to trigger the symptoms of functional dyspepsia.[12] Furthermore, CCK has also been shown to be involved in the pathogenesis of panic disorder, anxiety and pain[13] and triggers the release of β-endorphin from the anterior pituitary.[14] CCK downregulates post-prandial local immunity in the gut, perhaps by its affect on stress-axis hormones,[15] protects against inflammation-induced intestinal hyperpermeability[16] and may discourage the development of food intolerances.[17]

The Cholinergic Anti-inflammatory Pathway (CAP)

Fine tuning inflammation

Beyond its control of classic physiological functions, the vagus nerve controls the excessive release of TNF, IL-1, and other pro-inflammatory cytokines.[18] The CAP, via nicotinic receptors and by deactivation of NF-KB, controls the level of cytokines produced by macrophages in the spleen, liver and elsewhere in the reticuloendothelial system. This pathway suppresses cytokine activity locally in specific sites, thereby preventing the release of disease-inducing cytokines into the blood. Unlike humoral mechanisms which can become systemic, vagal inflammatory modulation is organ-specific. It appears to be triggered by dietary fat which is also a releasing mechanism for CCK. It has been speculated that the presence of the CAP and CCK explain why trillions of enteric microorganisms do not stimulate an exaggerated cytokine response.[19]

According to this theory, if there were dysfunction of the CAP, the risk of inflammatory bowel disease would be increased. This idea gains credence from data showing a therapeutic effect of nicotine for some patients with ulcerative colitis.[20] This may be due to the prevention of excessive colonic cytokine production. The binding of nicotine to receptors on gut immune cells might mimic the functions of the CAP, thereby suppressing cytokine production. Nicotine is not effective, however, in Crohn's disease and passive smoking does not have a significant effect on children with UC.[21] Likewise, fish oil is therapeutic in patients with ulcerative colitis, but not in those with Crohn's disease.[22] Early enteral feeding in trauma and surgery patients has been found to significantly reduce mortality from sepsis and organ damage. This may be another example of dietary fat activating the CAP.[23]

Adipocytokines

Blood sugar, insulin sensitivity, and endothelial health

Adipocytes produce both anti-inflammatory as well as pro-inflammatory peptides. Those which predominantly down-regulate inflammation include adiponectin, omentin-1, apelin, SFRP5 (secreted frizzled-related protein 5), and vaspin (visceral adipose tissue-derived serine protease inhibitor). Those predominantly up-regulating inflammation include leptin, resistin, tumor necrosis factor-α (TNF-α), interleukin-6 (IL-6), chemerin, CCL2 (CC-chemokine ligand 2), CCR5 (CC-chemokine receptor type 5), RBP4 (retinol binding protein 4), and ANGPTL2 (angiopoietin-like protein 2).[52] These secretions are regulators of body weight, insulin sensitivity/resistance and endothelial function/dysfunction. The mesentery is a rich source of these cells and an increase in abdominal girth triggers insulin resistance syndrome. Injection of a supernatant of Lactobacillus into rat CNS leads to a decrease in body weight and an increase in leptin concentrations in specific areas of the brain and retroperitoneal adipose.[24] Although the implications are unclear, it appears that entry of intestinal microflora or their products into the bloodstream may centrally modulate leptin.

Secretin

Neutralizing the duodenum

In 1902 Bayliss and Starling discovered secretin making it the first gastrointestinal hormone to be identified. Its major function is to buffer the effects of gastric acid-infused chyme as it enters the duodenum, and does this by stimulating the secretion of hepatic, cholecystic, pancreatic and duodenal bicarbonate. It also complements the action of CCK by increasing insulin and digestive enzyme secretion, delaying gastric emptying, inhibiting gastrin release and supporting pancreatic growth.[25]

Somatostatin

The break pedal for all GI peptides

This hormone downregulates the flow of all GI neuropeptides. There are cases of regression of large malignant gastrinomas by the use of Sandostatin, a long-acting somatostatin analogue.[26] In the CNS, somatostatin has an antiseizure effect with major influence in the hippocampus and the dentate nucleus.[27,28]

Motilin

Mobilizes the migrating motor complex

Motilin's main function is to initiate and control the migrating motor complex which sweeps chyme from the pylorus to the ileocecal valve during fasting.

Gastrin

Increasing gastric hydrochloric acid

Gastrin's main function is to increase hydrochoric acid release. Gastrin production tends to be excessive in many patients. The primary mechanism of hypergastrinemia is gastric acid hyposecretion. Examples include chronic use of proton pump inhibitors and chronic atrophic gastritis. The seventh edition of *Robbin's Pathology* states "...in the Western world, the prevalence of histologic changes indicative of chronic gastritis in the later decades of life is higher than 50%".[29] Hypergastrinemia has been associated with a possible increase in risk of gastric and colorectal cancers.[30,31,32] (see Chapter 13)

Melatonin

Regulator of circadian rhythm

The gastrointestinal EEC are the major source of extra-pineal melatonin. Melatonin in the gastrointestinal tissues is 10-100 fold higher than blood levels and there is 400 times more melatonin in the gastrointestinal tract than in the pineal gland. Melatonin prevents GI ulceration by antioxidant, acid modulating, immune enhancing, epithelial regenerating, and mucosal blood flow increasing effects.

An antagonistic relationship with serotonin has been suggested and may be related to periodicity of food intake. It may be the reason pancreatic tissue and plasma concentrations of melatonin increase with fasting. This speeds gastrointestinal transit via the migrating motor complex of the small bowel. Pharmacological doses of melatonin delay gastric emptying. Melatonin or its precursor L-tryptophan protects the pancreas against ischemia/reperfusion induced damage and therefore these are beneficial in acute pancreatitis. Night-time melatonin levels are significantly related to night-time insulin in subjects with metabolic syndrome, but not in controls.[33] Supplementation of 10 mg melatonin and 50 mg zinc acetate was found to decrease fasting glucose and glycosylated hemoglobin levels in type 2 diabetics.[34] Mechanisms offered include free radical scavenging, activation of antioxidative enzymes and modulation of cytokine production. Due to these effects as well as its kinetic and circadian regulatory activity, melatonin may be involved in the prevention or treatment of colorectal cancer, ulcerative colitis, gastric ulcers and irritable bowel syndrome.[35,36,37]

Serotonin

GI Motility and so much more

The large majority of serotonin (>90%) is produced by the enteroendocrine cells and acts on the receptors of the enteric nervous system. A paracrine hormone, serotonin has a major effect on the regulation of gut motility, vascular tone, secretion and pain perception in normal gut physiology and in IBS.[38] It is released from enterochromaffin cells and neurons by luminal distension and chemical signals. The serotonin receptors 5-HT_2 and 5-HT_4 are believed to be involved in the development, maintenance and lifespan of enteric neurons.[39] Of note, most of the effects of estrogen are brought about by this steroid hormone's influence on the various serotonin receptors.[40] In rat studies, estrogen, progesterone and testosterone all influence serotonin receptors and metabolism.[41,42,43] In the liver, serotonin modulates hepatic blood flow, innervation and wound healing.[44]

Seven types of serotonin receptors have been discovered with the 5-HT_3 and 5-HT_4 in the gut being the most widely researched GI types. In the GI mucosa 5-HT_3 receptors modulate visceral pain and assist in peristalsis. These same receptors within the CNS appear to influence the emotional component of visceral stimulation. Gut 5-HT_4 receptors are involved in peristalsis, gastric emptying, colonic secretion, and either contraction of smooth muscle or relaxation depending upon the GI location.[45]

Table 2.1 Serotonin Receptors And Their Known Functions	
5-HT$_{1A}$	CNS: nerve inhibition, thermoregulation, anxiety, sleep, hunger
5-HT$_{1B}$	CNS: similar to 1A plus vascular and pulmonary vasoconstriction
5-HT$_{1D}$	CNS: locomotion and cerebral vasoconstriction
5-HT$_{2A}$	CNS: nerve stimulation, sleep, hunger, smooth muscle contraction, blood vessel dilatation and constriction, platelet aggregation
5-HT$_{2B}$	Gastric muscle contraction
5-HT$_{2C}$	CNS: cerebrospinal fluid secretion
5-HT$_{3}$	CNS and PNS: nerve stimulation, anxiety, emesis GI: modulation of visceral pain and motility
5-HT$_{4}$	CNS: nerve stimulation, memory, depression, appetite GI: gastric emptying, colonic secretion, motility
5-HT$_{5, 6, 7}$	6 and 7- CNS: associated with learning and memory

Inflammation decreases Serotonin Reuptake Transporter Gene (SERT), a transmembrane 5-HT transporter, raising serotonin levels in the gut. This may explain the pain and diarrhea of IBS-D. Serotonin receptor desensitization over time may cause constipation.[46] IBS patients have less expression of SERT than healthy controls.[47] Drug research has revealed that 5-HT$_3$ receptor antagonists treat nausea and emesis associated with chemotherapy and treat functional disorders associated with diarrhea. In addition, 5-HT$_4$ receptor agonists are used as promotility agents, enhancing gastric emptying and relieving constipation.

Serotonin levels in both whole blood and in platelets are significantly higher in autistic spectrum disorder (ASD) patients vs. controls.[48] In contrast, low serotonin levels are found in ASD brains.[53] Vitamin D may be responsible for controlling these central and peripheral values. Ulcerative colitis is found in higher rates in mothers of children with infantile autism than in the mothers of neurotypical children.[49,50]

Table 2.2 Selected GI Paracrines

Name	Where Produced	Stimulus	Actions
Somatostatin	D cells in the pancreatic islets and gastric duodenal mucosa	Gastric acid Vagus nerve inhibits	Inhibits gastrin secretion Inhibits gastric secretion Inhibits growth hormone
Histamine	EEC	Gastrin	↑ Acid secretion Potentiates gastrin and acetylcholine
Pancreatic Polypeptide	PP cells of the pancreatic islets	Meals containing protein	↑ Gastric acid secretion ↑ Intestinal secretion
Serotonin	EEC and mast cells (platelets only store GI produced serotonin —they do not produce it)	Meals Food sensitivity reactions GI infections	Excitatory to neurons (↑depolarization) Accelerates gastric emptying ↑ Gastric accommodation May suppress acetylcholine release
Melatonin	EEC	Meals containing tryptophan	Mucosal antioxidant Enhances immunity Regenerates epithelium Increases mucosal blood flow Decreases gastric acid

Table 2.3 Selected GI Hormones			
Name (Year Discovered)	**Where Secreted**	**Stimuli**	**Actions**
Cholecystokinin (1924)	Duodenum & jejunum (I cells)	Peptides Amino Acids Fatty acids Peptic acid	↑Gastric & intest. motility ↑Gastric acid secretion ↑GB contraction Relaxes sphincter of Oddi ↑Pancreatic enzyme/bicarb ↑Pancreatic growth Inhibits gastric emptying
Secretin (1902)	Duodenum (S cells)	Peptic acid Fat	↑GB contraction/bicarb ↑Pancreatic enzyme/bicarb ↑Pancreatic growth ↑Insulin release Inhibits acid secretion Inhibits gastrin Inhibits gastric emptying Inhibits gastric & intest. motility
Gastric Inhibitory-Protein [aka. enterogastrone] (1969).	Duodenum & jejunum	Glucose Amino Acids Fat	↑Insulin secretion Inhibits acid secretion Inhibits gastrin secretion Inhibits gastric emptying Inhibits gastric motility
Motilin (1970s)	Duodenum & jejunum	Vagal input Fat Peptic acid	↑Gastric and intestinal motility Inhibits acid secretion Inhibits gastric emptying
Ghrelin (1999)	Fundal P/D1 cells, hypothalamus, pituitary, kidney, and placenta	Fasting	↑Growth hormone release ↑Hunger, food intake ↑Gastric motility ↑Cardiac output Opposes leptin's effects

Table 2.4 Selected GI Neurocrines			
Name	**Where Secreted**	**Stimulus**	**Actions**
Vasoactive Intestinal Peptide	D1 pancreatic islet cells Nerves in GI smooth muscle Nerves in GI mucosa		Relaxes GI smooth muscle (via nitric oxide) Vasodilates splanchnics ↑ Pancreatic secretion ↑ Intestinal secretion ↑ Glycogenolysis inhibits gastric secretion
Gastrin Releasing Peptide (bombesin)	Gastric mucosal nerves	Vagal input Peptides in the stomach	Neurotransmitter for vagal fibers innervating G cells ↑ Gastrin secretion
Enkephalins	Nerves of the GI mucosa and muscles		↑ Smooth muscle tone Mediates sphincter contraction (LES, pylorus and ileocecal)

1 Barlow, AJ *Development* 2008 Apr 2.
2 Schmidt, LD J *Neuroimmunol.* 2007 Apr;185(1-2):20-8.
3 Tixier, E *Biochem Biophys Res Commun* 2006 Jun 2;344(2):554-61.
4 Schreiber, KL *J Neuroimmune Pharmacol.* 2007 Dec;2(4):329-37.
5 Vulchanova, L *J Neuroimmunol.* 2007 Apr;185(1-2):64-74.
6 Sachs, GS *Nutr Clin Pract.* 2003 Dec;18(6):483-8.
7 Spindler-Vesel A *J Parenter Enteral Nutr.* 2007 Mar-Apr;31(2):119-26.
8 Falcao del Arruda, IS *Clin Sci (Lond).*2004 Mar;106(3):287-92.
9 Weikert, MO *J Clin Endocrinol Metab.* 2008 Mar 25
10 Bisjvoet, SJ et al *Neth J Med.* 1993 Feb;42(1-2):36-44.
11 Krauss, RM *Am J Med.* 1977 Jan;62(1):144-9.
12 Chua, AS *World J Gastroenterol.* 2006 May 7;12(17):2688-93.
13 Chua, AS *World J Gastroenterol.* 2006 May 7;12(17):2688-93.
14 Holden, RJ *Med Hypotheses.* 1999 Feb;52(2):155-62.
15 Greisen, MH *Behav Brain Res.* 2005 Jun 20;161(2):204-12.
16 Luyer, MD *J Exp Med.* 2005 Oct 17;202(8):1023-9.
17 Alverdy, J et al *Surgery.* 1997 Aug;122(2):386-92
18 Tracey, K.J. *Nature.* 2002 420:853–859.
19 Tracey, KJ *J Exp Med.* 2005 Oct 17;202(8):1017-21
20 Pullan, RD *N. Engl. J. Med. 1994* 330:811–815.
21 Jones, D et al *Am J Gastroent* 2008 Aug 28;103(9):2382-2393.
22 Endres, S *Curr. Opin. Clin. Nutr. Metab. Care.* 2:117–120.
23 Ward, N *Nutr. J 2003.* 2:18.
24 Sousa, R *BMC Complement Altern Med.* 2008 Feb 19;8:5.
25 L Gullo, P Priori, P L Costa, G Mattioli, and G Labò Action of secretin on pancreatic enzyme secretion in man. Studies on pure pancreatic juice. *Gut.* 1984 August; 25(8): 867–873.
26 Granberg, D *Digestion.* 2008 Mar 29;77(2):92-95
27 Qiu C *J Neurosci.* 2008 Apr 2;28(14):3567-3576.
28 Tallent, MK *Mol Cell Endocrinol.* 2007 Dec 14
29 Cotran, Kumar *Robbin's Pathological Basis of Disease,* Elsevier Press, 2005.
30 Watson, SA *Br J Cancer* 2002;87(5):567-73.
31 Kinoshita, Y et al *J Gastroenterol* 2004;39(6):507-13.
32 Ellison, EC et al *Am J Surg* 2003;186(3):245-8.
33 Robeva, R et al *J Pineal Res.* 2008 Jan;44(1):52-6.
34 Hussain, SA *Saudi Med J.* 2006 Oct;27(10):1483-8.
35 Thor, PJ, et al. *J Physiol Pharmacol.* 2007 Dec;58 Suppl 6:97-103.
36 Bubenik, GA *Dig Dis Sci.* 2002 Oct;47(10):2336-48.
37 Jaworek, J, et al. *J Physiol Pharmacol.* 2007 Dec;58 Suppl 6:65-80.
38 Gershon, MD *Aliment Pharmacol Ther* 1999; 13 Suppl 2: 15-30
39 Camilleri, M *Neurogastroenterol Motil.* 2008 Apr;20(4):418-29.
40 Ostlund H, Keller E, Hurd YL. Estrogen receptor gene expression in relation to neuropsychiatric disorders. *Ann N Y Acad Sci.* 2003 Dec;1007:54-
41 Ostlund, H et al *Ann N Y Acad Sci.* 2003 Dec;1007:54-63.
42 Simon, NG et al *Neurosci Biobehav Rev.* 1998;23(2):325-36.
43 Truitt, W et al *Brain Res. 2003 Jun 6;974(1-2):202-11.*
44 Ruddell RG, Mann DA, Ramm GA. The function of serotonin within the liver. 130*J Hepatol.* 2008 Apr;48(4):666-75.

45 Gershon, MD *Aliment Pharmacol Ther* 1999; 13 Suppl 2: 15-30
46 Gershon, MD *J Clin Gastroenterol.* 2005 May-Jun;39(4 Suppl 3):S184-93.
47 Cates, MD et al *Gastroenterology* 2004; 126: 1657-1664
48 Minderaa, RB, et al. *Biol Psychiatry.* 1987 Aug;22(8):933-40.
49 Mouridsen, SE, et al. *Dev Med Child Neurol.* 2007 Jun;49(6):429-32.
50 MacNamara, IM *Brain Res.* 2008 Jan 16;1189:203-14.
51 Iacono, G, et al. *Clin Gastroenterol Hepatol.* 2007 Mar;5(3):361-6.
52 Kwon H, Pessin JE, Adipokines mediate inflammation and insulin resistance. *Front Endocrinol* (Lausanne). 2013 Jun 12;4:71.
53 Patrick RP, Ames BN, Vitamin D hormone regulates serotonin synthesis. Part 1: relevance for autism. *FASEB J.* 2014 Jun; 28(6):2398-413.

Chapter 3
Flora And The Gastrointestinal Tract

It may be said that the purpose of the human body is to be a vessel for the intestinal flora. Another way to frame it is to say that intestinal flora regulate the human genome and therefore most of human metabolism.

Over a surface estimated to be 250 square meters, 1000–2000 trillion organisms (1–2 quadrillion) are found. This is 10–20 times the number of mammalian cells in the human body![1] The microflora is of 17 families, 45 types, and 400–500 species. 97% are anaerobic—Bacteroides, Bifidobacteria, Eubacteria, Fusobacteria, and Clostridia. The aerobes/facultative microbes are Lactobacilli, E. coli, Enterococci, Staphylococci, and Streptococci as well as multiple fungi.[2] The esophageal bacterial microbiota are similar in character to oral flora, the predominance being Streptococcus, but at least four other genera are also common.[89]

With polymerase chain analysis, the idea of a sterile stomach has been disproven. The population is diverse and includes 128 phylotypes, including *Proteobacteria*, *Firmicutes*, *Actinobacteria*, *Bacteroidetes* and *Fusobacteria*. Among these is the phylum *Deinococcus* which was previously thought to be found only in radioactive waste disposal sites.[90] The viral/bacteriophage component is just beginning to be studied.[91] According to Chehoud, et al:

> The human fecal virome is immense in the numbers of viruses present—comparable to the number of bacteria, which is 10^{11} per g of feces—and the number of different types. Gut bacteriophages are so numerous and diverse that sequence databases contain only a small fraction of the global population.

Role Of The Gut Microflora

This ecosystem, our largest metabolic "organ," is essential to the development of the mucosal immune system, the absorption of complex macromolecules, the synthesis of amino acids and vitamins and the maintenance of the mucosal barrier in its role of excluding antigens and pathogenic microorganisms. Distribution of gastrointestinal flora is lowest in the esophagus and gradually increases toward the colon. Disruption of the flora may lead to allergies, luminal and systemic inflammation, diabetes, cancer and inflammatory bowel disease.

Research strongly supports the following functions of the gastrointestinal flora via probiotic supplements/foods:

1. Prevention and treatment of C. difficile/antibiotic associated diarrhea
2. Protection against non-C. difficile diarrhea and dysbiosis post-antibiotic use[3]
3. Prevention of necrotizing enterocolitis in newborns
4. Prevention and treatment of rotavirus induced diarrhea
5. Improvement in the symptoms of lactose intolerance
6. Reduction in bacterial putrefactive metabolites in the gut
7. Reduction of cancer promoting enzymes in the gut

8. Improvement in non-specific GI complaints in healthy individuals
9. Modulation of enterocyte defensin expression[4]
10. Modulation of gut mucosal cytokine expression[5,6]
11. Improvement in inflammatory bowel disease (IBD)[7]
12. Improvement in irritable bowel syndrome (including in vitro normalization of smooth muscle motility)
13. Enhancement in treatment outcomes in H. pylori and bacterial overgrowth
14. Normalization of stool passage and consistency in constipation and IBS
15. Prevention/improvement of allergies and atopic diseases in infants
16. Prevention of respiratory tract infections
17. Treatment of urogenital infections
18. Reduction in social anxiety with the inclusion of fermented foods in the diet[92]

Preliminary evidence supports the following effects of probiotics:

1. Lowering of serum cholesterol levels
2. Improvement of small intestinal hyperpermeability in IBS-D
3. Prevention of dental caries[8]
4. Prevention and treatment of ischemic heart disease
5. Treatment of autoimmune diseases
6. Improvement in SSRI resistant depression[93]
7. Improvement in digestion and social functioning in autism[94]

A probiotic is a microbe that protects its host and prevents disease.

A prebiotic is "a selectively fermented ingredient that allows specific changes, both in the composition and/or activity in the gastrointestinal microflora that confers benefits upon host well being and health."

A symbiotic is a combination of probiotics and prebiotics.

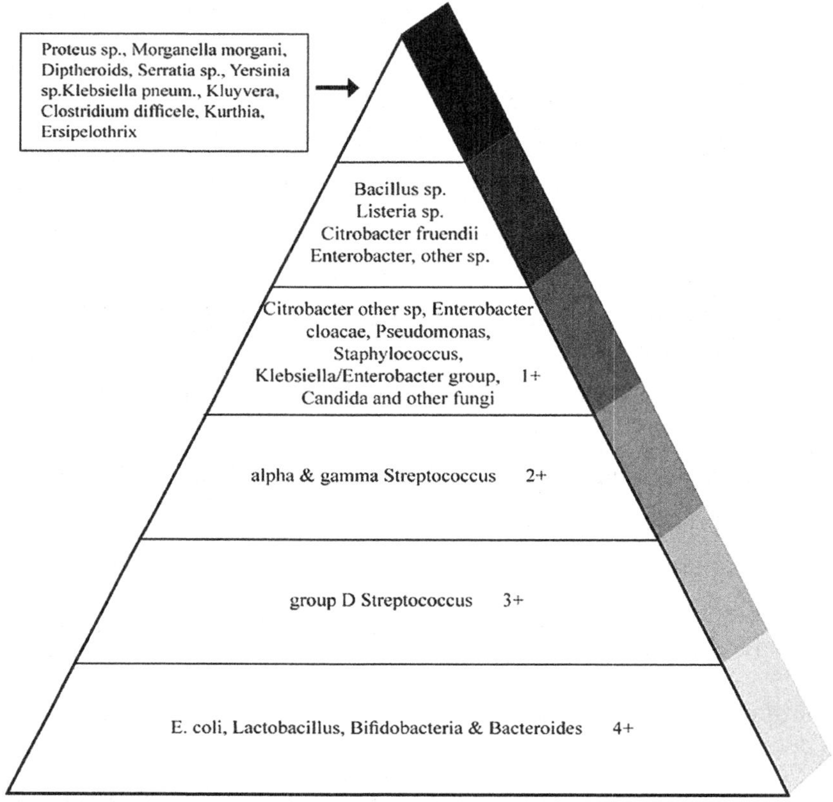

Figure 3.1 Organisms Comprising The Flora In stool

Is Stool Flora Representative Of The Totality Of Intestinal Flora?

No, stool cultures are indicative of lower colonic flora only. For example, testing a stool sample will not tell you anything about the possibility of small intestinal bacterial overgrowth. Flora vary with the location in the tract.

The esophagus and stomach have low levels of Streptococci, Lactobacilli and others—10^3 to 10^5/gram.

The small bowel has moderate levels of Lactobacilli, Streptococci, Enterobacteria and Bacteroides—10^3 to 10^{12}/gram.

The large intestine essentially contains the flora shown in Figure 3.1 above.

When And How Do The Intestinal Microflora Develop?

Humans are not born with a sterile intestinal tract. According to Koleva et al:

> The pioneer microbiota of the neonatal gut is essential for gut maturation, and metabolic and immunologic programming. Recent research has shown that early bacterial colonization may impact the occurrence of disease later in life (microbial programming). Despite early conflicting evidence, it has long been considered that the womb is a sterile environment and human microbial colonization begins at birth. In the last few years, several findings have reiterated the presence of microbes in infant first stool (meconium) and pointed to the existence of in utero microbial colonization of the infant gut. The dominant bacterial taxa detected in meconium specimens belong to the Enterobacteriaceae family (Escherichia genus) and lactic acid bacteria (notably members of the genera Leuconostoc, Enterococcus, and Lactococcus). Maternal atopy promotes dominance of Enterobacteriaceae in newborn meconium, which in turn may lead to respiratory problems in the infant. This microbial interaction with the host immune system may in fact, originate during fetal life.[95]

The first postnatal transfer of bacteria is from maternal vaginal and fecal flora (not so with Cesarean birth). The mouth to anus position of non-breech birth facilitates this colonization. E.coli, Enterococci, Enterobacteria, Streptococci and Staphylococci make up the flora on day one (in full term neonates). Breastfeeding introduces the Bifidobacteria, and by the end of the first week they predominate. A review of six studies showed that intestinal bacterial colonization of beneficial flora is delayed in preterm infants.[10] A systematic review of 7 studies concluded that lower diversity and numbers of Actinobacteria and Bacteroidetes as well as increases in Firmicutes were seen in Cesarean born vs vaginally birthed infants.[96] Firmicutes:Bacteroidetes ratio is related to childhood obesity because of increased short chain fatty acid and carbohydrate metabolism.[97] Chu et al found that by the first 6 weeks of life, there was significant alteration in infant flora depending on body site. Contrary to other studies they did not find that mode of delivery (vaginal vs. Cesarean) was a significant factor in make-up of the flora.[98]

Intestinal Flora, Antibiotics, Breastfeeding And The Newborn

A review of research done at Warwick Medical University investigated the effect of probiotics and peripartum antibiotics on the health of infants.[11] It is clearly proven that administering probiotics to newborns reduces the incidence of allergies later in life.[12,13,14,15] Prebiotics are also effective in preventing allergy and infection in the first two years of life.[16] Animal studies have linked autoimmune disease with early-life alterations in intestinal flora.[17] Gao et al report that gut microbiota play multiple roles in protecting against allergic reactions, inflammation, cardiac pathologies and malignancies in humans.[99] Administration of ampicillin to prevent neonatal group B Strep infection significantly increases resistant coliform infection in newborns.[18] Amoxicillin-clavulinate given to mothers at 36 weeks of pregnancy increases the risk of neonatal necrotizing enterocolitis.[19] Several studies suggest that the administration of probiotics may prevent this life threatening disease and may reduce morbidity and mortality rates for low birth weight infants.[20,21] Many preterm infants receive prophylactic antibiotics at birth which further delays the colonization of normal intestinal flora.[22] The general use of broad-spectrum antibiotics in hospital maternity units increases antibiotic resistance and nosocomial transmission of infection.[23]

The first organisms to colonize the newborn intestinal tract have profound effects on lifelong immunity. The flora creates a two-way crosstalk with the mucosa, influencing induction of gene expression which controls immunity and mucosal epithelial function.[24,25,26,27] Perinatal probiotics (and flora implanted from nursing) have been shown to have the most extended colonization of intestinal flora compared to those acquired after six months of age.[28,29] Several studies from the Ukraine show that, in infants, oligosaccharides stimulate the growth of Bifidobacteria and Lactobacilli, reduce pathogen growth, lower the fecal pH, improve stool consistency and modulate the immune system.[30]

Breastfeeding has an essential role in the maturation of the newborn's GI flora and general immunity. The volume of the thymus in exclusively breastfed infants is over twice that of formula fed infants at four months of age.[31]

Leukocytes, Lactoferrin, Lysozyme, And Immunoglobulins In Human Milk

Bacterial and viral associated diarrheal disease claims 5 million children per year in the developing world. Breastfeeding could reduce the risk of dying from diarrhea by a factor of twenty-four.[32] Human milk contains macrophages and neutrophils, which actively phagocytize bacteria-IgA complexes, and activated T cells.[33] Monoglycerides and short chain fatty acids which control bacterial, viral and fungal growth are more abundant in breast-fed infants.[34] Human whey protein contains lactoferrin, lysozyme and immunoglobulins IgE, IgA, IgM and IgG.[35,36] In 1983 Benno et al, found Bifidobacteria in both breast-fed and bottle-fed infants, while counts of other bacteria, such as Bacteroides, Eubacteria, Peptococci, Veillonella, Clostridia, Enterobacteria, Streptococci, and Bacillus were significantly higher in the bottle-fed group.[37] Both raw and processed bovine and human milk were cultured with Listeria by Chen et al, in 2001.[38] Up to 99% of the Listeria innocua were killed and growth was inhibited in both refrigerated raw and pasteurized human milk for at least 60 days. IgA antibodies against Listeria and E. coli antigens were found in some of the human milk samples, but not in the bovine samples.

Systemic Immunity, GI Immunity And The Microflora

In the absence of gut flora, the development of oral tolerance does not proceed.[39] The "hygiene hypothesis" is a popular theory which explains that immune dysregulation may stem from failure of induction of the gut and systemic immunity when people in highly developed countries attempt to create an ultra-clean environment for their newborns. Colonization of the gut primes the mucosal immune system. A major aspect of this priming effect is increasing the number of intraepithelial lymphocytes and development of the Peyer's patches.[40] A product produced by Bacteroides fragilis in mice also controls development of non-GI lymph tissue and splenic architecture, and prevents excessive Th2 and B-cell follicular thymic hyperplasia.[41] Research has shown that production and modulation of regulatory T cells depends on neonatal bacterial flora.[42] In human studies, dysregulation of regulatory T cells increases allergic sensitization.[43] Colonization by commensals creates a low level of physiological inflammation which is essential for the development of immune tolerance.[44,45,46]

Stress, Nutrition And Host-microorganism Interactions

Changes in the microflora of the intestinal tract are a potent example of the naturopathic 'terrain' concept, explaining factors which permit the development of virulent infectious processes. Psychological stress alters bacterial adherence (to the GI mucosa) and coadherence (bacterium to bacterium).[47] Adherence is a primary step in infection and microbial colonization. According to John Alverdy, MD, a researcher at the University of Chicago, four phenotypes of intestinal commensals are expressed based on levels of stress and nutrition.[48]

Chronic-colonizing Phenotype: Under normal conditions, the flora feed on luminal nutrients and are separated from the epithelia by a thick mucus coat.

Self-protection Phenotype: In mild stress conditions, the flora create a protective biofilm above a partially eroded mucous coat.

***Nutrition Obtaining Phenotype*:** In conditions of stress and poor nutrition, the flora adhere and feed off the enterocytes.

***Barrier Dysregulating Phenotype*:** In conditions of extreme stress and poor nutrition, the flora are influenced by host-derived catabolic and inflammatory signals. The microflora invade the enterocyte which alters intestinal permeability and immunity.

Examples of factors influencing stress and nutrition in the above phenotypical stages in increasing significance are emotional and metabolic stress, oral antibiotics, intravenous feeding, hypoxia, medical life-support, and multiple antibiotics.

With regard to emotional and metabolic stress, norepinephrine may be a major inducer of pathogen growth and virulence. In vitro, norepinephrine increases the growth and virulence of Pseudomonas aeruginosa, Yersinia enterocolitica, and Escherichia coli (enterotoxicogenic and enterohemorrhagic strains) with increasing production of Shiga-like toxin.[49] Increased growth of Salmonella is seen in mice with high norepinephrine levels.[50] The gut produces as much as 50% of total body norepinephrine.

Toll-like receptors (TLR) on enterocytes recognize intestinal flora as commensals or pathogens. Research shows that if activation of host TLR by the commensal flora is blocked, mucosal injury and even death ensue.

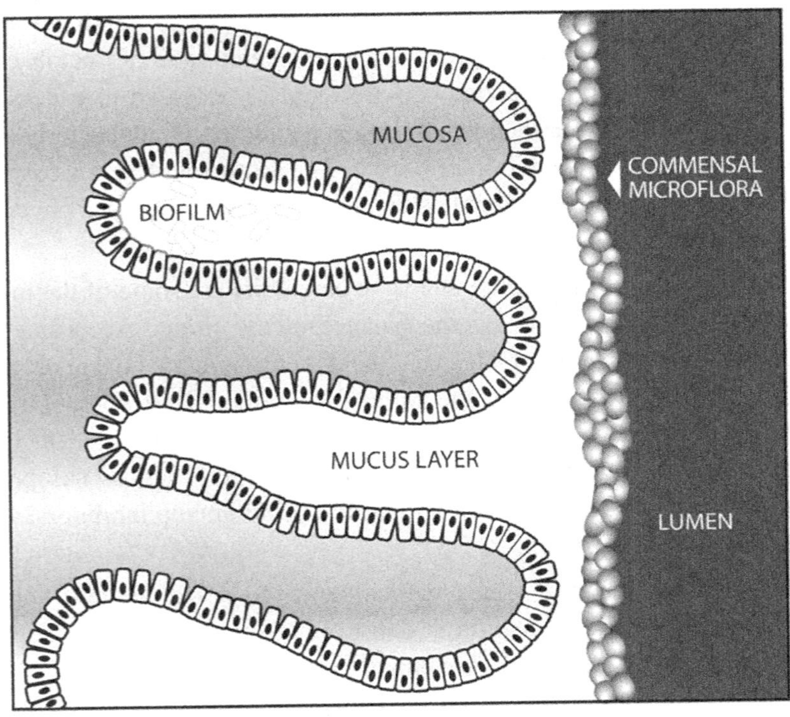

FIGURE 3.2 THE MUCOSA/FLORA RELATIONSHIP

Pathogenic organisms have developed the ability to produce bacteriocins, proteases, ureases (H. pylori), morphine (Ascaris), cytolethal distending toxin (Campylobacter and others), and other substances to overcome host immunity. Despite the adaptive physiology of these pathogens, host immune function generally prevails.

A fascinating study revealed that probiotic treatment of rat pups normalizes corticosterone release when triggered by the stress of maternal separation. The reduction in cortisol levels prevented the expected immediate and long-term colonic dysfunction induced by elevated stress hormone levels.[51] A decrease in Lactobacilli (not related to cortisol changes) and an increased risk of neonatal infection were found in newborn monkeys separated from their mothers for three days.[52] Pregnant monkeys exposed to periodic startling noise gave birth to neonates with decreased numbers of intestinal Bifidobacteria and Lactobacilli.[53]

Psychological stress also caused an overall decrease in enteric aerobes

(E. coli), an increase in the number of E. coli in the proximal small intestine (small intestinal bacterial overgrowth) and an altered ratio of Lactobacilli and E. coli. Russian test pilots who are regularly exposed to excessive physical, nervous and emotional strain had decreased Bifidobacteria and other undesirable changes in their flora.[54] The same held true for cosmonauts exposed to neuroemotional tension, hypokinesia, increased physical loads, isolation and thermal changes.[55]

Prolonged stays in hospital intensive care units are some of the most stressful situations influencing the balance of the flora. According to Alverdy at the University of Chicago "the disruption in the host microbial interaction that occurs during the care of the critically ill is potentially lethal."[56] In addition to the psychological upheaval, additional factors include the use of vasoactive drugs (epinephrine, terlipressin, vasopressin, dopamine, dobutamine, etc.), antibiotics, proton pump inhibitors, and parenteral nutrition (see Figure 3.3).

It is hypothesized that acne patients' increased risk of anxiety, anger, depression and suicidal ideation is due to nutritional factors, decreased anti-oxidant status and altered intestinal flora.[57]

Despite the elegance of the host immunity, there are chronic low-grade states that allow for changes that predispose to acute and chronic disease. When nutrient levels are low, other alterations in both host and bacteria may occur. Bacteria may proliferate at a slowed rate. At the same time, the enterocytes may reduce cell proliferation, protein synthesis and metabolic rate.

Human iron deficiency may lead to a decrease in some enteric infections, since a higher level of host iron is a cue for some pathogens to express virulence. Lactoferrin, present in breast milk and gastrointestinal secretions, is an iron binding protein, which decreases local iron levels for the purpose of reducing bacterial virulence. In addition, lactoferrin has potent antiviral, antifungal and antiparasitic activity.[58]

The effect of ICU stress was discussed above with respect to the invasiveness and virulence of commensal GI flora. In addition, the medications given to these patients add an extra dose of harm to the microflora. Antibiotics are administered in the ICU almost routinely, altering the enteric commensals. In addition, proton pump inhibitors are given to prevent the likely gastritis or peptic ulceration common in the ICU. Increasing gastric pH to >3.8 allows for bacterial overgrowth[59] including Clostridium difficile associated diarrhea.[60] Opiates administered for pain relief increase intestinal transit time, thereby decreasing the removal of pathogens. Some vasoactive drugs (epinephrine, norepinephrine) may cause luminal hypoxia, thereby promoting dysbiosis.[61]

Intestinal Flora And Obesity/Insulin Resistance

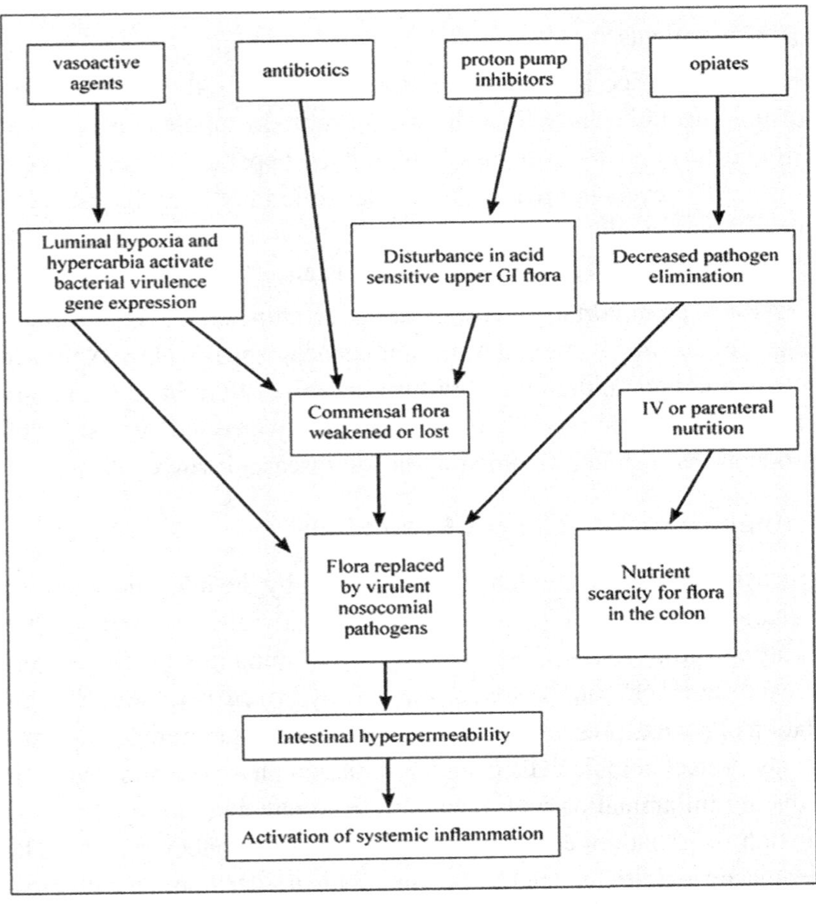

FIGURE 3.3 DYSBIOSIS IN THE INTENSIVE CARE UNIT PATIENT

(AFTER ALVERDY, ZABORINA AND WU)[62]

A profound example of the metabolic regulation of humans by the intestinal flora is seen in the bacterial phylum Firmicutes. Excess caloric intake in obese humans (and rodents) leads to greater numbers of Firmicutes which promote enhanced absorption of nutrients and weight gain. Feeding cultures of Firmicutes flora to mice promotes obesity.[63] Inflammation induced by the lipopolysaccharides from these bacteria into the portal circulation is thought to be a factor in the pathophysiology of insulin resistance and non-alcoholic fatty liver disease. Inhibition of fasting-induced adipocytokines may be a factor driving insulin resistance and atherogenesis in these patients.[64]

Insulin resistance is the major mechanism driving the pathophysiology of non-alcoholic fatty liver disease. Probiotic supplementation has been found to improve liver histology, reduce hepatic fatty acid levels, and lower ALT levels in mice with non-alcoholic fatty liver disease. The mechanism is thought to be reduction of a TNF-regulated kinase (Jun N-terminal kinase) that promotes insulin resistance.[65]

PPAR-γ is an important nuclear receptor on adipocytes. It has a major regulatory effect on inflammation and adipogenesis and is widely expressed in colonic mucosal epithelium.[66] In turn, intestinal flora have regulatory effects on PPAR-γ and it is thought that immunity directed against bacterial products, as seen in inflammatory bowel disease, involves PPAR-γ.

Intestinal Flora And Cancer Prevention

Butyric acid is a short-chain fatty acid produced by the intestinal flora via fermentation of soluble fiber. Colonic epithelial cells cultured in vitro with butyrate produce less COX-2 (reducing inflammatory processes) and more catalase (improving detoxification of hydrogen peroxide).[68] This regulation of gene expression by fermentation products of human intestinal flora may protect colonic cells from the initiation phase of carcinogenesis by reducing inflammation and oxidation. Butyrate also up-regulates the production of glutathione S-transferase in human colonocytes.[69,70] The antineoplastic activity induced by feeding pomegranate to mice with prostate cancer is dependant on the ability of microflora to convert ellagic acid to active metabolites.[71]

Intestinal Flora And The Liver

High levels of facultative microbes, particularly the Enterobacteriaceae, and low levels of anaerobes such as Bifidobacteria, produce higher levels of ammonia, endotoxins and other compounds. These are absorbed into the blood stream causing direct liver damage, as well as indirect damage from proinflammatory cytokines such as TNF-α.[72] There is evidence that melatonin may help prevent the GI motility changes induced by intestinal absorption of bacterial lipopolysacharides.[73] Probiotics, by modifying the intestinal flora, decrease the urease producing gram negatives and increase the anaerobic population. Clinical findings indicate that some strains of Lactobacilli may be useful in reducing the postoperative infection rate in critically ill patients post orthotopic liver transplant and in severe pancreatitis.[74] In 2008 the PROPATRIA trial warned of the harmful effects of probiotics on severe acute pancreatitis. A 2014 systematic review found no such danger and concluded that "The current data are not sufficient to draw a conclusion regarding the effects of probiotics on patients with predicted SAP (severe acute pancreatitis). Carefully designed clinical trials are needed to validate the effects of particular probiotics given at specific dosages and for specific treatment durations."[101]

Intestinal Flora, Prebiotics And Bone Health

Human and animal studies have shown the positive effects of prebiotics on mineral absorption and metabolism as well as bone composition and architecture.[75] These include inulin, fructooligosaccharides, galactooligosaccharides, soybean oligosaccharide, resistant starches, sugar alcohols, and difructose anhydride. High dietary calcium intake and an optimum amount and composition of prebiotics work together to produce this effect on bone.

Several mechanisms are likely to create this salutary effect of oligosaccharides and/or probiotics on bone:

1. increased solubility of minerals secondary to increased bacterial production of short-chain fatty acids
2. proliferation of enterocytes and improved absorptive surface
3. increased expression of calcium-binding proteins
4. an overall improvement in gut health

5. degradation of phytic acid
6. activation of factors such as phytoestrogens from foods
7. strengthening of the intestinal flora and improved gut ecology
8. stabilization of the intestinal mucus
9. provision of growth factors

A Japanese study found that mice genetically predisposed to early aging had decreased bone loss if fed a lactobacillus strain.[76] A Finnish study showed that L. helveticus fermented milk prevented bone loss in female rats by decreasing bone turnover and increasing bone mineral density.[77]

Intestinal Flora And Cholesterol Metabolism

The microflora have the capacity to convert luminal cholesterol into coprostanol. This reduces serum cholesterol, because coprostanol is not absorbed. This conversion most often occurs by two years of age. In Europe, the percentage of the population which can convert cholesterol to coprostanol ranges from 55%–74%. This conversion is often disturbed by standard antibiotic therapy.[78]

GI Flora And The Metabolism Of Botanical Medicines

The phytoestrogens in soy are metabolized into active isoflavones by the intestinal microflora.[79] Children treated with oral antibiotics who ingested soy had decreased urinary excretion of active isoflavonoids.[80] The GI flora produces beta-glycosidase which activates the glycosides in Salix alba (willow bark), Cassia senna (senna), Rheum palmatum (rhubarb), Harpagophytum procumbens (devil's claw), Trifolium pretense (red clover), Panax (ginseng) and Glycyrrhiza (licorice.)[81,82] Ellagic acid from pomegranate is activated by intestinal flora.[83]

GI Flora And Nutrition

A study done in Belgium showed that high fat diets decrease Bifidobacteria levels in rats. This effect was prevented by adding prebiotics (fructooligosaccharides) to the high fat diet.[84] Almonds (but not defatted almonds) were found to increase colonic butyrate levels and the growth of Bifidobacteria and Eubacterium.[85] Food-derived polyphenols alter the growth of microflora and adhesion to the mucus layer. Naringenin (from orange and grapefruit), quercetin (from capers, apples, green tea, onions, red grapes, citrus, broccoli, cherries, raspberry, cranberry, prickly pear fruit and honey), phloridzin (from apples) and rutin (from buckwheat, citrus, black tea, apple peel, Rheum species, and Ruta graveolens) were the most active. These effects included inhibition of Salmonella typhinurium and enhancement of Lactobacillus rhamnosus.[86]

The artificial sweetener Splenda™, (a combination of sucralose, maltodextrin and glucose, has been shown to alter the microflora of the gut. For twelve weeks, rats were fed Splenda™ at dosages comparable to human usage. The number of total fecal anaerobes, Bifidobacteria and Lactobacilli was significantly decreased compared to controls. In addition Phase I P450 enzymes (CYP3A4 and CYP2D1) were elevated.[87] A year later an expert panel refuted these results.[100] Calcium, but not zinc or magnesium, significantly increased the binding of Lactobacilli to enterocytes. Supplemental calcium may enhance the adhesion and effectiveness of probiotic cultures.[88]

---

1 Gibson, G University of Redding, UK—NPR interview 2006 July

2 Probert HM, Gibson GR. *Curr Issues Intest Microbiol.* 2002;3:23-7

3 Koning, CJ; Jonkers, DM; Stobberingh, EE; Mulder, L; Rombouts, FM; Stockbrugger, RW, The effect of a multispecies probiotic on the intestinal microbiota and bowel movements in healthy volunteers taking the antibiotic amoxycillin. *Am J Gastroenterol.* 2008 Jan; 103(1): 178-89

4 Schlee, M; Harder, J; Koten, B; Stange, E. F; Wehkamp, J; Fellermann, K. Probiotic lactobacilli and VSL#3 induce enterocyte beta-defensin 2. *Clin-Exp-Immunol.* 2008 Mar; 151(3): 528-35

5 Gackowska L, Michalkiewicz J, Krotkiewski M, Helmin-Basa A, Kubiszewska I, Dzierzanowska D. Combined effect of different lactic acid bacteria strains on the mode of cytokines pattern expression in human peripheral blood mononuclear cells. *J Physiol Pharmacol.* 2006 Nov;57 Suppl 9:13-21.

6 Borruel N, Casellas F, Antolín M, Llopis M, Carol M, Espíin E, Naval J, Guarner F, Malagelada JR. Effects of nonpathogenic bacteria on cytokine secretion by human intestinal mucosa. 2003 Apr;98(4):865-70.

7 Roediger,WE Review article: nitric oxide from dysbiotic bacterial respiration of nitrate in the pathogenesis and as a target for therapy of ulcerative colitis. *Aliment-Pharmacol-Ther.* 2008 Apr 1; 27(7): 531-41

8 Twetman, S; Stecksen-Blicks, C Probiotics and oral health effects in children. *Int J Paediatr Dent.* 2008 Jan; 18(1): 3-10.

9 De Vrese, M *Adv Biochem Eng Biotechnol.* 2008;111:1-66.
10 Westerbeek, EA et al *Clin Nutr.* 2006 Jun;25(3):361-8.
11 Bedford Russell, AR *BJOG* 2006;113:758-765.
12 Kalliomaki, M *Lancet* 2001:357:1076-9.
13 Murch, SH *Lancet* 2001;357:1057-9.
14 Kalliomaki, M *Lancet.* 2003;361:1869-71.
15 Lodinova-Zadnikova, R *Int Arch Allergy Immunol.* 2003;131:209-11.
16 Arslanoglu, S *J Nutr.* 2008 Jun;138(6):1091-5.
17 Bach, JF *NEJM.* 2002;347:911-20.
18 Stoll, BJ *NEJM.* 2002;347:240-7.
19 Kenyon, SL *Lancet.* 2001;357:979-94.
20 Gaul, J *Neonatal Netw* 2008 Mar-Apr;27(2):75-80
21 Barclay, AR *J Pediatr Gastroenterol Nutr.* 2007 Nov;45(5):569-76.
22 Westerbeek, EA et al *Clin Nutr.* 2006 Jun;25(3):361-8
23 Isaacs, D *Arch Dis Child Fetal Neonatal Ed* 2006;91:F72-4.
24 Hooper, LV *Science* 2001;291:881-4.
25 Hooper, LV *Trends Microbiol* 2004;12:129-34.
26 Sonnenburg, JL *Nat Immunol* 2004;5:569-73.
27 Xu, J *Proc Natl Acad Sci USA* 2003;100:10452-9.
28 Favier, CF *Appl Environ Microbiol* 2002;68:219-26.
29 Heilig, HG *App Environ Microbiol* 2002;68:114-23.
30 Nyankovskyy, S *Georgian Med News.* 2008 Mar;(156):40-6.
31 Hasselbalch, et al *Acta Paediatr.* 1996 Sep;85(9):1029-32.
32 Brandtzaeg, P et al *Vaccine.* 2003 Jul 28;21(24):3382-8.
33 Field, CJ *J Nutr.* 2005 Jan;135(1):1-4.
34 Siigur, U et al *Acta Paediatr.* 1993 Jun-Jul;82(6-7):536-8.
35 Davies, MC e al *Iran J Immunol.* 2006 Dec;3(4):181-6.
36 Smith-Norowitz, TA et al *Ann Clin Lab Sci.* 2008 Spring;38(2):168-73.
37 Benno, Y et al *Microbiol Immunol.* 1984;28(9):975-86.
38 Chen, HY et al *Adv Exp Med Biol.* 2001;501:341-8..
39 Sudo, N *J Immunol* 1997 159;1739-45.
40 Sebra, JJ *Am J Clin Nutr* 1999;69:(supp):1046S-51S.
41 Mazmanian, SK *Cell* 2005;122:107-18.
42 Sutmuller, RP *J Clin Invest* 2006;116:485-94.
43 Van den Biggelaar, AH *Lancet* 2000;356:1723-7.
44 Rook, GA *Gut* 2005;54:317-20.
45 Perez-Machado, MA *Eur J Immuno* 2003;33:2307-15.
46 Karlsson, MR *J Exp Med* 2004;199:1679-88.
47 Bosch, J et al *Psychosomatic Medicine* 2003;65:604-612.
48 Alverdy, J *Curr Opin in Clin Nutr Metab Care* 2005;8:205-209.
49 Reading, NC *J Bacteriol.* 2007 Mar;189(6):2468-76
50 Methner, U *Int J Med Microbiol* 2008 Jul;298(5-6):429-39.
51 Gareau, MD *Gut* 2007 Nov;56(11):1522-8.
52 Bailey, MT *Dev Psychobiol.* 1999 Sep;35(2):146-55.
53 Bailey, MT *J Pediatr Gastroenterol Nutr.* 2004 Apr;38(4):414-21.
54 Kafarskaia, LI *Zh Mikrobiol Epidemiol Immunobiol.* 1992 Apr;(4):12-4.
55 Liz'ko, NN *Antibiot Med Biotekhnol.* 1987 Mar;32(3):184-6.
56 Alverdy, J *Curr Opin in Clin Nutr Metab Care* 2005;8:205-209.

57 Katzman, M *Med Hypotheses*. 2007;69(5):1080-4.
58 Orsi, N *Biometals* 2004 Jun;17(3):189-96.
59 Thiesen, J *J Gastrointest* Surg 2000 Jan-Feb;4(1):50-4.
60 Aseeri, M et al *Am J Gastroent* 2008, Aug 12;103(9):2308-2313.
61 Holmes, CL *Curr Opin Crit Care* 2005 Oct;11(5):413-7.
62 Alverdy, J *Curr Opin in Clin Nutr Metab Care* 2005;8:205-209.
63 Yazigi, A. *Presse Med.* 2008 May 2.
64 He, ZQ *Med Hypotheses*. 2008;70(4):808-11.
65 Li, Z *Hepatology* 2003 Feb;37(2):343-50.
66 Rousseaux, C *J Soc Biol* 2006;200(2):121-31.
67 Adachi, M *Gut* 2006 Aug;55(8):1104-13.
68 Sauer, J *J Nutr Biochem* 2007 Nov;18(11):736-45.
69 Ebert, MN *Carcinogenesis*. 2003 Oct;24(10):1637-44.
70 Pool-Zobel, BL *Carcinogenesis* 2005 Jun;26(6):1064-76.
71 Seeram, NP et al *J Agric Food Chem* 2007 Sep 19;55(19):7732-7.
72 O'Sullivan, DJ *Curr Pharm Des* 2008;14(14):1376-81
73 De Fillipis, D et al *J Pineal Res*. 2008 Jan;44(1):45-51.
74 Lombardo, L *Minerva Gastroenterol Dietol.* 2008 Sep;54(3):287-93.
75 Schoz-Ahrens, KE *Nutr Rev* 2007 Jun;65(6 Pt 1):282-5.
76 Kimoto-Nira, H *Br J Nutr.* 2007 Dec;98(6):1178-86.
77 Narva, M *Ann Nutr Metab.* 2007;51(1):65-74.
78 Norin, E *Ann Nutr Metab* 2008:52(suppl 1):12-14.
79 Headlund, TE *J Nutr.* 2005 Jun;135(6):1400-6.
80 Halm, BM *Nutr Cancer.* 2008 Jan-Feb;60(1):14-22.
81 Hawrelak, JA and Myers, SP *Altern Med Rev* 2004 9(2):180-193.
82 Kim, YS et al *J Microbiol Biotechnol.* 2008 Jun;18(6):1109-14.
83 Seeram, NP et al *J Agric Food Chem* 2007 Sep 19;55(19):7732-7.
84 Cani, PD 2007 Nov;50(11):2374-83.
85 Mandalari, G et al *Appl Environ Microbiol.* 2008 Jul;74(14):4264-70.
86 Parkar, SG et al *Int J Food Microbiol.* 2008 Jun 10;124(3):295-8.
87 Abou-Donia, MB et al *J Toxicl Environ Health A.* 2008;71(21):1415-29.
88 Larsen, N et al *Int J Food Microbiol.* 2007 Feb 28; 114(1): 113-9.
89 Walker MM, Talley NJ, Review article: bacteria and pathogenesis of disease in the upper gastrointestinal tract--beyond the era of Helicobacter pylori. *Aliment Pharmacol Ther.* 2014 Apr;39(8):767-79.
90 Bik EM et al, Molecular analysis of the bacterial microbiota in the human stomach. *Proc Natl Acad Sci U S A*. 2006 Jan 17;103(3):732-7.
91 Chehoud C et al, Transfer of Viral Communities between Human Individuals during Fecal Microbiota Transplantation. MBio. 2016 Mar 29;7(2):e00322.
92 Hilimire MR et al, Fermented foods, neuroticism, and social anxiety: An interaction model. *Psychiatry Res*. 2015 Aug 15;228(2):203-8.
93 Bambling M et al, A combination of probiotics and magnesium orotate attenuate depression in a small SSRI resistant cohort: an intestinal anti-inflammatory response is suggested. *Inflammopharmacology*. 2017 Feb 2.
94 Navarro F et al, Can probiotics benefit children with autism spectrum disorders? *World J Gastroenterol.* 2016 Dec 14;22(46):10093-10102.
95 Koleva PT et al, Microbial programming of health and disease starts during fetal life. Birth Defects Res C *Embryo Today*. 2015 Dec;105(4):265-77.

96 Rutayisire E et al, The mode of delivery affects the diversity and colonization pattern of the gut microbiota during the first year of infants' life: a systematic review. *BMC Gastroenterol.* 2016 Jul 30;16(1):86.

97 Goffredo M et al, Role of Gut Microbiota and Short Chain Fatty Acids in Modulating Energy Harvest and Fat Partitioning in Youth. *J Clin Endocrinol Metab.* 2016 Nov;101(11):4367-4376.

98 Chu DM et al, Maturation of the infant microbiome community structure and function across multiple body sites and in relation to mode of delivery. Nat Med. 2017 Jan 23. doi: 10.1038/nm.4272. [Epub ahead of print]

99 Gao J et al, Importance of gut microbiota in health and diseases of new born infants. *Exp Ther Med.* 2016 Jul;12(1):28-32. Epub 2016 Apr 11.

100 Brusick D et al, Expert panel report on a study of Splenda in male rats. *Regul Toxicol Pharmacol.* 2009 Oct;55(1):6-12. doi: 10.1016/j.yrtph.2009.06.013. Epub 2009 Jun 28.

101 Gou S et al, Use of probiotics in the treatment of severe acute pancreatitis: a systematic review and meta-analysis of randomized controlled trials Crit Care. 2014; 18(2): R57. Published online 2014 Mar 31. doi: 10.1186/cc13809 PMCID: PMC4056604

Chapter 4

Stress And Digestion

How Is Stress Induced In Digestive Research?

GI stressors that have been used in murine, rabbit and canine research include fear conditioning, loud noise, restraint, cold exposure, water avoidance, swimming without a perceived escape, inescapable foot or tail shocks, and exposure to endotoxins. GI stressors that have been used in human studies include math calculation, anagram solving, the Stroop test, dichotomous listening (listening through headphones to two separate conversations simultaneously), intermittent bursts of white noise, watching upsetting video footage, intermittent hand immersion in cold water, driving in traffic and stressful interviews.

What Is The Neurology Of Stress Reactions In The GI Tract?

When exposed to emotional stress, both healthy subjects and those with IBS have decreased heart rate variability (a measure of decreased parasympathetic vagal tone) and increased heart rate and skin conductance (measures of increased sympathetic tone.)[1] Positron Emission Tomography (PET) and functional magnetic resonance imaging (fMRI) have illuminated central mechanisms of visceral hypersensitivity in FGID. Healthy control subjects show activation of the anterior cingulate gyrus (ACG), in contrast to IBS subjects. The ACG is an important opiate binding center which modifies incoming sensory input. Failure of ACG activation in patients with IBS permits increased pain perception in response to actual or anticipated painful stimuli.[2,3] In addition, an enhanced activation of the prefrontal cortex occurs in IBS which is associated with hypervigillance and facilitation of recall for emotionally charged memories.

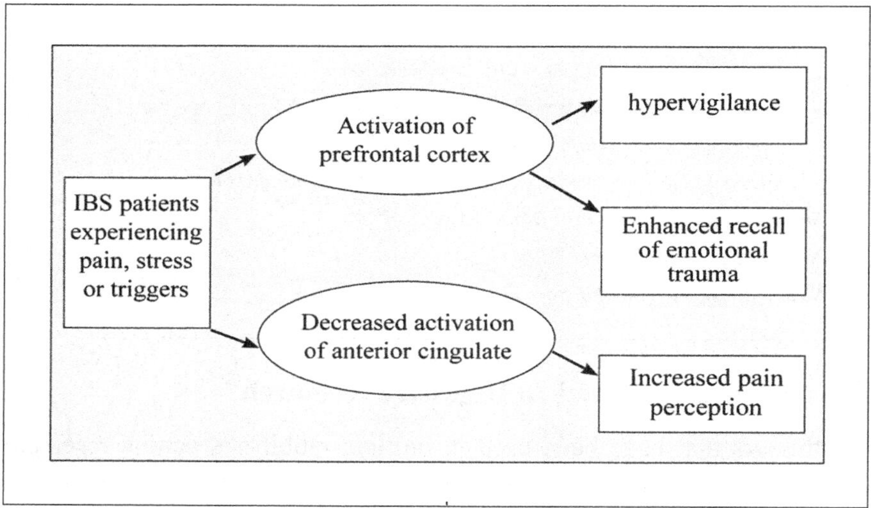

FIGURE 4.1 CENTRAL STRESS CIRCUITRY—PET AND FMRI FINDINGS IN IBS

Motility

Peristaltic contractions are controlled by stellate shaped fibroblast/neuron-like interstitial cells of Cajal (ICC) situated within the myenteric plexus.[4] These cells generate pacemaker potentials which are modified by neural input.[5]

Normal Esophageal Motility

A progressive, distally propagated peristaltic wave is triggered by swallowing a food bolus. The smooth muscle of the esophagus undergoes reflex peristaltic contraction as it is stretched by the bolus. The upper esophageal sphincter prevents excessive air from being swallowed and the lower esophageal sphincter prevents excessive gastric secretions from entering the esophagus. Between swallows the sphincters are closed. Peristalsis is normally involuntary and imperceptible.

Stress-induced Changes In Esophageal Motility

Esophageal spasms are present in a high percentage of patients with non-cardiac chest pain.[6] Esophageal contraction amplitudes and levels of anxiety-related behaviors are significantly greater during stress.[7,8] Owing to the proximity and innervation of the esophagus and the heart, esophageal spasm, gastroesophageal reflux or hiatal hernia can manifest as symptoms similar to a cardiac source of chest pain. Up to 64% of patients with gastroesophageal reflux disease (GERD) reported aggravation of reflux symptoms by stress. Possible mechanisms by which stress exacerbates heartburn include a change in the diaphragmatic support of the lower esophageal sphincter (LES) due to altered breathing patterns, altered esophageal chemosensitivity, and delayed gastric emptying.[9] The term "irritable esophagus" has been used to note a generalized alteration in esophageal pain threshold.[10] Esophageal spasms are frequently triggered by both physiological and psychological stressors. Anxiety increases the perception of reflux symptoms in susceptible patients, but not the actual volume or extent of acid reflux. Relaxation therapy decreases both reflux symptoms and total esophageal exposure to acid.[11] Although the relationship is not clear, there is an increased incidence of psychiatric diagnoses in patients with esophageal motility disorders and a high incidence of anxiety and depression in patients referred for esophageal motility testing.[12,13,14]

Subjects with reflux esophagitis showed the presence of simultaneous waves (non-peristaltic contractions) when exposed to stress (cold water hand emersion), but this was not seen in subjects without esophagitis.[15] Patients with globus sensation also have a high rate of psychiatric disorders.[16]

Normal Gastric Motility

The three layers of gastric muscles contract in a fascinating way—like a sleeve being partially turned inside out and then right side out. The first response to food filling the stomach is receptive relaxation. The proximal stomach accommodates incoming food by smooth muscle relaxation. The fundus and the body have thin muscles which easily accommodate 1.5 liters of food.

There is little contraction of the gastric fundus and body. Contents in the proximal stomach can remain unmixed for as long as an hour. Constrictor (mixing) waves are concentric rings of contraction that begin in the mid-stomach (pacemaker region) in response to food. On average there are three contractions/minute of the gastric smooth muscle which increase in force and velocity as they approach the pylorus. The resulting mixture of food and stomach secretions is called chyme. Lipids form an oily layer on top and exit the stomach last. Hypochlorhydria delays gastric emptying, whereas hyperchlorhydria speeds it. Duodenal activity inhibits gastric emptying by neural reflex and hormonal mechanisms. When hydrochloric acid, non-isotonic solutions and undigested fats enter the duodenum, receptors are stimulated. These trigger vagal reflexes and the release of hormones to inhibit gastric emptying.

Stress-induced Changes In Gastric Motility

With sympathetic dominance under stress, the gastric contractions decrease to one per minute. The character is entirely different, without the mixing action. The entire stomach has a weaker, more simultaneous contraction which has the function of blanching the mucosal circulation—moving blood to the brain and extremities where it is deemed more autonomically essential during a shift to sympathetic dominance. Fear, anger, painful stimuli, pre-operative anxiety, or intense exercise all delay gastric emptying but increase colonic peristalsis.[17] Other evidence points to depression and fear causing the stomach to empty slowly (related to hypochlorhydria), while anger and aggression may cause the stomach to empty quickly (related to hyperchlorhydria). Gastric emptying may be assessed by ultrasonography,[18] but the standard method involves x-ray tracing of a radiolabeled meal. Gastric emptying is inhibited by CRH acting on the CRH-2 receptor during stress.[19,20]

Normal Small Intestinal Motility

In the setting of optimal parasympathetic tone ("rest and digest"), peristalsis moves food along the small bowel at about 1 cm per minute. The migrating motor complex or MMC ("housekeeping wave") engages every 90 minutes between meals. The MMC begins about 4 hours after eating and ceases when food is eaten. This is a major difference between small and large bowel motility reflexes. Small bowel motor peristaltic activity is stimulated by fasting whereas colonic peristaltic activity is stimulated by eating or drinking. Segmentation (mixing waves) occur 2-3 times per minute.

Stress-induced Changes in Small Intestinal Motility

As in the stomach, small intestinal motility significantly slows with stress.[21,22] The altered motility in IBS may lead to small intestinal bacterial overgrowth and mucosal damage.[23] Luminal levels of CCK and VIP also decrease with psychological stress.[24] Acupuncture with electrical stimulation at the knee point ST-36 (Zusanli) significantly improves the stress-induced reductions in small intestinal motility.[25] Feeding tryptophan to rats increases ileal motility and ileal serotonin levels.[26]

Normal Colonic Motility

The non-stressed large intestine forms transient haustrations at the rate of 2 per minute in order to mix the colonic contents. Mass movements occur 1-3 times per day (a 10-30 minute cycle in which contractions develop every two to three minutes). These move stool through to the sigmoid at 30 second intervals.

Stress-induced Changes In Colonic Motility

Stress-induced colonic motility is increased in normal individuals and in IBS-D with hyper-responsiveness to CRH on the CRH-1 receptor.[27,28] Intraluminal serotonin levels may also mediate stress-induced rapid transit time in mice.[29] In severe ulcerative colitis mass movements may be relatively continuous day and night.[30] Research on rats suggests that neonatal stress alters intestinal smooth muscle responses to acute stress in adulthood.[31] If this proves to be true for humans, being born into a stressful environment with interruptions in bonding may predispose to IBS later in life. Daily intake of a high-fiber diet may be effective in preventing stress- and CRH-induced acceleration of colonic transit and diarrhea (murine research).[32]

Anxiety is believed to increase pelvic floor muscle tension in patients with constipation.[33] Patients with IBS show a greater change in colonic and ileal motility during stress than healthy controls. These patients also have higher salivary cortisol levels *in anticipation of pain* induced by rectal distention (anticipatory anxiety).[34] Decreased coping skills plus increased depression and anxiety were found in IBS subjects with functional constipation.[35] Acupuncture with electrical stimuation also reduces stress-induced colonic hypermotility by modifying serotonin levels.[36]

Disease behavior may be learned in childhood. As discussed by W. E. Whitehead at the Division of Digestive Diseases, University of North Carolina at Chapel Hill:

> A characteristic of many patients who consult gastroenterologists for IBS and other motility disorders is a tendency to report multiple somatic complaints (including many nongastrointestinal complaints) and to overuse medical resources. This pattern of behavior is referred to as somatization or abnormal illness behavior. One source of abnormal illness behavior is childhood social learning, which occurs (1) when parents provide gifts or special privileges to a child who reports somatic symptoms or (2) when parents model abnormal illness behaviors themselves.

Your patients who have been trained in these ways will require a high degree of focus on changing these long held patterns in order to improve their digestion.

Secretion

Stress-induced Changes In Salivary Secretion

Salivary flow decreases with sympathetic dominance and amylase levels increase under stress (public speaking or mental math calculations). The increased amylase may correlate with elevated cortisol or catecholamine levels.[37, 38]

Normal Gastric Mucosal Protection

Mucosal integrity is maintained by surface epithelial cells connected by tight junctions which produce:

- Bicarbonate, mucus, and phospholipids
- Prostaglandins
- Heat shock proteins
- Cell renewal by proliferation of progenitor cells
- Continuous blood flow through mucosal microvessels
- Nitric oxide

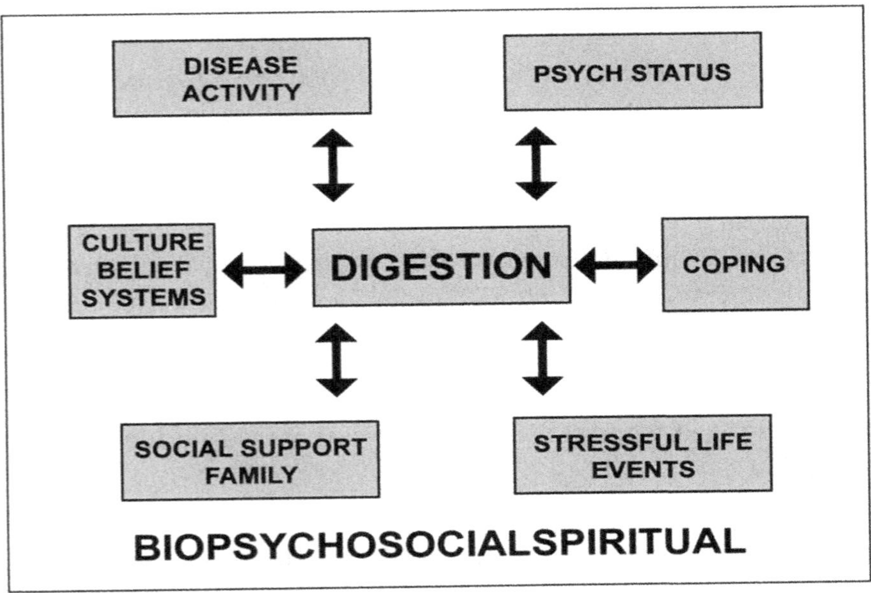

Reprinted with permission by K. Sandberg-Lewis.

FIGURE 4.2 BIOPSYCHOSOCIALSPIRITUAL DIGESTION MODEL

Stress-induced Changes In Gastric Digestion

The development of stress ulcers is well recognized and prophylaxis is routinely instituted in ICU units.[39] The etiology is loss of defensive gastric secretions.[40] Stress ulcers are one of the major findings in Hans Selye's (1907-1982) "general adaptation to stress" (GAS) in which he describes the changes seen in rats exposed to prolonged stress.

The GAS includes:

- Multiple gastric and duodenal ulcers
- Adrenal cortex hypertrophy
- Atrophy of the thymus, spleen and lymph nodes

Selye went on to explain these findings by the alterations in the hypothalamic-pituitary-adrenal axis. Prolonged elevations of gastrin, insulin and cortisol lead to degradation of the mucus/bicarbonate barrier.[41,42] Momordin, an oleanolic acid oligoglycoside isolated from the fruit of Kochia scoparia (Mexican fireweed or mock cypress) has shown gastroprotective properties against murine stress ulcers.[43] This is also true for Mangifera indica (mango flower infusion),[44] quebrachitol, a component from Magonia glabrata (soapberry) fruit extract,[45] centipedic acid—a diterpene from Egletes viscose (maceta),[46] boswellic acid (a leukotriene inhibitor from Boswellia serrata),[47] and 1-methylnicotinamide (a major derivative of nicotinamide).[48] Melatonin taken in 5 mg. doses or its precursor L-tryptophan taken in 500 mg. doses 30 minutes prior to ulcerogenic aspirin exposure significantly reduces gastric mucosal lesions.[49] Glycyrrhiza glabra has been found to protect against indomethacin-induced ulcers by reducing acid and leukotriene levels, while increasing mucin secretion and prostaglandin E2 release.[50]

Stress-induced Changes In Pancreatic And Gallbladder Secretion

Mental stress (arithmetic and anagram solving) caused chymotrypsin to significantly increase during—and significantly decrease following—30 minutes of stress.[51] Stress-induced sympathetic activity inhibits insulin secretion. There is evidence that the autonomic nervous system is one of the important regulators of pancreatic regeneration and pancreatic carcinogenesis.[52] Acoustic stress inhibits cholecystokinin and meal-induced gallbladder contraction in dogs. Restraint stress inhibits both CCK and secretin and is therefore a highly significant inhibitor of gall bladder and pancreatic secretion. Inhibitory responses were also produced by cerebral injection of corticotropin-releasing hormone. These effects of stress and exogenous CRH were simulated by intravenous infusion of norepinephrine.[53]

Stress and Gastric Mucosal Blood Flow

Acute stress ulcers are caused by reduced gastric mucosal blood flow (GBF), nitric oxide and prostaglandin synthesis in addition to increased free radical activation. Both melatonin, abundant in the gastrointestinal tract, and L-tryptophan have been shown to inhibit gastric acid secretion, augment GBF and scavenge free radicals, providing protection from stress-induced gastric lesions.[54,55]

Normal Intestinal Permeability

The intestinal epithelium is a single layer of columnar cells. These enterocytes secrete mucus, water, ions, defensins, enzymes and SIgA. The secretions serve to wash out irritants and toxins and prevent microbes from binding to the mucosal surface. Junctional complexes are composed of tight junctions, intermediate junctions and desmosomes (the paracellular space) which form a selective barrier against larger molecular weight molecules.[56] Pro-inflammatory cytokines, such as interferon-γ and tumor necrosis factor-β, increase paracellular permeability. Those that lead to resolution of inflammation, such as transforming growth factor-β, normalize paracellular permeability.[57]

Transcellular permeability allows absorption from the brush border through the cytoplasm. Pinocytosis may be a mechanism here and some of the antigens absorbed may be digested in lysosomes. Others may reach the lamina propria and create an immune response. M cells are specific for this transcellular conveyance of bacteria and antigens allowing for immune sampling in the Peyer's patches.[58] The M cells and dendritic cells, which can express tight junction proteins, influence intestinal permeability.

Stress Altered Permeability

Acute and chronic exposure to stressors can lead to changes in enteric physiology, including altered ion secretion, water secretion and increased epithelial permeability by both transcellular and paracellular pathways. Experimental acute stress has been shown to lead to increased secretion of water and the onset of diarrhea in mice and humans.[59,60] Prolonged exposure to stress can create low-grade inflammation, gross epithelial abnormalities, and altered bacterial-host interactions, allowing greater microbial translocation. These changes lead to increased hypersensitivity reactions and systemic inflammation.[61] IBS, as well as Crohn's disease, ulcerative colitis and food allergies seem to be associated with intestinal hyperpermeability.[62]

Rats exposed to one hour of acute restraint stress developed intestinal paracellular and transcellular hyperpermeability in the small and large bowel.[63] Visceral hyperalgesia (increased intestinal pain sensitivity) also occurred and persisted up to 24 hours. Rodents exposed to 10 days of stress had visceral hyperalgesia that persisted for 30 days.[64]

Heart rate variability is a well accepted method of measuring vagus nerve tone.[65] For research or clinical purposes, software can calculate the beat to beat heart rate variability, a measure of the variations in time between individual heart beats. These changes cannot be measured with manual pulse taking. The better the parasympathetic tone, the higher the heart rate variability. Think of this as an indicator of improved vascular elasticity and tone. Your patients can purchase home biofeedback devices which train them to improve this function. Examples include the inner balance phone app, emWave 2, or emWave Pro www.heartmath.com

If a physician is interested in further pursuing biofeedback for stress management (skin conductance, peripheral temperature, neurofeedback, etc.), see *Biofeedback—A Practitioner's Guide*, fourth edition edited by Mark S. Schwartz and Frank Andrasik, Guilford Press, New York, NY, 2016.

Figure 4.3 Practical In-Office/Home Measures Of GI Stress
Heart rate variability
Skin conductance (electrodermal response)
Digital (finger) peripheral temperature

The following questions in Figure 4.4 may reveal underlying stressors and negative influences on the digestive process.

Figure 4.4 Interviewing A Patient

What was mealtime like in your family of origin?

- Did people eat together?
- How would you characterize the general atmosphere of meal-times?

Describe your mealtimes now.

- Describe the preparation of your meals
- Do you sit down to eat or do you eat "on the run"?
- Do you eat alone?
- Do you attend meals as part of your employment?
- Do you eat in front of the television?
- Do you eat while at the computer?
- Is the radio on? What content?
- Do you eat while driving?
- Do you eat while reading? What kind of literature?
- Do you tend to eat quickly?
- Do you enjoy your meals?

Do you consider yourself a perfectionist? If not, why not?

Do you regularly wear:

- Tight panty hose?
- Tight jeans?
- A girdle (spanx™)?

When you remove your clothes at the end of the day, are there pressure marks around your waist?

Watch and listen to your patient's breathing patterns

- Is there breath holding?
- Mouth breathing? Air gulping?

Questionnaire developed by K. Sandberg-Lewis. Used with permission.

The family of origin issues having to do with mealtimes may give you clues to patterns that were formed in childhood but continue to exist years or decades later. Perhaps a parent grilled and berated the children at the dinner table. The hard wired memory of that fight or flight response may come up every time the patient eats a meal. Emotional clearing techniques, Bach Flower remedies or homeopathy may be used to change these learned association patterns.

The questions (Figure 4.4) concerning present mealtime patterns will illustrate the level of focus (or lack thereof), speed and emotional setting of meals. Rushing or feeling rushed during meals reduces parasympathetic tone. Watching upsetting images on television (news programs, etc.) induces fight or flight responses. Eating in a relaxing atmosphere and chewing food until liquid (Fletcherizing) improves digestive motility, and secretion, while normalizing mucosal permeability and blood flow.

Perfectionism, especially in the extreme, perpetuates sympathetic dominance. Many perfectionists are unaware of this trait and will tell you that they are not perfect, or do not do things perfectly and therefore do not fit this pattern. If the expectation of perfection is one that they hold, the effect is often there and reduced parasympathetic tone will degrade the digestive process. Letting go of perfectionist beliefs is a complex process, but your patients can gradually learn to decrease the focus on unrealistic expectations.

Tight clothing over the waist and abdomen impede diaphragmatic breathing, thereby increasing sympathetic tone.

Breath holding ramps up the sympathetics. Obligate mouth breathing makes it impossible to breath while chewing—leading to breath holding and the increase in fight or flight responses. Air gulping (aerophagia) may be the cause of abdominal bloating and pain due to swallowing an excessive volume of air into the digestive tract.

1 Spetalen, S et al *Dig Dis Sci.* 2008 Jun;53(6):1652-9.
2 Silverman, DH et al *Gastroenterology.* 1997 Jan;112(1):64-72.
3 Mertz, H et al *Gastroenterology.* 2000 May;118(5):842-8.
4 Sanders, KM *Gastroenterology.* 1996 Aug;111(2):492-515.
5 Shea-Donohue, T et al *Neurogastroenterol Motil.* 2005 Oct;17 Suppl 3:20-40.
6 Minocha, A Joseph, AS *J Ky Med Assoc.* 1995 May;93(5):196-201.
7 Cook, IJ et al *Gastroenterology.* 1987 Sep;93(3):526-32.
8 Anderson, KO et al *Dig Dis Sci.* 1989 Jan;34(1):83-91.
9 Bradley, LA et al *Am. J. Gastroenterol.* 1993; 88: 11–19.
10 Castell, DO *Am J Med.* 1992 May 27;92(5A):2S-4S.
11 Richter JE, Bradley LC, *Semin Gastrointest Dis.* 1996 Oct;7(4):169-84.
12 Kane, FJ Jr *South Med J.* 1991 Jul;84(7):847-52.
13 Whitehead, WE *Gastroenterol Clin North Am.* 1996 Mar;25(1):21-34.
14 Clouse, RE *Med Clin North Am.* 1991 Sep;75(5):1081-96.
15 Johnston, BT et al *Gut.* 1996 Apr;38(4):492-7.
16 Moser, G et al *Arch Intern Med.* 1998;158:1365-73.
17 Tache, Y et al *Ann. NY Acad. Sci.* 1993; 697: 233–63.
18 Haruma, K et al *Digestion.* 2008;77 Suppl 1:48-51.
19 Monnikes, H et al *Dig Dis.* 2001;19(3):201-11.
20 Stengel A, Tache Y, *Annu Rev Physiol.* 2008 Oct 17.
21 Wang, SX et al *World J Gastroenterol.* 2005 Apr 7;11(13):2016-21.
22 Kellow, JE et al *Scand J Gastroenterol.* 1992;27(1):53-8.
23 Dobronte, Z et al *Orv Hetil.* 2006 Oct 29;147(43):2077-80.
24 Cao, SG et al *World J Gastroenterol.* 2005 Feb 7;11(5):737-40.
25 Tabosa, A et al *Braz J Med Biol Res.* 2002 Jun;35(6):731-9.
26 Ozer, C et al *Amino Acids.* 2007;32(3):453-8.
27 Tache, Y et al *Dig Dis.* 2001;19(3):201-11.
28 Spiller, R *Neurogastroenterol Motil.* 2006 Dec;18(12):1045-55.
29 Tsukamoto, K et al *Am J Physiol Regul Integr Comp Physiol.* 2007, Jul;293(1) R64-9.
30 Bassoltti, G et al *Int J Colorectal Dis.* 2004 Sep;19(5):493-7.
31 Lopez, LV et al *J Proteomics.* 2008 Apr 30;71(1):80-8.
32 Takahashi, T et al *Dig Dis Sci.* 2008 May;53(5):1271-7.
33 Whitehead, WE *Gastroenterol Clin North Am.* 1996 Mar;25(1):21-34.
34 Walter, SA et al *Neurogastroenterol Motil.* 2006 Dec;18(12):1069-77.
35 Chan, AO et al *World J Gastroenterol.* 2005 Sep 14;11(34):5362-6.
36 Tian, XY et al *Brain Res.* 2006 May 9;1088(1):101-8.
37 Nater, UM et al *Psychoneuroendocrinology.* 2006 Jan;31(1):49-58.
38 Nater, UM et al *Int J Psychophysiol.* 2005 Mar;55(3):333-42.
39 Heidelbaugh JJ, Inadomi JM, *Am J Gastroenterol.* 2006 Oct;101(10):2200-5.
40 Sesler, JM *AACN Adv Crit Care.* 2007 Apr-Jun;18(2):119-26.
41 Vakhrushev IaM *Klin Med (Mosk).* 1999;77(2):28-31.
42 Domschke, W et al *Acta Hepatogastroenterol (Stuttg).* 1977 Feb;24(1):34-7.
43 Matsuda, H et al *Life Sci.* 1999;65(2):PL27-32.
44 Carvalho, AC et al *Planta Med.* 2007 Oct;73(13):1372-6.
45 De Olinda, TM et al *Phytomedicine.* 2008 May;15(5):327-33.
46 Guedes, MM et al *Biol Pharm Bull.* 2008 Jul;31(7):1351-5.

47 Singh, S et al *Phytomedicine.* 2008 Jun;15(6-7):408-15.
48 Brzozowski, T et al *J Pharmacol Exp Ther.* 2008 Jul;326(1):105-16.
49 Konturek PC, Celinski K, Slomka M, Cichoz-Lach H, Burnat G, Naegel A, Bielanski W, Konturek JW, Konturek SJ. Melatonin and its precursor L-tryptophan prevent acute gastric mucosal damage induced by aspirin in humans. *J Physiol Pharmacol.* 2008 Aug;59 Suppl 2:67-75.
50 Khayyal, MT, el-Ghazaly, MA, Kenawy, SA, Seif-el-Nasr M, Mahran LG, Kafafi YA, Okpanyi, SN. Antiulcerogenic effect of some gastrointestinally acting plant extracts and their combination. *Arzneimittelforschung.* 2001;51(7):545-53.
51 Holtman, G et al *Dig Dis Sci.* 1989 Nov;34(11):1701-7
52 Kiba, T, *Pancreas.* 2004 Aug;29(2):e51-8.
53 Lens, HJ et al *J Clin Invest.* 1992 Feb;89(2):437-43.
54 Brzozowski, T et al *J Physiol Pharmacol.* 2007 Dec;58 Suppl 6:53-64.
55 Brzozowski, T et al *J Pineal Res.* 2005 Nov;39(4):375-85.
56 Baumgart, DC et al *Curr Opin Clin Nutr Metab Care.* 2002 Nov;5(6):685-94.
57 Utech, M et al *Methods Mol Biol.* 2006;341:185-95.
58 Man, AL et al *J Immunol.* 2008 Oct 15;181(8):5673-80.
59 Kiliaan, AJ et al *Am J Physiol.* 1998 Nov;275(5 Pt 1):G1037-44.
60 Barclay, JR et al *Gastroenterology* 1987; 93: 91–7.
61 Gareau, MG et al *Curr Mol Med.* 2008 Jun;8(4):274-81.
62 Chichlowski M, Hale LP, *Am J Physiol Gastrointest Liver Physiol.* 2008 Oct 16.
63 Kiliaan, AJ et al *Am J Physiol Gastrointest Liver Phsyiol.* 1998;275:G1037-G1044.
64 Bradesi, S et al *Am J Physiol Gastrointest Liver Phsyiol.* 2005 Jul;289(1):G42-53.
65 Lu, CL, *Dig Dis Sci.* 1999 Apr;44(4):857-61.

Chapter 5

The ENS-CNS Axis, The Holobiome, And The GI Metabolome

Evolving vocabulary
Neurons, mechanoreceptors and taste receptors
Microbial lipopolysaccharides, cytokines and inflammation
How LPS is metabolized
The ENS, Microbiome and Neurotransmitter Synthesis
Short Chain Fatty Acids—a major class of ENS to CNS cross-talk molecules
SCFAs, Microbes, Diabesity and CNS Inflammation

I strongly feel that it is the engagement of the gut and its microbiome that plays a major role in determining the intensity duration and uniqueness of our emotional feelings.

—**Emeran A Mayer, MD, PhD**
Director, Oppenheimer Center for Neurobiology of Stress
Professor, Medicine, Physiology & Psychiatry,
UCLA School of Medicine

While many of us have intuited the importance of helping our patients modulate the gut-brain axis via treatments aimed at the microbiota, the HPA axis and the nervous system, there is now a significant and growing body of evidence indicating that the gut microbiome plays a dominant role in this conversation. This chapter reviews the gut-brain axis via the vagus nerve and microbial metabolic products including endotoxin and short chain fatty acids, hormones, neuropeptides and adipokines. Two-way communication between the gut brain (enteric nervous system or ENS) and the central nervous system (CNS) is a continuous process which optimizes functioning in both systems. The gut microbiota can be thought of as a distinct "organ" which initiates and modifies much of this cross-talk.

To address this material, I will use an evolving vocabulary:

The gut **microbiota**—includes oral, esophageal, gastric, small intestinal and colonic flora

The gut **microbiome**—the genome of the gut flora which consists of about 4 million genes

The **holobiome** is defined as the sum of the approximately 26,000 human genes plus the 4 million microbial genes.

The gastrointestinal **metabolome**—the sum of all metabolic products produced by the microbiome

When one considers the immensity of the microbiome compared to the human genome, it becomes clear that humans are getting a free ride. We rely on the gut flora to modify our genetic functions. In fact, there are 360 microbial genes for every 1 human gene and the metabolome comprises about 40% of the total metabolities in human blood. Leo Galland, MD puts it succinctly in his 2014 review article: "The gut microbiome can be viewed as an anaerobic bioreactor programmed to synthesize molecules which direct the mammalian immune system, modify the mammalian epigenome and regulate host metabolism".[1] The gut microbiome is essential for the maturation and development of the enteric nervous system. These effects include both density and proper activity of the enteric neurons.

Neurons, Mechanoreceptors And Taste Receptors

Cross talk between the gut and brain occurs through the vagus nerve and the metabolome. The autonomic nervous system is the major anatomical connection between the enteric nervous system and the central nervous system. 90% of the impulses are sensory from ENS to CNS. This information includes the shape and consistency of the bolus as well as the pressure that the bolus exerts against the gut mucosa. Mechanoreceptors are stimulated by shearing forces as the bolus moves through the gut and stimulates the enteroendocrine cells (EEC) to release serotonin which modifies both vagal and ENS function. This data is transmitted through the vagus nerve. Additional information about food composition, levels of inflammation and quality of the microbiota is transmitted. This feedback helps to fine tune eating behavior, mood, blood glucose, digestive secretion, absorption and gut motility via the production of serotonin and other neuropeptides by EEC. Taste receptors throughout the length of the gut respond to food and stimulate production of various neuropeptides which have local and distant effects. These receptors are located on EEC and dendritic cells scattered throughout the mucosa. For example, the stimulation of bitter receptors triggers release of ghrelin which upregulates appetite when it reaches the CNS. As Emeran Mayer, MD states—"the gut is the NSA (analogous to the National Security Agency); the vagus nerve is the information highway for gut-brain traffic". The ENS optimizes motility, secretion, and mucosal blood flow as well as detecting toxins and irritants. One of the most significant ways that the microbiome acts on this gut-brain axis is via some key metabolites discussed below.

Microbial Lipopolysaccharides, Cytokines and Inflammation

Remarkably, 40% of the circulating metabolites in human blood are microbiota derived.[2] One such metabolite, lipopolysaccharide (LPS or endotoxin), is a component of the outer membrane of gram negative bacterial cell walls. When intestinal gram negative bacteria are present in normal levels, the liver is able to clear excess LPS—preventing wide-ranging effects on mood, cognition, intestinal permeability and inflammation.[3]

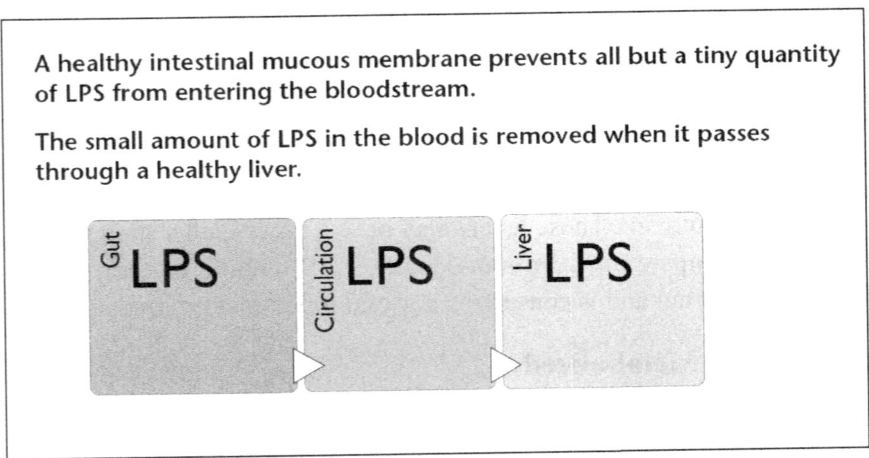

FIGURE 5.1 NORMAL LOW LEVEL LPS IN THE CIRCULATION

There are 1 million copies of LPS in each gram negative microbe[4] and these are released from both growing and dead bacteria.[6] Release may also be triggered by antibiotic therapy. Adults have approximately one gram of gut LPS.[5] Locally LPS is a significant stimulus for the zonulin pathway which induces intestinal hyperpermeability. When absorbed into the portal vein, LPS has major effects on the liver and, when excessive, LPS serum levels rise and have far reaching effects. LPS and inflammatory cytokines in serum can upregulate TNF-α, IL-1B, and IL-6 in the brain.[4] Clearly, intestinal bacteria do not need to cross the blood brain barrier to influence the CNS.

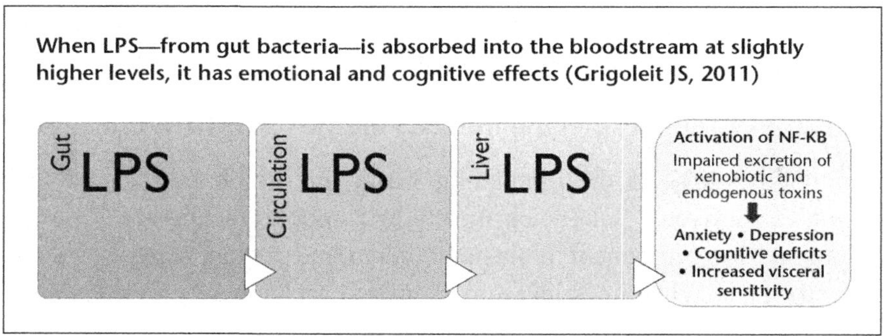

FIGURE 5.2 ELEVATED LPS IN THE CIRCULATION

It is important to note, however, that not all bacterial LPS is the same. For example Enterobacter derived LPS may be 1000 times more potent than that derived from other gram negative bacteria.[2] Other research shows that the microbial balance affects body habitus, and while the exact mechanisms are still being elucidated, one is clear—obesity multiplies the volume of endotoxin. These levels may be 2-3 times higher in the obese population compared to lean individuals. LPS binding protein can be measured in serum and is considered a useful inflammatory marker.

How LPS Is Metabolized

Humans have several pathways to metabolize LPS and limit its systemic impact. In the neonate, it is bound and inactivated by CD14, a bacterial pattern recognition receptor found in human breast milk. CD14 is not detectable in commercial cow's milk or infant formula, but is found in bovine colostrum. Lactoferrin in breast milk also binds to LPS.[6] After weaning, LPS binds to Toll-like receptor 4 (TLR-4) on intestinal epithelial cells. In addition, endosomal SIgA inactivates LPS, thereby reducing the NF-KB pathway and its cascade of proinflammatory cytokines—interferon, IL-6, and TNF-α.[7,8,9] Mucins (from goblet cells) and antimicrobial peptides such as defensins (from Paneth cells) act on gram negative bacteria and therefore reduce exposure of intestinal epithelia to LPS. Defensins also alter the structure of developing bacterial cell walls to weaken the gram negative microbes.[10]

Intestinal alkaline phosphatase is a brush border enzyme secreted into blood and the intestinal lumen. It regulates lipid absorption, duodenal pH and removal of LPS. Alkaline phosphatase is also produced in the liver, where it helps reduce LPS arriving via the portal vein. When endotoxin from gut bacteria is absorbed into the bloodstream at slightly higher levels, alkaline phosphatase may not adequately clear endotoxin, leading to increased systemic inflammation. This systemic inflammation can trigger CNS inflammation by activating microglia.[11] The ensuing inflammatory cascade affects emotion & cognition by stimulating anxiety, depression and memory loss. In addition, this pathway can cause visceral hypersensitivity. When CNS inflammation is initiated it is difficult to turn off.[12] Excessive levels of LPS upregulate activity in the amygdala, the seat of emotional memory, anxiety and fear.[3]

The ENS, Microbiome And Neurotransmitter Synthesis

Neurotransmitter synthesis is another significant mechanism of the gut-brain axis. The composition of the microbiota largely determines the levels of tryptophan in the systemic circulation and hence, indirectly, the levels of serotonin in the brain. Bacteria may synthesize neurotransmitters directly (e.g., gamma-amino butyric acid) or may modulate the synthesis of neurotransmitters (e.g., dopamine, norepinephrine, and brain-derived neurotropic factor). The composition of the microbiota determines the level and nature of tryptophan catabolites which in turn have profound effects on epithelial barrier integrity. These metabolites determine whether there will be an inflammatory or tolerogenic environment in the gut and other organs.[13,1]

There is evidence that gut bacteria are involved in the production of the following functionally active neurotransmitters:

- Serotonin
- Dopamine
- Gamma-aminobutyric acid
- Acetylcholine
- Epinephrine[14]

These neurotransmitters strongly affect the function of the ENS and CNS, as well as the peripheral nervous system.

Short Chain Fatty Acids—A Major Class Of ENS To CNS Cross-talk Molecules

Short chain fatty acids (SCFAs) are produced by anaerobic bacterial fermentation of either dietary soluble fiber or intestinal mucin. The major SCFAs—butyrate, propionate and acetate—are small organic acids with less than 6 carbon atoms. Butyrate is an energy source for colonocytes via β–oxidation. Butyrate decreases appetite and reduces the risk of immune modulated disease by balancing inflammation. **Inflamm-age-ing** is a term for the chronic inflammatory state affecting many tissues including the brain.[15] Butyrate is essential in neuroprotection, modulating microglial NF-KB signaling and optimizing apoptosis.[16]

Clostridia (Firmicutes phylum) is the most studied SCFA-producing microbe[17] yet Lactobacillus and Bifidobacter species also produce butyrate by "complex interspecies cross-feeding mechanisms".[18] Significant quantities of butyrate are also present in human breast milk as well as butter, full fat cow's milk and most cheeses. Parmesan, as well as goat and sheep derived cheeses may be especially rich in butyrate.[19] Measurement of fecal SCFAs may not fully represent concentrations in the colon because much is quickly absorbed into colonocytes. In addition, new research is showing that certain Clostridia adhere tenaciously to the colonic mucin and therefore are not often present in stool samples, so neither assay of the organism nor its product are likely indicative of intestinal levels.

SCFAs are absorbed into the systemic circulation and cross the blood brain barrier. A unique liver-specific transporter carries SCFAs into hepatocytes.[20] Other SCFA transporters are present on the luminal aspect of enterocytes. Two types, monocarboxylate transporters and sodium coupled monocarboxylate transporters are also located on brain neurons,[21] astrocytes, microglia, oligodendrocytes, and the endothelia of the blood brain barrier.[22] In the CNS these fatty acids modulate the inflammatory cascade.[23] The effects of SCFAs in the gut and the brain are due to G protein coupling receptor signaling and inhibition of histone deacetylases, promoting gene expression in human cells.[24] A recent study suggests that butyrate is a major factor controlling the permeability of the blood brain barrier via its effect on levels of the tight junction proteins claudin and occludin.[25]

Butyric acid is also partially responsible for the modest acidity of the colon (pH 5.7-6.7). β–hydroxybutyric acid and lactic acid are related molecules. A ketogenic diet induced by very low carbohydrate intake may raise the blood and cerebrospinal fluid content of β–hydroxybutyric acid and mimic some of the effects of butyric acid.[26]

SCFAs are mediators of the cross talk among microbes, mitochondria and the host. Along with microbially deconjugated secondary bile metabolites, the SCFAs react with receptors on EECs. This influences serotonin levels and therefore modulates colonic motility,[27,28] mood (anxiety), sleep and pain sensitivity.

SCFAs, Microbes, Diabesity And CNS Inflammation

Microbial metabolites including butyrate have crucial regulatory effects on the health of nearly every organ system.[29] In experimental animals on a high-fat diet there is a reduction in obesity and insulin resistance after dietary supplementation with butyrate.[30] This decrease in diabesity is likely due to down-regulation of the peroxisome proliferator-activated receptor-γ.[31] This down regulation promotes a shift from lipid synthesis to lipid oxidation. The SCFAs butyrate and propionate have been shown to have the most significant effects on this mechanism.[32] When visceral adiposity enlarges, it increases production of free fatty acids, adipokines such as tumor necrosis factor-α (TNF-α), resistin, and interleukin-6 (IL-6) and decreases levels of insulin sensitizing adiponectin. The adipokines stimulate a tenfold increase in the percentage of macrophages in obese visceral fat. In turn, these macrophages produce pro-inflammatory cytokines, inducing more chronic inflammation; exacerbating insulin resistance, as well as systemic and CNS inflammation. High carbohydrate diets and small intestine bacterial overgrowth feed this cycle of systemic inflammation. Chronically high normal range blood glucose levels are associated with neurodegeneration of the hippocampus and amygdala.[33] Following high carbohydrate meals, rapid fluctuations in blood glucose deplete serotonin, dopamine, B vitamins and magnesium. These changes contribute to glycation, insulin resistance, depression and neurodegeneration.[34,35]

Among the neurodegenative diseases, Parkinson's disease (PD) stands out as having a clear gastrointestinal etiology. According to Mulak, et al:

> Dysregulation of the brain-gut-microbiota axis in PD may be associated with gastrointestinal manifestations frequently preceding motor symptoms, as well as with the pathogenesis of PD itself, supporting the hypothesis that the pathological process is spread from the gut to the brain.[36]

This complex relationship between microbial metabolites, local and systemic inflammatory responses and changes in CNS functionality, illustrates the significance of our expanding understanding of the gut-brain axis. The microbiome, and more specifically, the metabolome, is the major influence on cross-talk between the ENS and CNS. As described above, LPS, neurotransmitters, SCFAs, and adipokines impact mental-emotional health and disease states through a complex series of mechanisms stemming from, in part, microbial balance in the gut. By understanding these relationships we can allow for more informed decision making and success in holistic patient care.

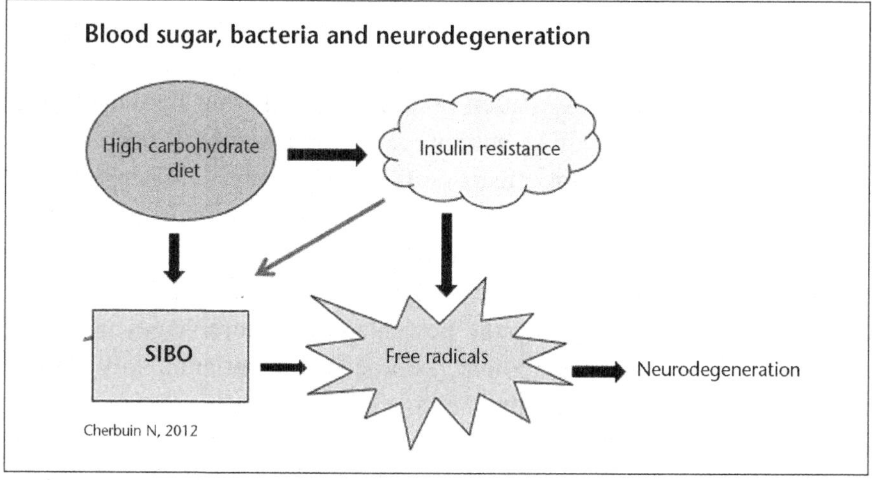

FIGURE 5.3 BLOOD SUGAR, BACTERIA, AND NEURODEGENERATION

1 Galland, L, The gut microbiome and the brain. Dec 2014, *J Med Food*, Vol. 17(12), pp. 1261-72.

2 Mayer, E. The Mind-Gut Connection. New York : Harper Collins, 2016.

3 Grigoleit, JS, Dose-dependent effects of endotoxin on neurobehavioral functions in humans. 6(12):e28330, *PLoS One*. 2011, Vol. 2.

4 The GI Metabolome. Quig, D. Seattle, WA : www.clinicaleducation.org, 2016.

5 Erridge, C, A high-fat meal induces low-grade endotoxemia: evidence of a novel mechanism of postprandial inflammation. (5) 1286-92, *Am J Clin Nutr*. 2007, Vol. 86.

6 Guerville, M, Gastrointestinal and hepatic mechanisms limiting entry and dissemination of lipopolysaccharide into the systemic circulation. (1):G1-G15, *Am J Physiol Gastrointest Liver Physiol*. 2016, Vol. 311.

7 Boullier, S, Secretory IgA-mediated neutralization of Shigella flexneri prevents intestinal tissue destruction by down-regulating inflammatory circuits. (9):5879-85, *J Immunol*. 2009, Vol. 183.

8 Fernandez, MI, Anti-inflammatory role for intracellular dimeric immunoglobulin a by neutralization of lipopolysaccharide in epithelial cells. (6):739-49., *Immunity*. 2003, Vol. 18.

9 Morris, G, The Role of the Microbial Metabolites Including Tryptophan Catabolites and Short Chain Fatty Acids in the Pathophysiology of Immune-Inflammatory and Neuroimmune Disease. *Mol Neurobiol*. 2016, Vol. Epub ahead of print.

10 Sass, V, Human beta-defensin 3 inhibits cell wall biosynthesis in Staphylococci. 6):2793-800., *Infect Immun*. 2010, Vol. 78.

11 Hannestad, J, Endotoxin-induced systemic inflammation activates microglia: [^{11}C] PBR28 positron emission tomography in nonhuman primates. (1):232-9, *Neuroimage*. 2012, Vol. 63.

12 Fenn, AM, Immune activation promotes depression 1 month after diffuse brain injury: a role for primed microglia. (7):575-84, *Biol Psychiatry*. 2014, Vol. 76.

13 LecLercq, S, Posttraumatic Stress Disorder: Does the Gut Microbiome Hold the Key? (4):204-13., *Can J Psychiatry*. 2016, Vol. 61.

14 Bailey, MT, Exposure to a social stressor alters the structure of the intestinal microbiota: implications for stressor-induced immunomodulation. (3):397-407, *Brain Behav Immun*. 2011, Vol. 25.

15 Cevenini, E, Inflamm-ageing. (1):14-20, s.l.: *Curr Opin Clin Nutr Metab Care*. 2013, Vol. 16.

16 Sun, J, Clostridium butyricum pretreatment attenuates cerebral ischemia/reperfusion injury in mice via anti-oxidation and anti-apoptosis. 613:30-5., *Neurosci Lett*. 2016, Vol. 2.

17 Barcenilla, A, Phylogenetic relationships of butyrate-producing bacteria from the human gut. Barcenilla, A. (4):1654-61., *Appl Environ Microbiol*. 2000, Vol. 66.

18 Rios-Covian, D, Enhanced butyrate formation by cross-feeding between Faecalibacterium prausnitzii and Bifidobacterium adolescentis. (21). pii: fnv176, *FEMS Microbiol Lett*. 2015, Vol. 362.

19 Jaeggi, JJ, Hard ewe's milk cheese manufactured from milk of three different groups of somatic cell counts. (10):3082-9., *J Dairy Sci*. 2003, Vol. 86.

20 Shin, HJ, Novel liver-specific organic anion transporter OAT7 that operates the exchange of sulfate conjugates for short chain fatty acid butyrate. (4):1046-55., *Hepatology*. 2007, Vol. 45.

21 Vijay, N, Role of monocarboxylate transporters in drug delivery to the brain. (10):1487-98., *Curr Pharm Des.* 2014, Vol. 20.
22 Immunogold cytochemistry identifies specialized membrane domains for monocarboxylate transport in the central nervous system. Bergersen, L. (1-2):89-96., *Neurochem Res.* 2002, Vol. 27.
23 Targeting microbiota-mitochondria inter-talk: Microbiota control mitochondria metabolism. Y, Saint-Georges-Chaumet. (4):121-4., Cell Mol Biol (Noisy-le-grand). 2015, Vol. 61.
24 Stilling, RM, The neuropharmacology of butyrate:The bread and butter of the microbiota-gut-brain axis? 110-32, *Neurochem Int.* 2016, Vol. 99.
25 Braniste, V, The gut microbiota influences blood-brain barrier permeability in mice. (263):263ra158, *Sci Transl Med.* 2014, Vol. 6.
26. Iriki, T, Concentrations of ketone body and antidiuretic hormone in cerebrospinal fluid in response to the intra-ruminal administration of butyrate in suckling calves. (6):655-61., *Anim Sci J.* 2009, Vol. 80.
27. Yano, JM, Indigenous bacteria from the gut microbiota regulate host serotonin biosynthesis. (2):264-76., *Cell.* 2015, Vol. 161.
28. Reigstad, CS, Gut microbes promote colonic serotonin production through an effect of short-chain fatty acids on enterochromaffin cells. (4):1395-403., *FASEB J.* 2015, Vol. 29.
29. Clarke, G,. Minireview: Gut microbiota: the neglected endocrine organ. (8):1221-38., *Mol Endocrinol.* 2014, Vol. 28.
30. Gao, Z, Butyrate improves insulin sensitivity and increases energy expenditure in mice. (7):1509-17., *Diabetes.* 2009, Vol. 58.
31. Den Besten, G, Short-Chain Fatty Acids Protect Against High-Fat Diet-Induced Obesity via a PPARγ-Dependent Switch From Lipogenesis to Fat Oxidation. (7):2398-408, *Diabetes.* 2015, Vol. 64.
32. Lin, HV, Butyrate and propionate protect against diet-induced obesity and regulate gut hormones via free fatty acid receptor 3-independent mechanisms. (4):e35240., *PLoS One.* 2012, Vol. 7.
33. Cherbuin, N, Higher normal fasting plasma glucose is associated with hippocampal atrophy: The PATH Study. (10):1019-26, *Neurology.* 2012, Vol. 79.
34. Geroldi, C, Insulin resistance in cognitive impairment: the InCHIANTI study. (7):1067-72., *Arch Neurol.* 2005, Vol. 62.
35. Perlmutter, D, *Grain Brain.* New York : Little, Brown and Co., 2013.
36. Mulak, A, Brain-gut-microbiota axis in Parkinson's disease. (37):10609-20., *World J Gastroenterol.* 2015, Vol. 21.

Chapter 6

Small Intestine Bacterial Overgrowth: Dysfunction Begins In The Small Bowel*

*This chapter was co-authored by Alison Siebecker, ND, MSOM

Many patients with bloating, abdominal pain, constipation or diarrhea are diagnosed with irritable bowel syndrome and never get adequate responses to treatment. Others are given no diagnosis at all for their suffering which leads to even less chance of recovery. Our experience is that many of these perplexing patients have commensal microbial overgrowth. This chapter details the complex issue of small intestine bacterial overgrowth.

Small intestine bacterial overgrowth (SIBO) is a condition in which abnormally large numbers of commensal bacteria (or archaea) are present in the small intestine. SIBO is a common cause of IBS—in fact it is involved in over half the cases of IBS[1] and as high as 84% in one study using breath testing as the diagnostic marker.[2] It accounts for 37% of cases when endoscopic cultures of aerobic bacteria are used for diagnosis.[3] Eradication of this overgrowth leads to a 75% reduction in IBS symptoms.[4] Either bacterial overgrowth or the overgrowth of methanogenic archaea leads to impairment of digestion and absorption and produces excess quantities of hydrogen, hydrogen sulfide or methane gas. Hydrogen and methane are not produced by human cells but are the products of carbohydrate fermentation by intestinal organisms. When commensals (oral, small intestine or large intestine flora) multiply in the small intestine to excessive numbers, IBS is likely. Hydrogen/methane breath testing is the most widely used diagnostic method for this condition. Stool analysis has no value in diagnosing SIBO.

Symptoms Of SIBO

- Bloating/abdominal gas
- Flatulence, belching
- Abdominal pain, discomfort or cramps
- Constipation, diarrhea or a mixture of the two
- Heartburn
- Nausea
- Malabsorption—steatorrhea; iron, vitamin D, A, E or B_{12} deficiency with or without anemia; and osteoporosis[5]
- Systemic symptoms—headache, fatigue, joint/muscle pain and certain dermatology conditions

- A partial list of other diseases associated with SIBO includes hypothyroidism,[6] lactose intolerance,[7] gallstones,[8] Crohn's disease, systemic sclerosis,[10] celiac disease,[11] chronic pancreatitis,[12] diverticulitis,[13] diabetes with autonomic neuropathy,[14] fibromyalgia and chronic regional pain syndrome,[15] hepatic encephalopathy,[16] non-alcoholic steatohepatitis,[17] interstitial cystitis,[18] restless leg syndrome,[19] acne rosacea,[20] erosive esophagitis,[21] and deep vein thrombosis.[1] Based on clinical experience, we suspect that biliary dyskinesia and lymphocytic colitis may also be associated with SIBO.

As mentioned above, malabsorption is a major concern and many of our patients are underweight based on their body mass index scores. In the developing world this may be a major factor in failure to thrive and increased pediatric mortality. According to Donowitz et al:

> Recent data show that SIBO is also found in children living in unsanitary conditions that do not have access to clean water. SIBO leads to impaired micronutrient absorption and increased GI permeability, both of which may contribute to growth stunting in children. SIBO also disrupts mucosal immunity and has been implicated in oral vaccination underperformance and the development of celiac disease. SIBO in the setting of the impoverished human habitat may be an under recognized cause of pediatric morbidity and mortality in the developing world.[2]

In our practices we have found that the following indicators increase the chances that a patient's IBS is caused by SIBO:

- When a patient develops IBS following a bout of acute gastroenteritis (post-infectious IBS)
- When a patient reports dramatic transient improvement in IBS symptoms after antibiotic treatment
- When a patient reports worsening of IBS symptoms from ingesting probiotic supplements which also contain *pre*biotics
- When a patient reports that eating more fiber increases constipation and other IBS symptoms
- When a celiac patient reports insufficient improvement in digestive symptoms even when carefully following a gluten-free diet

- When a patient develops constipation type IBS (IBS-C) after taking opiates
- When a patient has a chronic low ferritin level with no other apparent cause
- When abdominal imaging reveals a large gas accumulation partially obscuring the pancreas
- When small bowel follow through imaging reveals areas of "flocculation"[22]

Mechanisms By Which Overgrowth Is Prevented

An important protective mechanism against SIBO is proper small intestine motility via the migrating motor complex (MMC)[23] because stasis promotes bacterial growth. Also key in prevention are gastric, pancreatic, and gall bladder secretions, since hydrochloric acid, enzymes, and bile are bactericidal/static.[24] Conditions that disrupt the glycocalyx and microvillus portions of the brush border may fuel overgrowth. The pathophysiology involved is the loss of disaccharidases in these areas and the resulting carbohydrate malabsorption which provides excess substrate for microbial growth. The role of proper ileocecal valve function in preventing cecoileal reflux of colonic bacteria into the small intestine may also be important.[25,26] Surprisingly, a recent study suggests that surgical removal of the gall bladder reduces the risk as well[27] although it is likely that adhesions from any surgery may slow the MMC and promote overgrowth. Mucosal biofilms may be preventive or may be a risk.[28,29] Heavy drinking, as well as moderate use of alcohol, is significantly associated with increased SIBO risk.[30] The use of proton pump inhibitors encourages overgrowth, especially of the hydrogen producing type.[31,32]

Definition

Traditionally, $\geq 10^5$ colony-forming units (CFU) per mL of proximal jejunal aspiration has been the definition of SIBO in culturing studies. More recent studies reveal that $\leq 10^3$ CFU's is the normal level in healthy controls.[33,34] The bacteria which are most commonly overgrown are both commensal anaerobes—*Bacteroides* 39%, *Lactobacillus* 25%, and *Clostridium* 20% as well as commensal aerobes—*Streptococcus* 60%, *Escherichia coli* 36%, *Staphylococcus* 13%, and *Klebsiella* 11%.[35] A more recent study found the aerobes to be *Escherichia coli* 37%, *Enterococcus spp* 32%, *Klebsiella pneumonia* 24%, and *Proteus mirabilis* 6.5%.[36] Colonic hydrogen production is believed to be anti-inflammatory and anti-neoplastic[37] whereas excessive small intestine hydrogen causes the symptoms and signs of diarrhea type irritable bowel syndrome (IBS-D.) In addition to bacteria, the source of methane generation in SIBO is the archaeon Methanobrevibacter smithii. This organism has been linked to obesity in humans.[38] In addition, sulphate reducing bacteria, such as Desulfovibrio species are anaerobes that reduce sulfate to hydrogen sulfide (H_2S). Beyond its role in SIBO, H_2S is being studied as a possible etiologic factor in ulcerative colitis and colonic carcinogenesis.[39] In health, low level H_2S has a protective function in the gastrointestinal tract.[40]

When reviewing the results of SIBO research it is essential to note the type of testing used to make the diagnosis. Duodenal/jejunal sampling and glucose breath testing measure proximal SIBO only. Lactulose breath testing measures bacterial overgrowth anywhere in the small bowel.[3]

Pathophysiology Of SIBO—Autoimmunity

Post-infectious IBS (PI-IBS) has been shown to have an autoimmune etiology in both murine and human studies. Infectious gastroenteritis is the most significant environmental risk factor for IBS.[41] Organisms that trigger PI-IBS include Campylobacter, Salmonella, Shigella, E. coli,[42,43] viruses,[44] and Giardia.[45]

Cytolethal distending toxin B (CDT-B) is produced by enteric pathogens that cause PI-IBS. Campylobacter jejuni is the prototypical bacteria that produces CDT-B.[46] Other bacteria that produce it include *Haemophilus ducreyi* (chancroid), *Aggregatibacter actinomycetemcomitans* (periodontitis), *Escherichia coli* (traveler's diarrhea), *Shigella dysenteriae* (dysentery), *Salmonella enterica* (typhoid fever), and *Campylobacter upsaliensis* (enterocolitis).

The interstitial cells of Cajal (ICCs) are fibroblast-like cells that act as pacemakers for the migrating motor complex (MMC). A key underlying cause of SIBO is thought to be deficiency of the MMC, which when properly functioning is responsible for moving debris and bacteria down to the ileocecal valve during fasting at night and between meals.[47] In a landmark study by Pokkunui, et al the number of ICCs were reduced in Campylobacter jejuni infected rats that eventually developed SIBO.[48] Three months after *C. jejuni* gastroenteritis, 27% of rats had SIBO. These rats had a lower number of ICCs in the jejunum and ileum than controls (0.12 ICC/villus was the threshold for developing SIBO).

CDT-B may contribute to a slowed MMC by stimulating the production of autoantibodies against a cytoskeletal protein known as vinculin. The antigen-antibody complexes between anti-vinculin antibodies and CDT-B lead to autoimmune destruction of ICCs.[49,50]

Living in unsanitary conditions with frequent exposure to food and water-bourne infection is a likely cause of SIBO in children in the developing world. In 90 Bangladeshi 2 year-olds from impoverished neighborhoods, SIBO was significantly related to both growth stunting and proximity to an open sewer. 16.7% of these children had hydrogen SIBO based on glucose breath testing.[133] Growth stunting is associated with reduced cognitive development as well as an increased risk of death prior to 5 years of age.

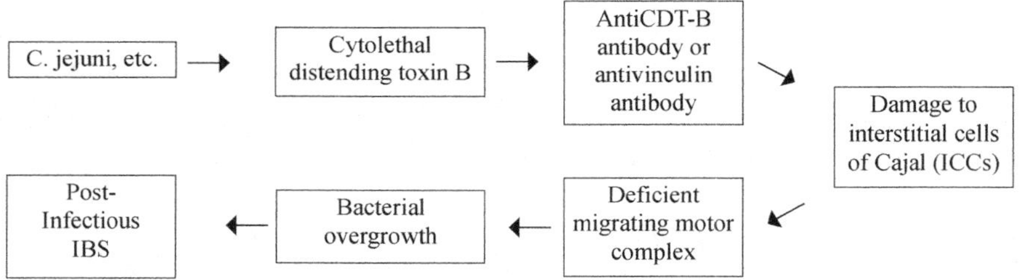

FIGURE 6.1 AUTOIMMUNE PATHOPHYSIOLOGY OF PI-IBS

Additional Underlying Etiologies For SIBO

Patients and physicians often ask if SIBO is curable. At times, a course marked by frequent recurrence and serial treatment is seen. The key is to uncover the predisposing cause. When the underlying cause can be removed or at least controlled, relapsing SIBO can be prevented. In other cases, SIBO may be a chronic condition that requires management. The good news is that there are many options for control and treatment which will be discussed below.

Some of the key underlying causes in our experience are factors that alter the structure or function of collagen, alter the tone of the ileocecal valve, elevate tissue glucose levels, decrease immune competence, create blind loops or decrease migrating motor complex activity or create compression or obstruction (medications, thickening of the bowel wall or adhesion/stricture formation). Trauma and lifestyle factors such as traumatic brain injury, alcohol consumption and overtraining are also important considerations.

Altered Collagen—Ehlers-Danlos Syndrome/Joint Hypermobility Type (EDS/JHT)

EDS/JHT is a collagen variant affecting about 5% of Americans. The Beighton score is a 9 point scale used to determine the presence of EDS-JHT on physical exam. Joint hypermobility is rated at the knees, elbows, first and fifth metacarpophylangeal joints, and lumbar spine (see http://www.ehlers-danlos.org/about-eds/getting-a-diagnosis/beighton-score/). Dystrophic scars, easy bruising and bleeding, soft-velvety skin, subcutaneous spheroid masses, chronic joint and limb pain, recurrent joint subluxations and fatigue are common findings.

Gastrointestinal manifestations of EDS-JHT include hiatal hernia, reflux, post-operative hernias, colonic redundancy and prolapse, anal prolapse and ileocecal valve dysfunction. All these changes may lead to GI symptoms, but most important for SIBO is the finding of irritable bowel syndrome in 48-62% of patients. 36% report functional constipation and GERD is reported in 68.7%.[135] Delayed gastric emptying which is exacerbated by opioids may increase the incidence of gastroesophageal reflux (GERD) in these patients which may be non-responsive to high dose proton pump inhibitors.[103] Proton pump inhibitors and opioids therefore may be additional triggers for SIBO since opioids decrease activity of the migrating motor complex and hypoacidity increases bacterial overgrowth. The decreased tone of the collagen may also permit prolapse and kinks to form in the small intestine. Mitral valve prolapse (MVP) is more common in these individuals. MVP and arrhythmias are important considerations when prescribing prokinetic medications for the prevention phase of SIBO treatment because several agents of this type can have cardiac side effects. In a Swedish whole population-based study (n=28,631) the incidence of celiac disease was found to be increased 49% in EDS-JHT.[137] This collagen variant is also associated with increased incidence of Crohn's disease.[9] Both celiac and Crohn's are also known to be SIBO associated diseases.

Theories for the increase in GI symptoms include: increased visceral hypersensitivity, autonomic dysmotility, underlying celiac disease and excessive use of analgesics including opiates, NSAIDS, and antidepressants which induce GI side effects. Whether SIBO is present or not, chronic gastritis as well as constipation, diarrhea and nausea are problematic for over 75% of persons with EHS-JHT.[138,139]

Altered Ileocecal Valve Function

A functional ileocecal valve prevents cecoileal reflux. Since the colon typically contains 100 billion bacteria per ml, reflux from the cecum through this valve may introduce huge numbers of organisms into the ileum.[140] If the migrating motor complex or other compensatory contractions cannot override this reflux, SIBO is likely. In a retrospective study of 23 patients ileocecal valve pressure was significantly lower in patients with a positive lactulose breath test compared to a negative test.[141]

Elevated Serum Glucose

SIBO incidence is significantly higher in patients with increased abdominal fat, metabolic syndrome and type 2 diabetes mellitus.[142] Type 1 diabetes mellitus has been shown to be associated with significantly higher rates of SIBO only when autonomic neuropathy was present. Higher insulin dosages were required in the management of the SIBO/autonomic neuropathy group.[143]

Gastroparesis, pancreatitis and non-alcoholic fatty liver disease (NAFLD) are all diabetes associated complications. SIBO is reported to be "very common" in patients with gastroparesis that have symptoms of abdominal pain and bloating. This is especially true for those who have had greater than a five year history of gastroparesis.[144] A meta-analysis of chronic pancreatitis and SIBO found that one third of these patients have SIBO which is significantly increased over controls and the treatment of SIBO was associated with clinical improvement.[145] Looking only at studies that employed lactulose as a test substrate rather than glucose yielded a much higher prevalence of 73.3%. In a case controlled trial of 372 patients, NAFLD was over twice as likely in SIBO positive patients compared to a SIBO negative control group.[146]

We suggest that tight glucose control in diabetics may be essential to prevent chronic relapsing SIBO.

Immunocompromised States

There is evidence that HIV/AIDS, IgA deficiency, and common variable immunodeficiency are associated with SIBO. In the case of HIV/AIDS, the mechanism may be related to hypochlorhydria.[147,148]

Blind Loops

Non-draining pockets of small intestine allow decreased clearance and increased replication of enteric microbes.[149] Examples include congenital anomalies such as duodenal duplication and small intestine diverticuli. Post-surgical causes include Roux-en-Y and other diversion surgeries.

Intestinal Compression

An uncommon cause of complete or partial obstruction of the upper small bowel is superior mesenteric artery (SMA) syndrome. We have seen several such cases marked by chronic duodenal compression leading to recurrent SIBO. There is a narrowing of the angle between the SMA and the aorta which can lead to compression of the third part of the duodenum. Rapid weight loss, abdominal trauma, aortic aneurysm repair, or spinal surgery (especially scoliosis surgery) may cause SMA syndrome to become symptomatic.[150] SMA syndrome is most often diagnosed by an upper GI barium series or abdominal CT.[151] We are not aware of an effective treatment for this. It may be helpful to lengthen the ligament of Trietz with myofascial therapy. Surgical treatment may reduce symptoms in more severe cases but, as in other surgical procedures, these interventions increase the risk of adhesion formation.[152]

Bowel Wall Thickening

Scleroderma (systemic sclerosis) has a strong association with SIBO because enteric wall collagen deposition stiffens the small bowel, leading to decreased motility. Breath testing has been found to be the most accurate test for SIBO in scleroderma[153] but elevated fecal calprotectin (especially above 275 ug/g—normal range is less than 50 ug/g) was significantly associated with SIBO in systemic sclerosis.[154] Transmural thickening in Crohn's as well as fistula formation are likely causes of SIBO. It is highly recommended that physicians rule out SIBO in patients with treatment resistant Crohn's.[155]

Adhesions/Strictures

By way of definition, adhesions are acquired serosal fibrous connections whereas strictures are fibrous connections within the enteric lumen. They may develop after physical injury, radiation or surgery, as a response to infection, ie. peritonitis following perforation of the appendix or in response to other inflammations, ie. endometriosis.[156]

As these bands of fibrotic tissue develop they may lead to compression or acute angle turns (kinks) in the structure of the small bowel. These can be seen on laparotomy or open surgery, so be sure to get any previous surgical notes and read them carefully. If surgical/laparoscopic direct visualization has not been performed, the best imaging for diagnosis of adhesions is a GI barium small bowel follow-though series. Most imaging centers perform a cursory version of this technique—so find a center willing to do the following: "Small bowel follow-through series with positional changes and multiple spot films to visualize individual loops of bowel and thoroughly investigate the possibility of adhesions". It takes more time and the imaging techs may complain, but you may find a radiologist in charge who is completely on board with your need for a thorough study. Don't rely on a CT or MRI to rule out adhesions. With the right operator, abdominal/pelvic ultrasound may be able to differentiate between the normal gliding of unimpeded tissue versus the fixation of adhesions.

Peritoneal adhesions are one of the more common underlying etiologies we have seen in our SIBO patients who relapse after treatment.

Traumatic Brain Injury

One of the factors that appears to trigger enteric dysmotility and therefore some of our cases of SIBO is traumatic brain injury (TBI). At one end of the spectrum a patient may have had severe trauma with intracranial hypertension and coma prior to the onset of their digestive problems.

At the other extreme there may have been little or no direct impact to the skull, but rather a mild TBI. To uncover these types of traumas the physician must understand that "shaking of the brain" within the rigid cranium is the key issue. "Heading" the ball in soccer, whiplash injuries, proximity to explosions (such as military IED blasts) and shaken baby syndrome can all lead to motility changes in the gut. Decreases in murine intestinal motility and mucosal blood flow occur early in TBI.[176] In human patients with brain trauma and coma, gastric dysrrhythmias and inability to tolerate food was significant. Prokinetics were recommended to improve motility as patients were advanced to enteral feedings.[157]

Traumatic brain injury induces intestinal paracellular hyperpermeability in humans and other mammals.[158] TBI in rodents decreases expression of the tight junction proteins occludin and ZO-1 and increases TNF-α.[159]

Another study found that patients with Ehlers-Danlos Syndrome-Joint Hypermobility Type (discussed above), had consistent and specific brain lesions involving white matter tracts. They suggest that "the record of a physical trauma in a substantial proportion of cases suggests that these lesions could be post-trauma consequences. Therefore, physical trauma could be a triggering factor in EDS".[160]

Alcohol Consumption

Alcoholism is a risk factor for SIBO, but moderate intake of alcohol may be as well. In a retrospective review of 210 patients who had lactulose breath testing, moderate consumption of alcohol (1 drink per day for women and 2 drinks a day for men) was a strong risk factor for SIBO.[161] Obese children have increased endogenous intestinal production of alcohol which is associated with an increased risk of hepatic steatosis, intestinal hyperpermeability and SIBO based on glucose breath testing and lactulose mannitol urine assays.[162]

Medication Use

As discussed above, the migrating motor complex (MMC) is an important enteric reflex controlling bacterial growth in the small bowel. In rats, the MMC was found to be disrupted by a continuous 3 day infusion of morphine. Morphine was found to increase duodenal bacterial overgrowth and bacterial translocation.[163] Single bolus injections of morphine were not found to have these effects. In mice, morphine increases ileal MMC circular muscle contractions, but dramatically decreases longitudinal muscle contraction.[164] In humans, short time infusion of morphine may actually increase phase III MMC contractions, but it is not clear that this has a promotility effect as circular versus longitudinal muscle activity was not specified.[165] In dogs, feeding of casein (compared to soy) was followed by a statistically significant decrease in amplitude and frequency of enteric contractions. The authors suggest that stimulation of opioid receptors by β-casomorphin is the likely mechanism.[166]

Findings of proton pump inhibitor (PPI) administration and the risk of SIBO vary greatly by study. A recent meta-analysis concluded that PPI use statistically increased SIBO risk, but only when duodenal or jejunal aspirate cultures were the diagnostic markers.[167] This effect was not found using glucose breath testing and studies which employed lactulose as the substrate were not included.

Overtraining

Runners have a high incidence of bloating, diarrhea and flatulence. This may or may not be related to an increase in SIBO. In various studies rates vary from 20% up to 71%. Additional digestive symptoms in long distance runners include nausea, vomiting, heartburn, bloody diarrhea and fecal incontinence.[168] In a study of 606 runners, cyclists and triathletes who responded to a questionnaire of GI symptoms, cyclists reported both upper (67%) and lower (64%) digestive symptoms.[169] In a small study of seven long distance runners with diarrhea only one was found to have SIBO. The study used glucose breath testing, which is known to result in false negatives for all but the most proximal of SIBO cases. Proposed mechanisms for GI symptoms in long-distance runners include prolonged reduction in mesenteric blood flow[170] altered motility from mechanical irritation,[171] and increased intestinal permeability due to excessive ibuprofen use.[172]

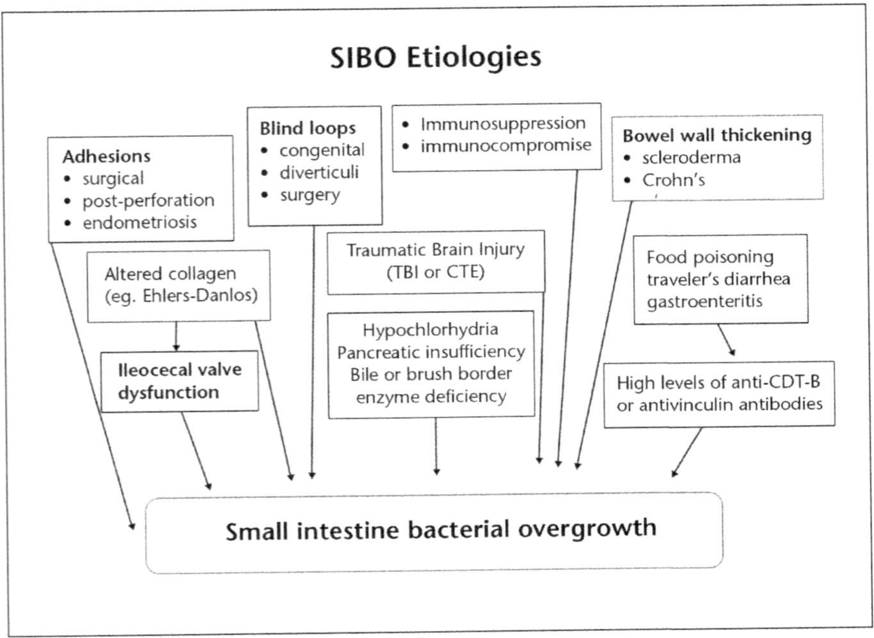

FIGURE 6.2 SIBO ETIOLOGIES

Below is a checklist to assess risk of SIBO recurrence due to an underlying risk factor.

History of:

- Food poisoning, traveler's diarrhea or gastroenteritis?
- Abdominal or pelvic surgery or radiation therapy?
- Inflammation or perforation affecting the peritoneal structures (endometriosis, appendicitis, especially if perforated; perforated peptic ulcer)?
- History of small bowel obstruction or pseudo-obstruction?
- Use of opiates, proton pump inhibitors, anticholinergics, anti-spasmotics or immunosuppressive medications?
- Diagnosis of prediabetes or diabetes?
- HIV or other immunocompromised state?
- Physical trauma to the abdomen or pelvis? Traumatic brain injury, "shaken" brain or concussion?
- Diagnosis of superior mesenteric artery syndrome?

- Joint hypermobility, "double jointed", excessively flexible joints or skin? (Screen with Beighton scale)
- Thickening of the GI tract due to scleroderma, Crohn's disease, cancer?

Biopsy Findings In SIBO

Although biopsy is not a standard procedure in SIBO, it is wise to be aware of the types of histological changes likely to be found should your SIBO patients have duodenal biopsy for some other reason. The morphology may resemble that found in the revised Marsh 1 criteria for celiac disease. Half the biopsies in one series were normal. The other half had modest, often patchy, villous blunting and increased lamina propria neutrophils and/or lymphocytes.[173] Plasma cells may also be increased in the lamina propria.

How SIBO Causes The Symptoms Of IBS

There are two main pathophysiological issues involved in SIBO. First, bacteria are able to ferment carbohydrates and consume other nutrients ingested by the host simply by their inappropriate location in the small intestine. This allows them premature exposure to host nutrition before there is time for absorption. Bacterial fermentation produces hydrogen and/or hydrogen sulfide gas. In addition M. smithii converts hydrogen to methane.[51] M. smithii may be present in the intestinal tracts of between 44%–95.7% of humans.[52] Microbial gas leads to the IBS symptoms of bloating, pain, altered bowel movements, eructation and flatulence (Figure 6.3).

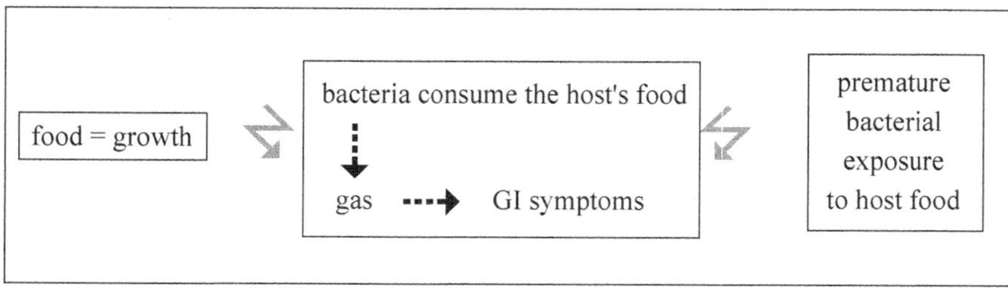

Figure 6.3 The Cycle Of SIBO

The quantity of gas may be extensive, causing severe bloating and distention.[53] It is estimated that with normal levels of enteric flora, the quantity of lactose in an ounce of milk fuels the production of 50 cc of gas. With microbial overgrowth, gas levels produced from one ounce of milk may approach 5000 cc.[54] Excess gas can then exit the body as flatulence or eructation. A portion is also absorbed into the blood and eventually filters through the pulmonary alveolus to exit on exhalation. The intestines are sensitive to pressure and therefore the pressure of distention can lead to abdominal pain. In addition, visceral hypersensitivity, a feature of IBS, may create a lower threshold for pain/discomfort[55] and a hyperesponsiveness of muscular contraction to the gaseous distention leading to cramps.[56] The gases also affect bowel motility. Hydrogen has a greater association with diarrhea and methane has an almost exclusive association with constipation.[57,58] Methane has been shown to slow gastrointestinal motility by 59% in animal studies,[59] and the volume of methane overproduction correlates with the severity of constipation.[60] When both hydrogen and methane are present, diarrhea, constipation, or a mixture of the two can occur based on the relative amounts of these gases.[61] It appears that the pressure created by either gas or the decreased gastric motility may lead to gastric distention resulting in gastroesophageal reflux.[62] The bacterial consumption and uptake of host nutrients, such as B12 and iron, can lead to macrocytic and/or microcytic anemia or chronic low ferritin levels in addition to general malabsorption and malnutrition in more severe cases.[63,64] The increased motility of diarrhea may also induce malabsorption. Finally, continuous fermentation of host nutrition by repeated exposure to daily meals, perpetuates bacterial overgrowth and IBS symptoms, creating a vicious cycle (Figure 6.4).

The second mechanism is microbial damage to the digestive and absorptive function of the small intestine. Unlike the colon, the small intestine is not designed for heavy bacterial colonization. Commensal organisms may synthesize glycosidase leading to damage of glycocalyx or disaccharidases. The gastrointestinal and systemic symptoms induced by these changes are listed in Figure 6.4. Key factors include bacterial deconjugation of bile which induces fat malabsorption, steatorrhea and fat soluble vitamin deficiencies,[65] bacterial digestion of disaccharidase enzymes which furthers carbohydrate malabsorption, fermentation, and

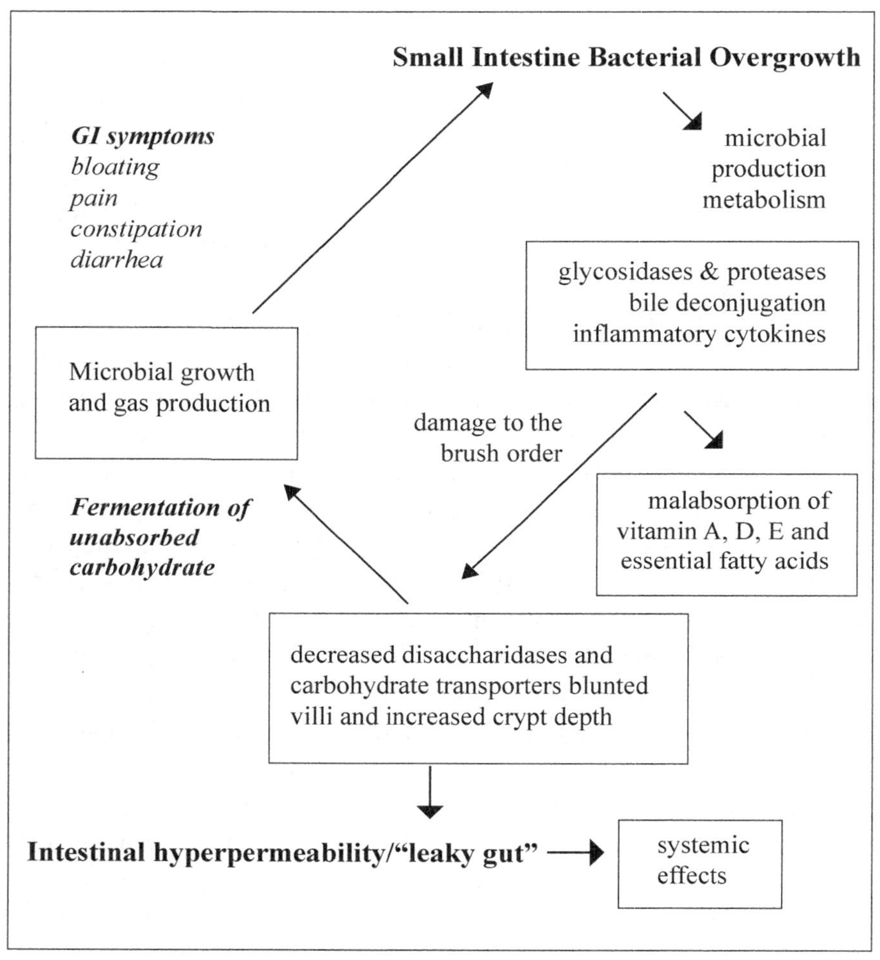

Figure 6.4 The Pathophysiology Of GI And Systemic Effects In SIBO

gas,[66] and increased intestinal permeability (leaky gut) which often leads to systemic symptoms.[67, 68]

Diagnosis Of SIBO

As mentioned above, hydrogen/methane breath testing is the most common method of assessing SIBO. Instrumentation is available from Quintron Instrument Company in Milwaukie, Wisconsin. They build and distribute the Breathtracker, which is used to measure these gases following a 24-48 hour prep diet and an overnight fast. After collection of the fasting baseline specimen, a solution of lactulose—an unabsorbable synthetic sugar—is ingested as the substrate for bacterial fermentation. Lactulose is non-absorbable because only bacteria, not humans, produce the enzymes to digest it. Lactulose is a disaccharide solution of galactose and fructose in a base which also contains a minute quantity of lactose and epilactose.[69] Transit time for lactulose through the stomach and small bowel is approximately 120 minutes. Glucose may also be used as a test substance, but because of its rapid absorption in the proximal small intestine, it may fail to identify distal SIBO.[70] Serial breath specimens are taken every 20 minutes during this time and for a third hour as well. Breath may be sampled and immediately analyzed at a lab or these samples may be collected at the patient's home using a series of tubes and a transfer device for later analysis. Home breath samples are exhaled into special vials similar to a vacutainer tube which stores the labeled sample until it can be delivered to the lab. Not all labs have the equipment to test for methane. The methodology for hydrogen sulfide is currently being perfected and is therefore not yet available. Testing for methane in addition to hydrogen is important because treatment varies based on the type of gas. A unique symptom of H_2S production may be a "rotten egg" odor to the belching or flatus.

Preparation for the test varies from lab to lab, but a typical prep diet is limited to white rice, fish/poultry/meat, eggs, hard cheeses, clear beef or chicken broth (not bone broth or bouillon), oil, salt, and pepper. The purpose of the prep diet is to get a clear reaction to the lactulose solution by eliminating fermentable foods the day prior to testing. In cases of constipation, two days of prep diet may be needed to reduce baseline gases to negative. Antibiotics should not be used for at least 2 weeks prior to an initial test although some sources recommend 4 weeks.[71] Laxatives, including high dose magnesium and/or vitamin C, should be avoided for at least 4 days prior to the day of the test. If symptoms allow, proton pump inhibitors should also be eliminated for at least seven days before testing.[72]

Interpretation of the test varies among practitioners. The criteria provided by Quintron for a positive test are as follows:

A rise over baseline in hydrogen production of 20 parts per million (PPM) or greater within 120 minutes after ingesting the test substrate.

A rise over baseline in methane production of 12 PPM or greater within 120 minutes after ingesting the test substrate.

A rise over baseline in the sum of hydrogen and methane production of 15 PPM or greater within 120 minutes after ingesting the test substrate.

Additional testing and interpretation parameters:

Hydrogen sulfide SIBO may be suspected when the typical symptoms are present but the breath test shows low "flat-line" hydrogen and methane levels with none of the expected colonic rise in gases after 120 minutes.[73]

Modest levels of methane gas at any level equal or greater than 3 PPM at any sample on a 3 hour lactulose breath test may be a cause of methane-induced constipation.[74]

A single "spot methane" level may be used for follow-up testing in methane positive individuals. When testing methane alone there is no need for a preparatory diet and fasting is optional prior to this single breath sample. This is only available for direct patient testing. We know of no available mail-based spot testing.

We have found that the absolute level of gases, without consideration of the rise over baseline, correlates well with clinical SIBO. This is especially true for methane gas, which can have a pattern of elevated baseline which remains high for the duration of the test. In cases such as these, methane may only rise a few PPM over baseline, but the level is consistently above positive. Interpretation of elevated hydrogen or methane on the baseline specimen (pre-lactulose ingestion) is controversial, but at our center we prefer to consider a high baseline methane to be a positive test.[76]

The classic positive for SIBO has been considered to be a double peak, with the first peak representing the small intestine and the second peak representing the normal large intestine flora. It is not essential to have a second peak in order to have an accurate test. We find that a single peak which rises highest in the third hour may also represent distal SIBO followed by the normal colonic gas levels.

Breath testing may be used in pediatric cases, so long as the child can follow instructions to collect the samples. For those under 3 years old, testing is best done on site at a lab due to differences in collection methods versus at-home kits. Pediatric lactulose dosing is 1g/kg body weight with a maximum of 10 g. Children weighing 22 pounds and above receive the maximum adult dose of 10 g.[77] Lactulose is available only by prescription.

Treatment Of SIBO

In 2006, Dr. Pimentel shared his treatment algorithm for SIBO which included the use of antibiotics, elemental diet or both.[78] Our approach offers two additional options: diet and herbal antibiotics (see Figure 6.5 SIBO Treatment Algorithm).

Diet

We advise the use of the Specific Carbohydrate Diet™ or the SIBO Specific Foodguide.[79,80] The SIBO Specific Foodguide (see www.siboinfo.com/diet.html) is a combination of the Specific Carbohydrate Diet™, the Low FODMAP diet and the clinical experience of Dr. Siebecker in the treatment of SIBO with diet. Bacteria use carbohydrates as their energy source and ferment them to gases, therefore a low carbohydrate diet can directly reduce symptoms by decreasing the amount of gas produced.[81] Reducing carbohydrates may also decrease the overall microbial load, though formal studies to validate this are lacking. The Specific Carbohydrate Diet™ and the SIBO Specific Foodguide greatly reduce the intake of polysaccharides, oligosaccharides and disaccharides by eliminating all grains, starchy vegetables, lactose, and sweeteners other than honey, dextrose and liquid stevia. Legumes are often avoided in initial phases of these diets.

Many patients experience a rapid and significant decrease in symptoms after starting a SIBO diet. The Specific Carbohydrate Diet has been reported to have an 84% success rate for inflammatory bowel disease,[82] a condition commonly associated with SIBO.[83] Patients that find the Specific Carbohydrate Diet™ or SIBO Specific Foodguide approach to be too restrictive can follow the Cedars-Sinai diet as described at http://www.gidoctor.net/diet-ibs-sibo.php

The Low FODMAP Diet™ is a nutritional plan that greatly reduces the fermentable levels of carbohydrate containing foods and has a success rate of 76% in IBS.[84,85] The Low FODMAP Diet™ is not specifically designed for SIBO and therefore does not eliminate polysaccharide and disaccharide sources such as grains, starch, starchy vegetables, and sucrose. Eliminating these poly and disaccharides is helpful in SIBO because these carbohydrates—which normally feed the host—also feed the increased numbers of microflora in the small intestine (see Figure 6.4).

In our experience either the Low FODMAP or Cedars-Sinai diet is a better option for vegan or stricter vegetarian patients than the Specific Carbohydrate or SIBO Specific Foodguide diets.

Diet alone has proven successful for infants and younger children, but for older children and adults one or more of several treatment options are often needed to reduce bacteria quickly, particularly in cases in which the patient's diet becomes excessively limited in an attempt to obtain symptomatic relief. Additionally, any of the diets discussed above need to be customized to the individual by trial and error over time.

Low carbohydrate diets often induce weight loss. Particular attention must be paid to underweight patients. Increased intake of winter squash, glucose or honey may be recommended in these circumstances. White rice (jasmine/sticky variety is best) or white potato may also be needed to maintain weight along with medium chain triglyceride sources such as coconut and other oils.

Diet is also essential for prevention of relapse following successful SIBO eradication. Pimentel recommends postponing any dietary changes until after the effective treatment of the microbial overgrowth, rather than during the treatment phase.[86] Our clinical experience with the SIBO Specific Foodguide is that it is beneficial for both the treatment and prevention phases.

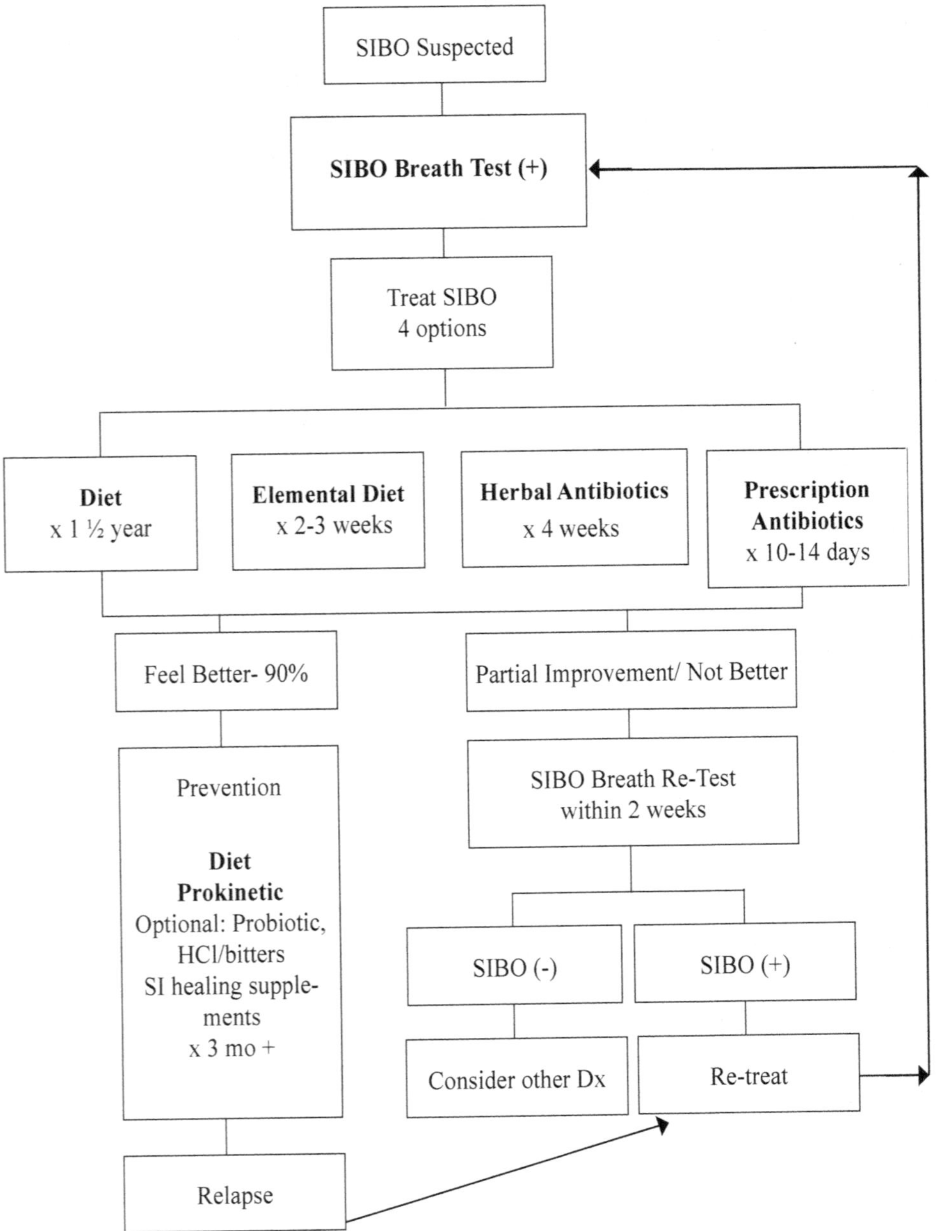

FIGURE 6.5 SIBO TREATMENT ALGORITHM

Elemental diet

An elemental diet can be used in place of prescription antibiotics or herbal antibiotics in order to rapidly decrease overgrowth. In the treatment of SIBO, elemental diet is used to the exclusion of all other food sources. These products are a powdered mix of free form amino acids, fat, vitamins and minerals as well as rapidly absorbed carbohydrates. The concept behind this treatment is that the nutrients will be absorbed before reaching the involved organisms, thus feeding the patient but starving the flora. It is used in place of all meals, for 2-3 weeks, and has a success rate of 80-85%[87] using the Nestle product Vivonex Plus™. Two versions of a homemade recipe for elemental diet can be found at http://www.siboinfo.com/elemental-formula.html Elemental diets are not protein powders or typical detoxification formulas. They are available over the counter and are not reimbursed by most insurance coverage, which can make this treatment costly. Patients should be warned that vivonex plus or homemade elemental diets are very bitter tasting. Elemental diet may not be suitable to underweight patients who cannot afford to lose weight. Weight maintenance can be achieved as long as the patient ingests the full recommended caloric intake of elemental diet powder. A new corn-free, pleasant tasting elemental formula (Physician's Elemental Diet) is now also available. Elemental formulas may also be used as "safe" foods while traveling or ingested in addition to other foods to add calories and nutrients to highly restricted diets. Due to high simple carbohydrate content of elemental formulas, yeast overgrowth may be a problem for some patients. Prophylactic antifungals may be included in the treatment of these patients.

Herbal Antibiotics

While there have only been two published reports of herbal antibiotics in the treatment of SIBO,[88,89] our experience is that they have similar effectiveness to antibiotics. Chedid et al studied patients with SIBO based on a positive lactulose breath test. A negative breath test after treatment was seen in 34% of the rifaximin or triple antibiotic treated group vs. 46% of the herbal treated group.

The herbal arm of the study employed one of two paired options. The dosage was 2 capsules of each bid for 30 days. The two paired options are listed following (FC cidal plus Dysbiocide *or* Candibactin-AR plus Candibactin-BR):

Table 6.1 Herbal Preparations For The Treatment Of Small Intestine Bacterial Overgrowth

FC Cidal	Dysbiocide	Candibactin-AR	Candibactin-BR
Proprietary Blend 500 mg: 1 capsule	Proprietary Blend 950 mg per 2 capsules	One Capsule 408 mg contains:	One Capsule 400 mg contains:
Tinospora cordifolia	Anthenum graveolens	Thymus vulgaris	Coptis chinensis
Equisetum arvense	Stemona sessilifolia	Origanum vulgare Salvia officinalis	Berberis aquafolium
Pau D'Arco Thymus vulgaris Urtica dioica Artemesia dracunculus Olea europaea	Artemisia absinthium Brucea javanica Pulsatilla chinensis Hedyotis diffusa Picrasma excelsa Acacia catechu Achillea millefolium	Melissa officinalis	Berberine HCl Scutellaria baicalensis Phellodendron chinense Zingiber officinale Glycyrrhiza uralensis Rheum officinale

At our center we have used the following botanicals: Allium sativum (garlic), Hydrastis canadensis and other berberine containing herbs, Origanum vulgare (oregano) and Azadirachta indica (neem). We have used these as both single agents and in various combinations at dosages that are at the upper end of label suggestions x 30 days. Specific single dosages we have used include allicin extract of garlic: 450mg bid-tid, goldenseal/Oregon grape/berberine combination: 5g qd in divided dosage, emulsified oregano: 100mg bid and a formula which contains 300 mg of neem plus a proprietary blend containing a total of 200 mg of the following: Emblica officinalis, Terminalia chebula, Terminalia belerica, Tinospora cordifolia, and Rubia cordifolia. The latter formula is dosed at 1 capsule tid. Researchers at Johns-Hopkins have studied other herbal combinations which are listed in Table 6.1. Our breath testing has validated the need for the longer treatment period of 30 days for herbal antibiotics compared to 14 days for prescription antibiotics. Note that although whole garlic is a high FODMAP food, we do not observe purified allicin to provoke symptoms in our patients. Allicin is the only herb we have noted so far that can reduce breath methane levels. We have also observed that some patients experience prolonged die-off reactions with herbal treatment which can last for the duration of the treatment course. More studies on herbal antibiotics for SIBO are needed, particularly to identify botanicals effective in reducing methane.

Another proprietary herbal product called Atrantil has been designed to be specific for methane reduction.

Prescription Antibiotics

The most studied and successful prescription antibiotic for SIBO is rifaximin (brand name Xifaxan). It has a broad spectrum of activity and is non-absorbable. Its luminal status allows it to act locally and it is therefore less likely to cause systemic side effects common to other antibiotics.[90] Some generic forms of rifaximin may have higher rates of systemic absorption which raises the concern for a higher side effect profile.[174] According to the FDA, other than a 1% increase in headache, standard Salix (American made) or Italian rifaximin have lower rates of side effects than placebo. Rifaximin has up to a 91% success rate[91] and is given at 550mg TID x 14 days.[92] Many physicians continue to prescribe a lower dosage of 1200 mg bid x 10 days although research shows a 22% increase in breath test normalization with the higher dosage. Suggested pediatric dosages are 200 mg TID x 7 days for ages 3-15[93]or 10-30 mg/Kg[94]

Additionally, rifaximin has several unique benefits: it purportedly does not cause yeast overgrowth[95]and it decreases antibiotic resistance in bacteria by reducing plasmids.[96] Antibiotic resistance does not develop to rifaximin, making it effective for re-treatments[97] and it has anti-inflammatory properties, decreasing intestinal inflammatory cytokines and inhibiting NF-Kβ via the PXR gene.[98] It is bile soluble so it typically crystalizes when entering the large intestine, which prevents it from lowering the normally high bacterial content of the colon. There is evidence that rifaximin increases Lactobacillus and Bifidobacter levels in the colon.[175] As a solo antibiotic it is best used for SIBO when only the hydrogen levels are elevated. When methane gas is also increased, double therapy of rifaximin plus neomycin (500mg bid x 14 days) is more effective.[99] Many gastroenterologists use metronidazole (250mg tid x 14 days) as an alternative to neomycin (unpublished). Since different antibiotic regimens are recommended based on the gas type, breath testing is necessitated when choosing a treatment regimen.

Furnari et al compared breath test normalization using rifaximin 1200 mg qd vs. rifaximin 1200 mg qd plus partially hydrolyzed guar gum (5 g qd) for 10 days. The combination treatment was proven to be 23% more effective than rifaximin monotherapy.[100]

If hydrogen sulfide SIBO is suspected the same treatments as those used for methanogen overgrowth may be tried. An alternative treatment is a prescription compounded medicine called Biosolve PA which is a combination of alpha lipoic acid, DMSA and bismuth subnitrate. It was developed by Paul Anderson, ND.

Biofilm Disruptors

Mucosal methanogenic organisms are able to elaborate biofilms.[101] The use of N-acetyl cysteine, nattokinase, serrapeptase, lumbrokinase or Biosolve may be considered in addition to herbal or prescription antibiotic treatment to provide mucolytic and biofilm disruption effects. As mentioned earlier in this chapter, there is evidence both for and against enteric mucosal biofilms and SIBO.

Prevention of SIBO Relapse

SIBO is a disease that relapses because eradication itself, does not necessarilly correct the underlying cause.[102,103] Pimentel's 2006 treatment algorithm includes 2 essential preventions: diet and a prokinetic (motility agent). Our approach offers additional options: hydrochloric acid, pancreatic enzymes, hepatic support, probiotics, and brush border healing supplements. Also worth consideration are physical exercises, breathing techniques, acetylcholine precursors and modulators of neural inflammation.

Prokinetics

A key underlying cause found in SIBO is deficient activity of the migrating motor complex (MMC). An intact MMC moves debris and bacteria to the ileocecal valve during fasting at night and between meals.[104] Prokinetics stimulate the MMC, symptomatically correcting this underlying cause. Iberogast is a German compound botanical tincture with possible prokinetic action.[105] This formula includes alcoholic extracts of *Iberis amara totalis recens, Angelicae radix, Cardui mariae fructus, Chelidonii herba liquiritiae radix, Matricariae flos, Melissae folium, Carvi fructus* and *Menthae piperitae folium*. It has been used to treat functional dyspepsia and IBS since the 1960s. One study found symptom improvement, but no increase in gastric emptying, which suggests that if this formula is prokinetic, it is likely not the only mechanism underlying its action in IBS.[106] A double blind controlled trial compared iberogast to cisapride (a prescription prokinetic with limited special use in the U.S. due to cardiovascular side effects). The herbal formula performed as well as the prokinetic drug for functional dyspepsia[107]and was superior to metaclopramide in a retrospective cohort study of 961 patients.[108] It has also been shown to be effective for undifferentiated IBS in children.[109,110]

Prescription prokinetics that have been studied for SIBO include: low dose naltrexone 2.5mg qhs for IBS-D or 2.5 mg bid for IBS-C,[111] low dose erythromycin 50mg qhs, and tegaserod 2-6mg qhs.[112] Tegaserod has a higher success rate for SIBO prevention versus erythromycin,[113] but has been withdrawn from the US for safety reasons. Prucalopride (resolor) 0.5-2mg qhs, is not yet available in the US but is a safer alternative to Tegaserod.[114] It is presently available in Canada and Europe. A trial removal of a prokinetic at ≥ 3 months is suggested but continued long term use may be needed for some patients.[115]

Diet

A lower carbohydrate diet is used in combination with a prokinetic to discourage a return of bacterial overgrowth. Once the breath test has normalized and small intestine damage has healed, the diet can be expanded beyond the strictness of the Specific Carbohydrate™ and SIBO Specific Foodguide. The timeframe for this is uncertain. Two studies have examined the rate of healing post-SIBO, and found that intestinal permeability normalized four weeks after successful SIBO eradication in 75-100% of patients.[116, 117] While these reports are very encouraging, they may or may not reflect the other repair needed post-SIBO. Therefore we currently suggest continuing a SIBO diet for one to three months post successful eradication. At this point, the Cedars-Sinai Diet,[118] Low FODMAP Diet,[119] or a similar diet may be adopted long term, as the patient tolerates. These diets allow more carbohydrates in the form of grains, gluten free grains, cane sugar, and soy, though they still limit overall carbohydrate load.

Spacing meals four to five hours apart, with nothing ingested but water, allows for activity of the MMC.[120] We have found this to be very helpful clinically. If a low carbohydrate SIBO diet does not correct hypoglycemia, this strategy will need to be altered to allow for more frequent meals.

Optional Supplementation

Hydrochloric acid or herbal bitter supplements, which encourage hydrochloric acid (HCl) secretion[121] may be used to decrease the load of incoming bacteria. When considering HCl supplementation, Heidelberg radiotelemetry testing for HCl levels and response to treatments is the gold standard. Heidelberg testing reveals achlorhydria, frank hypochlorhydria and hidden hypochlorhydria and allows individualization of dosing.

Probiotics are a controversial intervention in SIBO because lactobacillus has been cultured as the causative organism in some cases of SIBO[122] and there is also concern about adding to the bacterial overload. Despite this, the few studies that have focused directly on probiotics for treatment of SIBO have shown good results. Bacillus clausii as a sole treatment normalized the breath test in 47% of cases.[123] An 82% clinical improvement in SIBO was found using a combination of Lactobacillus casei and plantarum, Streptococcus faecalis, and Bifidobacter brevis.[124] Probiotic yogurt containing Lactobacillus johnsonii normalized cytokine responses thereby reducing the low grade chronic inflammation found in SIBO after 4 weeks.[125] We have used various multi-strain and single probiotics as well as lactose-free yogurt and cultured vegetables with our SIBO patients with good results. A key point for the use of probiotic supplements in SIBO is to avoid *pre*biotics as main ingredients. Prebiotics are fermentable food for bacteria which can exacerbate symptoms during active SIBO and encourage bacterial growth post-SIBO. Common prebiotics found in probiotic supplements include: FOS (fructooligosaccharide), inulin, arabinoglactan, MOS (mannoseoligosaccharide) and GOS (galactoligoosaccharide).

Prebiotics may be tolerated in small amounts used as base ingredients, but this depends on the individual.

Brush border healing supplements may be given to assist the repair of small intestine tissue. While mucilaginous herbs are traditionally employed for this purpose (licorice, slippery elm, aloe vera, marshmallow), their use is controversial post-SIBO, due to their high level of mucopolysaccharides which are fermentable and could encourage bacterial re-growth. Specific nutrients we have used include lactose-free colostrum: 2-6 g qd, L-glutamine: 375 mg-3000 mg qd, zinc carnosine: 75mg bid, vitamins A and D (often given as cod liver oil): 1 Tbsp qd, curcumin: 400mg-3 g qd, resveratrol: 250mg-2 g qd, glutathione (oral liposomal): 50-425mg qd or glutathione precursor N-acetyl cysteine 200-600mg qd. Supplements are given for one to three months, though these may be continued long term for general benefit if desired. Higher dosages of curcumin and resveratrol are given for two weeks for the purpose of down-regulating NF-KB, a mediator of increased intestinal permeability, and then reduced to maintenance levels.[126, 127, 128]

Herbal cholinergic support may include phosphatidyl choline, pantothenic acid, huperzine A (from Huperzia serrata), and N-aceytl L-carnitine.[129] Pranayama (yogic alternate nostril breathing) has been shown to have benefits in IBS-D by normalizing parasympathetic tone.[130]

If dampening of CNS inflammation is indicated consider the use of green tea catechins, Curcuma longa, bioflavonoids, Scutellaria, resveratrol, Chrysanthemum morifolium leaf and Matricaria chamomilla.[131]

In our practices we have found that the following circumstances increase the chances of an unsatisfactory patient outcome in SIBO:

- *Failure to continue treatment courses until SIBO is eradicated (negative breath test or patient ≥90% better*). This crucial process of successive treatment is indicated by the long go-back arrow on the right side of our algorithm (Figure 6.5).
- *Failure to use double antibiotic therapy (when choosing prescription Rx) for methane producers.* Methanogenic flora need different antibiotic treatment than hydrogen producing bacteria.
- *Failure to utilize breath testing to identify if the patient has SIBO, the type of gas pattern, and the overall level of gas.* This infor-

mation is necessary for diagnosis, treatment choice/duration and prognosis.

- *Failure to use a prokinetic immediately following treatment.* Prokinetics along with diet are needed to prevent relapse of this commonly recurring condition. Antibiotic treatment as a sole therapy typically leads to recurrence of hydrogen SIBO within three months and methane SIBO within one month.[127]
- *Failure to use a low carb preventative diet following treatment.* Diet along with prokinetics are needed to prevent relapse of this commonly recurring condition.
- *Failure to tailor diet to individual tolerances with personal experimentation.* No fixed diet can predict an individual's complex bacterial, digestive, absorptive, immunological and genetic circumstances and therefore customizing is necessary.
- *Failure to identify underlying causative conditions.* One report found the following conditions led to a poor response to antibiotics: anatomical abnormalities (adhesions, blind loops, diverticuli, superior mesenteric artery syndrome, etc.), chronic narcotic use, Addison's disease, scleroderma, colonic inertia, inflammatory bowel disease, and NSAID-induced intestinal ulceration.[128] If the underlying etiology is not responsive to treatment, some of these patients will need long term cyclical rotation of herbal treatments or, very rarely, a 550 mg single dose of rifaximin every other day in order to stay asymptomatic.
- Failure to find underlying causes in order to allow for repair or modulation of the MMC will lead to a less desirable outcome.

1 Peralta S et al, Small intestine bacterial overgrowth and irritable bowel syndrome-related symptoms: experience with Rifaximin. *World J Gastroenterol.* 2009 Jun 7;15(21):2628-31.

2 Lin HC, et al. Small intestinal bacterial overgrowth: a framework for understanding irritable bowel syndrome. *JAMA.* 2004 Aug 18;292(7):852-8.

3 Pyleris E et al, The prevalence of overgrowth by aerobic bacteria in the small intestine by small bowel culture: relationship with irritable bowel syndrome. *Dig Dis Sci.* 2012 May;57(5):1321-9.

4 Pimentel M, Chow EJ, Lin HC, Normalization of lactulose breath testing correlates with symptom improvement in irritable bowel syndrome. A double-blind, randomized, placebo-controlled study. Am J Gastroenterol. 2003 Feb;98(2):412-9.

5 Anantharaju A Klamut M, Small intestinal bacterial overgrowth: a possible risk factor for metabolic bone disease. Nutr Rev. 2003 Apr;61(4):132-5.

6 Lauritano EC et al, Association between hypothyroidism and small intestinal bacterial overgrowth. *J Clin Endocrinol Metab.* 2007 Nov;92(11):4180-4.

7 Almeida JA et al, Lactose malabsorption in the elderly: role of small intestinal bacterial overgrowth. *Scand J Gastroenterol.* 2008;43(2):146-54.

8 Kaur J, Prolonged orocecal transit time enhances serum bile acids through bacterial overgrowth, contributing factor to gallstone disease. *J Clin Gastroenterol.* 2014 Apr;48(4):365-9.

9 Klaus J et al, Small intestinal bacterial overgrowth mimicking acute flare as a pitfall in patients with Crohn's Disease. *BMC Gastroenterol.* 2009 Jul 30;9:61.

10 Marie I, Ducrotté P, Denis P, Menard JF, Levesque H. Small intestinal bacterial overgrowth in systemic sclerosis. *Rheumatology* (Oxford). 2009 Oct;48(10):1314-9. Epub 2009 Aug 20.

11 Rubio-Tapia A, et al, Prevalence of small intestine bacterial overgrowth diagnosed by quantitative culture of intestinal aspirate in celiac disease. *J Clin Gastroenterol.* 2009 Feb;43(2):157-61.

12 Mancilla AC et al, [Small intestine bacterial overgrowth in patients with chronic pancreatitis]. *Rev Med Chil.* 2008 Aug;136(8):976-80.

13 Tursi A, Assessment of small intestinal bacterial overgrowth in uncomplicated acute diverticulitis of the colon. *World J Gastroenterol.* 2005 May 14;11(18):2773-6.

14 Ojetti V et al, Small bowel bacterial overgrowth and type 1 diabetes. *Eur Rev Med Pharmacol Sci.* 2009 Nov-Dec;13(6):419-23.

15 Goebel HYPERLINK "http://www.ncbi.nlm.nih.gov/pubmed?term=Goebel%20A%5BAuthor%5D&cauthor=true&cauthor_uid=18540025" HYPERLINK "http://www.ncbi.nlm.nih.gov/pubmed?term=Goebel%20A%5BAuthor%5D&cauthor=true&cauthor_uid=18540025" A et al, Altered intestinal permeability in patients with primary fibromyalgia and in patients with complex regional pain syndrome. *Rheumatology* (Oxford). 2008 Aug;47(8):1223-7.

16 Gupta A et al, Role of small intestinal bacterial overgrowth and delayed gastrointestinal transit time in cirrhotic patients with minimal hepatic encephalopathy. *J Hepatol.* 2010 Nov;53(5):849-55.

17 Shanab AA et al, Small intestinal bacterial overgrowth in nonalcoholic steatohepatitis: association with toll-like receptor 4 expression and plasma levels of interleukin 8. *Dig Dis Sci.* 2011 May;56(5):1524-34.

18 Weinstock LB, Klutke CG, Lin HC, Small intestinal bacterial overgrowth in pa-

tients with interstitial cystitis and gastrointestinal symptoms. *Dig Dis Sci.* 2008 May;53(5):1246-51.

19 Weinstock LB, Walters AS, Restless legs syndrome is associated with irritable bowel syndrome and small intestinal bacterial overgrowth. *Sleep Med.* 2011 Jun;12(6):610-3.

20 Parodi A et al, Small intestinal bacterial overgrowth in rosacea: clinical effectiveness of its eradication. *Clin Gastroenterol Hepatol.* 2008 Jul;6(7):759-64.

21 Kim KM, Erosive esophagitis may be related to small intestinal bacterial overgrowth. *Scand J Gastroentero*l. 2012 May;47(5):493-8.

22 Pimentel M, Personal communication, 2014

23 Husebye E, The patterns of small bowel motility: physiology and implications in organic disease and functional disorders. *Neurogastroenterol Motil.* 1999 Jun;11(3):141-61.

24 Bures J, 2010 Small intestinal bacterial overgrowth syndrome. *World J Gastroenterol.* 2010 Jun 28;16(24):2978-90.

25 Machado WM et al, The small bowel flora in individuals with cecoileal reflux. *Arq Gastroenterol.* 2008 Jul-Sep;45(3):212-8.

26 Roland BC, Low ileocecal valve pressure is significantly associated with small intestinal bacterial overgrowth (SIBO). *Dig Dis Sci.* 2014 Jun;59(6):1269-77.

27 Gabbard SL, The impact of alcohol consumption and cholecystectomy on small intestinal bacterial overgrowth. *Dig Dis Sci.* 2014 Mar;59(3):638-44.

28 Chedid V, Herbal therapy is equivalent to rifaximin for the treatment of small intestinal bacterial overgrowth. *Glob Adv Health Med.* 2014 May;3(3):16-24.

29. Macfarlane S, Microbial biofilm communities in the gastrointestinal tract. *J Clin Gastroenterol.* 2008 Sep;42 Suppl 3 Pt 1:S142-3.

30 Gabbard SL, The impact of alcohol consumption and cholecystectomy on small intestinal bacterial overgrowth. *Dig Dis Sci.* 2014 Mar;59(3):638-44.

31 Pyleris E et al, The prevalence of overgrowth by aerobic bacteria in the small intestine by small bowel culture: relationship with irritable bowel syndrome. *Dig Dis Sci.* 2012 May;57(5):1321-9.

32 Jacobs C, Dysmotility and proton pump inhibitor use are independent risk factors for small intestinal bacterial and/or fungal overgrowth. *Aliment Pharmacol Ther.* 2013 Jun;37(11):1103-11.

33 Khoshini R, Dai SC, Lezcano S, Pimentel M. A systematic review of diagnostic tests for small intestinal bacterial overgrowth. *Dig Dis Sci.* 2008 Jun;53(6):1443-54.

34 Pimentel M. Webcast: Gut Microbes and Irritable Bowel Syndrome. July 20, 2012. Available at: http://www.gihealthfoundation.org/coe/ibs/webcast/2012/july/MPimentel/?link=2012/july/MPimentel&cme_proj_id=12&actionPage=topics/Gut_Microbes_and_IBS/request-for-credit.cfm?cme_proj_id=12. Accessed on October 27, 2012.

35 Bouhnik Y et al, Bacterial populations contaminating the upper gut in patients \ with small intestinal bacterial overgrowth syndrome. *Am J Gastroenterol.* 1999 May;94(5):1327-31.

36 Pyleris E et al, The prevalence of overgrowth by aerobic bacteria in the small intestine by small bowel culture: relationship with irritable bowel syndrome. *Dig Dis Sci.* 2012 May;57(5):1321-9.

37 Carbonero F, Microbial pathways in colonic sulfur metabolism and links with health and disease. *Front Physiol.* 2012 Nov 28;3:448.

38 Million M, Correlation between body mass index and gut concentrations of Lactobacillus reuteri, Bifidobacterium animalis, Methanobrevibacter smithii and Escherichia coli. *Int J Obes* (Lond). 2013 Nov;37(11):1460-6.
39 Medani M, Emerging role of hydrogen sulfide in colonic physiology and pathophysiology. *Inflamm Bowel Dis*. 2011 Jul;17(7):1620-5
40 Elsheikh W, Enhanced chemopreventive effects of a hydrogen sulfide-releasing anti-inflammatory drug (ATB-346) in experimental colorectal cancer. *Nitric Oxide*. 2014 Sep 15;41:131-7.
41 Rodríguez LA, Ruigómez A. Increased risk of irritable bowel syndrome after bacterial gastroenteritis: cohort study. *BMJ*. 1999 Feb 27;318(7183):565-6.
42 Rodríguez LA, Ruigómez A. Increased risk of irritable bowel syndrome after bacterial gastroenteritis: cohort study. *BMJ*. 1999 Feb 27;318(7183):565-6.
43 Beatty JK, Post-infectious irritable bowel syndrome: mechanistic insights into chronic disturbances following enteric infection. *World J Gastroenterol*. 2014 Apr 14;20(14):3976-85.
44 Zanini B, Incidence of post-infectious irritable bowel syndrome and functional intestinal disorders following a water-borne viral gastroenteritis outbreak. *Am J Gastroenterol*. 2012 Jun;107(6):891-9.
45 Hanevik K, Development of functional gastrointestinal disorders after Giardia lamblia infection. *BMC Gastroenterol*. 2009 Apr 21;9:27.
46 Pokkunuri V, Role of Cytolethal Distending Toxin in Altered Stool Form and Bowel Phenotypes in a Rat Model of Post-infectious Irritable Bowel Syndrome. *J Neurogastroenterol Motil*. 2012 Oct;18(4):434-42.
47 Pimentel M, Low-dose nocturnal tegaserod or erythromycin delays symptom recurrence after treatment of irritable bowel syndrome based on presumed bacterial overgrowth. *Gastroenterol Hepatol* (N Y). 2009 Jun;5(6):435-42.
48 Pokkunuri V, Role of Cytolethal Distending Toxin in Altered Stool Form and Bowel Phenotypes in a Rat Model of Post-infectious Irritable Bowel Syndrome. *J Neurogastroenterol Motil*. 2012 Oct;18(4):434-42.
49 Sung J, et al Effect of repeated Campylobacter jejuni infection on gut flora and mucosal defense in a rat model of post infectious functional and microbial bowel changes. *Neurogastroenterol Motil*. 2013 Jun;25(6):529-37
50 Pimentel M et al, Autoimmunity Links Vinculin to the Pathophysiology of Functional Bowel Changes Following Campylobacter jejuni Infection in a Rat Model. *Dig Dis Sci* 2014 Nov; Epub ahead of Print.
51 Kim G, Methanobrevibacter smithii is the predominant methanogen in patients with constipation-predominant IBS and methane on breath. *Dig Dis Sci*. 2012 Dec;57(12):3213-8.
52 Dridi B, High prevalence of Methanobrevibacter smithii and Methanosphaera stadtmanae detected in the human gut using an improved DNA detection protocol. *PLoS One*. 2009 Sep 17;4(9):e7063.
53 Youn YH, Park JS, Jahng JH, Lim HC, Kim JH, Pimentel M, Park H, Lee SI. Relationships among the lactulose breath test, intestinal gas volume, and gastrointestinal symptoms in patients with irritable bowel syndrome. *Dig Dis Sci*. 2011 Jul;56(7):2059-66.
54 Gottschall E, *Breaking the Vicious Cycle: Intestinal Health Through Diet*, 1994, Kirkton Press Ltd., Ontario, Canada.

55 Elsenbruch S. Abdominal pain in Irritable Bowel Syndrome: a review of putative psychological, neural and neuro-immune mechanisms. *Brain Behav Immun.* 2011 Mar;25(3):386-94. Epub 2010 Nov 20.
56 Pimentel, M. *A New IBS Solution.* Health Point Press, Sherman Oaks, Ca. 2006.
57 Pimentel M, Mayer AG, Park S, Chow EJ, Hasan A, Kong Y. Methane production during lactulose breath test is associated with gastrointestinal disease presentation. *Dig Dis Sci.* 2003 Jan;48(1):86-92.
58 Kunkel D et al, Methane on breath testing is associated with constipation: a systematic review and meta-analysis. *Dig Dis Sci.* 2011 Jun;56(6):1612-8.
59 Pimentel M, Lin HC, Enayati P, van den Burg B, Lee HR, Chen JH, Park S, Kong Y, Conklin J. Methane, a gas produced by enteric bacteria, slows intestinal transit and augments small intestinal contractile activity. *Am J Physiol Gastrointest Liver Physiol.* 2006 Jun;290(6):G1089-95.
60 Chatterjee S et al, The degree of breath methane production in IBS correlates with the severity of constipation. *Am J Gastroenterol.* 2007 Apr;102(4):837-41.
61 Pimentel M, Mayer AG, Park S, Chow EJ, Hasan A, Kong Y. Methane production during lactulose breath test is associated with gastrointestinal disease presentation. *Dig Dis Sci.* 2003 Jan;48(1):86-92.
62 Kim KM, Erosive esophagitis may be related to small intestinal bacterial overgrowth. *Scand J Gastroenterol.* 2012 May;47(5):493-8.
63 Singh VV, Toskes PP. Small Bowel Bacterial Overgrowth: Presentation, Diagnosis, and Treatment. *Curr Treat Options Gastroenterol.* 2004 Feb;7(1):19-28.
64 Leung Ki EL, Small intestine bacterial overgrowth. *Rev Med Suisse.* 2010 Jan 27;6(233):186-8, 190-1.
65 DiBaise JK. Nutritional consequences of small intestinal bacterial overgrowth. *Prac Gastroenterol.* 2008;69:15-28.
66 Prizont R. Glycoprotein degradation in the blind loop syndrome: identification of glycosidases in jejunal contents. *J Clin Invest.* 1981 Feb;67(2):336-44.
67 Lauritano EC, Valenza V, Sparano L, Scarpellini E, Gabrielli M, Cazzato A, Ferraro PM, Gasbarrini A. Small intestinal bacterial overgrowth and intestinal permeability. *Scand J Gastroenterol.* 2010 Sep;45(9):1131-2.
68 Resnick C. Nutritional Protocol for the Treatment of Intestinal Permeability Defects and Related Conditions. *Natural Medicine Journal.* March 2010.
69 Lactulose solution USP label, Pharmaceutical Assoc. Inc, Greenville, SC 29605.
70 Pimentel M, Report from the multinational irritable bowel syndrome initiative **HYPERLINK "http://www.ncbi.nlm.nih.gov/pubmed/23644078"2012** HYPERLINK "http://www.ncbi.nlm.nih.gov/pubmed/23644078". *Gastroenterology.* 2013 Jun;144(7):e1-5.
71 Eisenmann A et al, Implementation and interpretation of hydrogen breath tests. *J Breath Res.* 2008 Dec;2(4):046002.
72 Costa MB, Evaluation of small intestine bacterial overgrowth in patients with functional dyspepsia through H2 breath test. *Arq Gastroenterol.* 2012 Dec;49(4):279-83.
73 Pimentel M, Lecture at the SIBO Symposium, Portland OR, 2014
74 Pimentel M, Lecture at the SIBO Symposium, Portland OR, 2014
75 Attaluri A, Methanogenic flora is associated with altered colonic transit but not stool characteristics in constipation without IBS. *Am J Gastroenterol.* 2010 Jun;105(6):1407-11.

76 Quigley EM, Quera R. Small intestinal bacterial overgrowth: roles of antibiotics, prebiotics, and probiotics. *Gastroenterology*. 2006 Feb;130(2 Suppl 1):S78-90.

77 Quin Tron Instrument Company Inc. *Quin Tron Catalog and Information*. p. 22, 2012.

78 Pimentel, M. *A New IBS Solution*. Health Point Press, Sherman Oaks, Ca. 2006.

79 Gottschall E. *Breaking the Vicious Cycle*. Kirkton Press Ltd, Baltimore Ontario Canada, 1994.

80 Siebecker A, The SIBO Specific Foodguide

81 Ong DK, Manipulation of dietary short chain carbohydrates alters the pattern of gas production and genesis of symptoms in irritable bowel syndrome. *J Gastroenterol Hepatol*. 2010 Aug;25(8):1366-73.

82 Nieves R, Jackson RT. Specific carbohydrate diet in treatment of inflammatory bowel disease. *Tenn Med*. 2004 Sep;97(9):407.

83 Choung RS, Clinical predictors of small intestinal bacterial overgrowth by duodenal aspirate culture. *Aliment Pharmacol Ther*. 2011 May;33(9):1059-67.

84 Shepherd SJ, The role of FODMAPs in irritable bowel syndrome. *Curr Opin Clin Nutr Metab Care*. 2014 Nov;17(6):605-9.

85 Staudacher HM, Whelan K, Irving PM, Lomer MC. Comparison of symptom response following advice for a diet low in fermentable carbohydrates (FODMAPs) versus standard dietary advice in patients with irritable bowel syndrome. *J Hum Nutr Diet*. 2011 Oct;24(5):487-95.

86 Pimentel M, Constantino T, A 14-day elemental diet is highly effective in normalizing the lactulose breath test. *Dig Dis Sci*. 2004 Jan;49(1):73-7.

87 Pimentel M, Constantino T, A 14-day elemental diet is highly effective in normalizing the lactulose breath test. *Dig Dis Sci*. 2004 Jan;49(1):73-7.

88 Logan AC, Beaulne TM. The treatment of small intestinal bacterial overgrowth with enteric-coated peppermint oil: a case report. *Altern Med Rev*. 2002 Oct;7(5):410-7.

89 Chedid V, Herbal therapy is equivalent to rifaximin for the treatment of small intestinal bacterial overgrowth. *Glob Adv Health Med*. 2014 May;3(3):16-24.

90 Scarpignato C, Pelosini I. Experimental and clinical pharmacology of rifaximin, a gastrointestinal selective antibiotic. *Digestion*. 2006;73 Suppl 1:13-27.

91 Lombardo L, Increased Incidence of Small Intestinal Bacterial Overgrowth During Proton Pump Inhibitor Therapy. *Clinical Gastroenterology and Hepatology*. 2010 June; 8(6):504-508.

92 Pimentel M, Lembo A, TARGET Study Group. Rifaximin therapy for patients with irritable bowel syndrome without constipation. *N Engl J Med*. 2011 Jan 6;364(1):22-32.

93 Scarpellini E et al, Rifaximin treatment for small intestinal bacterial overgrowth in children with irritable bowel syndrome. *Eur Rev Med Pharmacol Sci*. 2013 May;17(10):1314-20

94 Muniyappa P et al, Use and safety of rifaximin in children with inflammatory bowel disease. *J Pediatr Gastroenterol Nutr*. 2009 Oct;49(4):400-4.

95 Scarpignato C, Pelosini I, Experimental and clinical pharmacology of rifaximin, a gastrointestinal selective antibiotic. *Digestion*. 2006;73 Suppl 1:13-27.

96 Debbia EA, Maioli E, Roveta S, Marchese A. Effects of rifaximin on bacterial virulence mechanisms at supra- and sub-inhibitory concentrations. *J Chemother*. 2008 Apr;20(2):186-94.

97 Yang J, Lee HR, Low K, Chatterjee S, Pimentel M. Rifaximin versus other antibiotics in the primary treatment and retreatment of bacterial overgrowth in IBS. *Dig Dis Sci*. 2008 Jan;53(1):169-74

98 Mencarelli A,. Inhibition of NF-κB by a PXR-dependent pathway mediates counter-regulatory activities of rifaximin on innate immunity in intestinal epithelial cells. *Eur J Pharmacol*. 2011 Oct 1;668(1-2):317-24.

99 Low K, Hwang L, Hua J, Zhu A, Morales W, Pimentel M. A combination of rifaximin and neomycin is most effective in treating irritable bowel syndrome patients with methane on lactulose breath test. *J Clin Gastroenterol*. 2010 Sep;44(8):547-50.

100 Furnari M, Clinical trial: the combination of rifaximin with partially hydrolysed guar gum is more effective than rifaximin alone in eradicating small intestinal bacterial overgrowth. *Aliment Pharmacol Ther*. 2010 Oct;32(8):1000-6

101 Bang C, Biofilm formation of mucosa-associated methanoarchaeal strains. *Front Microbiol*. 2014 Jul 8;5:353

102 Pimentel M, Morales W, Low-dose nocturnal tegaserod or erythromycin delays symptom recurrence after treatment of irritable bowel syndrome based on presumed bacterial overgrowth. *Gastroenterol Hepatol* (N Y). 2009 Jun;5(6):435-42.

103 Pimentel M. An evidence-based treatment algorithm for IBS based on a bacterial/SIBO hypothesis: Part 2. *Am J Gastroenterol*. 2010 Jun;105(6):1227-30.

104 Pimentel M, Morales W, Low-dose nocturnal tegaserod or erythromycin delays symptom recurrence after treatment of irritable bowel syndrome based on presumed bacterial overgrowth. *Gastroenterol Hepatol* (N Y). 2009 Jun;5(6):435-42.

105 Ochoa-Cortes F, Potential for developing purinergic drugs for gastrointestinal diseases. *Inflamm Bowel Dis*. 2014 Jul;20(7):1259-87.

106 Braden B, Clinical effects of STW 5 (Iberogast) are not based on acceleration of gastric emptying in patients with functional dyspepsia and gastroparesis. *Neurogastroenterol Motil*. 2009 Jun;21(6):632-8, e25.

107 Rösch W, A randomised clinical trial comparing the efficacy of a herbal preparation STW 5 with the prokinetic drug cisapride in patients with dysmotility type of functional dyspepsia. *Z Gastroenterol*. 2002 Jun;40(6):401-8.

108 Raedsch R, Assessment of the efficacy and safety of the phytopharmacon STW 5 versus metoclopramide in functional dyspepsia-a retrolective cohort study. *Z Gastroenterol*. 2007 Oct;45(10):1041-8.

109 Leichtle K. Experience reports of the application of Iberogast in children. Research report. Steigerwald: Arzneimittelwerk; 1999.

110 Gundermann KJ, Vinson B, Hänicke S. Die funktionelle Dyspepsie bei Kindern—eine retrospektive Studie mit einem Phytopharmakon. Päd. 2004;10:1–6.

111 Ploesser J, Weinstock LB, Thomas E. Low Dose Naltrexone: Side Effects and Efficacy in Gastrointestinal Disorders. *International Journal of Pharmaceutical Compounding*; March 2010.

112 Pimentel M, Morales W, Low-dose nocturnal tegaserod or erythromycin delays symptom recurrence after treatment of irritable bowel syndrome based on presumed bacterial overgrowth. *Gastroenterol Hepatol* (N Y). 2009 Jun;5(6):435-42.

113 Pimentel M, Morales W, Low-dose nocturnal tegaserod or erythromycin delays symptom recurrence after treatment of irritable bowel syndrome based on presumed bacterial overgrowth. *Gastroenterol Hepatol* (N Y). 2009 Jun;5(6):435-42.

114 Manabe N, Rao AS, Wong BS, Camilleri M, Emerging pharmacologic therapies for irritable bowel syndrome. *Curr Gastroenterol Rep*. 2010 Oct;12(5):408-16.

115 Pimentel, M, *A New IBS Solution*. Health Point Press, Sherman Oaks, Ca. 2006.

116 Lauritano EC, Small intestinal bacterial overgrowth and intestinal permeability. *Scand J Gastroenterol*. 2010 Sep;45(9):1131-2.

117 Riordan SM et al, Luminal bacteria and small-intestinal permeability *Scan J Gastroenterol* 1997 Jun;32(6):556-63.
118 Pimentel, M. *A New IBS Solution*. Health Point Press, Sherman Oaks, Ca. 2006.
119 Gibson PR, Shepherd SJ. Evidence-based dietary management of functional gastrointestinal symptoms: The FODMAP approach. *J Gastroenterol Hepatol*. 2010 Feb;25(2):252-8. Review.
120 Pimentel, M. *A New IBS Solution*. Health Point Press, Sherman Oaks, Ca. 2006.
121 Bowman, G. The Gut, the Brain and the Functional GI Disorders. *Functional Gastroenterology Seminar: Level 1*. Winter 2010, p. 19.
122 Bouhnik Y, Bacterial populations contaminating the upper gut in patients with small intestinal bacterial overgrowth syndrome. *Am J Gastroenterol*. 1999 May;94(5):1327-31.
123 Gabrielli M, Bacillus clausii as a treatment of small intestinal bacterial overgrowth. *Am J Gastroenterol*. 2009 May;104(5):1327-8.
124 Soifer LO, Peralta D, Dima G, Besasso H, Comparative clinical efficacy of a probiotic vs. an antibiotic in the treatment of patients with intestinal bacterial overgrowth and chronic abdominal functional distension: a pilot study. *Acta Gastroenterol Latinoam*. 2010 Dec;40(4):323-7.
125 Schiffrin EJ, Parlesak A, Bode C, Bode JC, van't Hof MA, Grathwohl D, Guigoz Y, Probiotic yogurt in the elderly with intestinal bacterial overgrowth: endotoxaemia and innate immune functions. *Br J Nutr*. 2009 Apr;101(7):961-6.
126 Ruland J, Return to homeostasis: downregulation of NF-κB responses. *Nat Immunol*. 2011 Jun 19;12(8):709-14. doi: 10.1038/ni.2055.
127 Al-Sadi RM, Ma TY. IL-1beta causes an increase in intestinal epithelial tight junction permeability. *J Immunol*. 2007 Apr 1;178(7):4641-9.
128 Csaki C, Mobasheri A, Synergistic chondroprotective effects of curcumin and resveratrol in human articular chondrocytes: inhibition of IL-1beta-induced NF-kappaB-mediated inflammation and apoptosis. *Arthritis Res Ther*. 2009;11(6):R165.
129 Kharazian D, *The Digestive Sessions*, Underground Radio Webinar, 2014.
130 Taneja I, Yogic versus conventional treatment in diarrhea-predominant irritable bowel syndrome: a randomized control study. *Appl Psychophysiol Biofeedback*. 2004 Mar;29(1):19-33.
131 Kharazian D, *The Digestive Sessions*, Underground Radio Webinar, 2014.
132 Fialho, A. Association between small intestinal bacterial overgrowth and deep vein thrombosis. (4):299-303, *Gastroenterol Rep* (Oxf)., 2016, Vol. 4.
133 Donowitz, JR, Pediatric small intestine bacterial overgrowth in low-income countries. (1):6-15, Trends Mol Med., 2015, Vol. 21.
134 Pimentel, M, Portland, OR, SIBO Symposium. National College of Natural Medicine, 2014.
135 Zeitoun, JD, Functional digestive symptoms and quality of life in patients with Ehlers-Danlos syndromes: results of a national cohort study on 134 patients. (11):e80321, *PLoS One*. 2013, Vol. 8.
136 Levy, HP, Ehlers-Danlos Syndrome, Hypermobility Type. Seattle, WA : Genereviews, 2016.
137 Laskowska, M, Nationwide population-based cohort study of celiac disease and risk of Ehlers-Danlos syndrome and joint hypermobility syndrome. (9):1030-4., *Dig Liver Dis*. 2016, Vol. 48.
138 Castori, M, Gastrointestinal and nutritional issues in joint hypermobility syndrome/

Ehlers-Danlos syndrome, hypermobility type: A characterization of the patients' lived experience. (1):54-75, *Am J Med Genet C Semin Med Genet.*2015, Vol. 169C .

139 Murray, B, (12):2981-8, *Am J Med Genet A*. 2013, Vol. 161A.

140 Machado, WM, The small bowel flora in individuals with cecoileal reflux. (3):212-8, *Arq Gastroenterol*. 2008, *PLoS Biol*. Vol. 45, p. 14(8): e1002533.

141 Rowland, BC, Low ileocecal valve pressure is significantly associated with small intestinal bacterial overgrowth (SIBO). (6):1269-77, *Dig Dis Sci*. 2014, Vol. 59.

142 Fialho, A, Higher visceral to subcutaneous fat ratio is associated with small intestinal bacterial overgrowth. (9):773-7., *Nutr Metab Cardiovasc Dis*. 2016, Vol. 26.

143 Ojetti, V, Small bowel bacterial overgrowth and type 1 diabetes. (6):419-23, *Eur Rev Med Pharmacol Sci*. 2009, Vol. 13.

144 Reddymasu, SC, Small intestinal bacterial overgrowth in gastroparesis: are there any predictors? (1):e8-13, *J Clin Gastroenterol*. 2010, Vol. 44.

145 Capurso, G, Systematic review and meta-analysis: Small intestinal bacterial overgrowth in chronic pancreatitis. (5):697-705, *United European Gastroenterol J*. 2016, Vol. 4.

146 Fialho, A, Small Intestinal Bacterial Overgrowth Is Associated with Non-Alcoholic Fatty Liver Disease. (2):159-65, *J Gastrointestin Liver Dis*. 2016, Vol. 25.

147 Belitson, PC, Association of gastric hypoacidity with opportunistic enteric infections in patients with AIDS. 2):277-84., *J Infect Dis*. 1992, Vol. 166.

148 Bures, J, Small intestinal bacterial overgrowth syndrome. (24):2978-90, *World J Gastroenterol*. 2010, Vol. 16.

149 Rana, SV, Small intestinal bacterial overgrowth. (9):1030-7, *Scand J Gastroenterol*. 2008, Vol. 43.

150 Naseem, Z, "Less is more": Non operative management of short term superior mesenteric artery syndrome. (4):428-30, *Ann Med Surg* (Lond). , 2015, Vol. 4.

151 Kaur, A, Superior Mesentric Artery Syndrome in a Patient with Subacute Intestinal Obstruction: A Case Report. (6):TD03-5, *J Clin Diagn Res*. 2016, Vol. 10.

152 Fraser, JD, Laparoscopic duodenojejunostomy for superior mesenteric artery syndrome. (2):254-9, *JSLS*. 2009, Vol. 13.

153 Braun-Moscovici, Y, What tests should you use to assess small intestinal bacterial overgrowth in systemic sclerosis? (4 Suppl 91):S117-22, *Clin Exp Rheumatol*. 2015, Vol. 33.

154 Marie, L, Fecal calprotectin in systemic sclerosis and review of the literature. (6):547-54, *Autoimmun Rev*. 2015, Vol. 14.

155 Sandborn, WJ, How to avoid treating irritable bowel syndrome with biologic therapy for inflammatory bowel disease. Suppl 1:80-4, *Dig Dis*. 2009, Vol. 27.

156 Peritoneal adhesions: etiology, pathophysiology, and clinical significance. Recent advances in prevention and management. Liakakos, T. (4):260-73., *Dig Surg*. 2001, Vol. 18.

157 Makkar, J K, Comparison of erythromycin versus metoclopramide for gastric feeding intolerance in patients with traumatic brain injury: A randomized double-blind study. 2016, *Saudi J Anaesth*. pp. 10(3): 308–313.

158 Hernandez, G, Splanchnic ischemia and gut permeability after acute brain injury secondary to intracranial hemorrhage. (1):40-4, *Neurocrit Care*. 2007, Vol. 7.

159 Liu, Y, ERK/Nrf2/HO-1 Pathway-Mediated Mitophagy Alleviates Traumatic Brain Injury-Induced Intestinal Mucosa Damage and Epithelial Barrier Dysfunction. doi: 10.1089/neu.2016.4764., *J Neurotrauma*. 2017.

160 Hamonet, C, Brain injury unmasking Ehlers-Danlos syndromes after trauma: the fiber print. 11:45, *Orphanet J Rare Dis*. 2016, Vol. Apr 22;.

161 Gabbard, SL, The impact of alcohol consumption and cholecystectomy on small intestinal bacterial overgrowth. (3):638-44., *Dig Dis Sci*. 2014, Vol. 59.

162 Guercio Nuzio, S, Multiple gut-liver axis abnormalities in children with obesity with and without hepatic involvement. *Pediatr Obes*. 2016, Vol. doi: 10.1111/ijpo.12164.

163 Nieuwenhuijs, VB, The role of interdigestive small bowel motility in the regulation of gut microflora, bacterial overgrowth, and bacterial translocation in rats. (2):188-93, *Ann Surg*. 1998, Vol. 228.

164 Powell, AK, Murine intestinal migrating motor complexes: longitudinal components. (3):245-56, *Neurogastroenterol Motil*. 2003, Vol. 15.

165 Lewis, TD, Morphine and gastroduodenal motility. (11):2178-86, *Dig Dis Sci*. 1999, Vol. 44.

166 Defilippi, C, Inhibition of small intestinal motility by casein: a role of beta casomorphins? (6):751-4, *Nutrition*. 1995, Vol. 11.

167 Lo, WK, Proton pump inhibitor use and the risk of small intestinal bacterial overgrowth: a meta-analysis. (5):483-90, s.l.: *Clin Gastroenterol Hepatol*. 2013, Vol. 11.

168 Riddoch, C, Gastrointestinal disturbances in marathon runners. (2):71-4, *Br J Sports Med*. 1988, Vol. 22.

169 Peters, HP, Gastrointestinal symptoms in long-distance runners, cyclists, and triathletes: prevalence, medication, and etiology. (6):1570-81, *Am J Gastroenterol*. 1988, Vol. 94.

170 Perko, MJ, Mesenteric, coeliac and splanchnic blood flow in humans during exercise. (Pt 3):907-13., *J Physiol*. 1998 Dec 15;513 , 1998, Vol. 513.

171 de Oliveira, EP, The impact of physical exercise on the gastrointestinal tract. (5):533-8, *Curr Opin Clin Nutr Metab Care*. 2009, Vol. 12.

172 Smetanka, RD, Intestinal permeability in runners in the 1996 Chicago marathon. (4):426-33, *Int J Sport Nutr*. 1999, Vol. 9.

173 Greenson, J, The biopsy pathology of non-coeliac enteropathy. (1):29-36, *Histopathology*. 2015, Vol. 66.

174 Scarpignato, C, SIBO Symposium III. Portland, OR: National College of Natural Medicine, 2016.

175 Scarpignato, C, Rifaximin in the Treatment of SIBO. Portland, OR: 2016. SIBO Symposium.

176 Wang, YB, Effects of intestinal mucosal blood flow and motility on intestinal mucosa. 2011, *World J Gastroenterol*. pp. 17(5): 657–661.

Chapter 7

Blood Sugar, Insulin, And The Gastrointestinal Tract

Effects of Altered Glucose on:

Mouth

Esophagus

Stomach

Gastroparesis

Diagnosis of Gastroparesis

Treatment of Gastroparesis

Autoimmune Gastritis and Achlorhydria

Metformin and B12 Deficiency

Small Intestine

Bariatric Surgery and Insulin Resistance

Liver

Non-Alcoholic Fatty Liver Disease and Non-Alcoholic Steatohepatitis

Celiac Disease and NASH

Treatment of NAFLD and NASH

Glycogenic Hepatopathy

Pancreas

Exocrine Pancreas

Endocrine Pancreas

Gall Bladder

Non-Alcoholic Fatty Gallbladder Disease

Biliary Dyskinesia//Functional Biliary Disorder

Treatment Options for Biliary Sludge and Cholelithiasis

Colon

The blood glucose level and associated insulin deficiency or resistance confer tremendous impact on the function of the gastrointestinal tract-from mouth to anus. This chapter will discuss the research relating to each level of the tract.

Mouth

The risk of oral Candidiasis increases with hyperglycemia and diabetes. In children with Type 1 diabetes, yeast overgrowth and increased salivary glucose concentrations are correlated with poor glycemic control.[1] In adults with diabetes, cigarette smoking, denture use and poor glycemic control increase the chance of thrush. This may be related to decreased salivary secretion.[2,3] Hypoguesia (diminished taste perception) also occurs in more than one-third of diabetics which may alter appetite and cause overeating.[4] Salivary amylase may be increased in diabetes, (perhaps a compensation for decreased pancreatic amylase secretion).[5] Salivary IgA levels are consistently found to be elevated in diabetics.[6]

Esophagus

In a Swedish study, 58% of diabetics had abnormal esophageal function and 68% had delayed gastric emptying. Abdominal fullness was the only symptom that related to any dysfunction, and it was associated with delayed gastric emptying.[7] When diabetic esophageal signs are present (esophageal dysmotility, dilatation and spasm), they are associated with concomitant cardiovascular disease.[8] Changes include delayed transit of food, decreased esophageal peristaltic amplitude and velocity and a higher rate of gastro-esophageal reflux disease due to laxity of the lower esophageal sphincter. Subjects with over a five year history of diabetes had more exposure of the esophagus to acid due to reflux when compared to those with less than a five year history of diabetes.[9]

Stomach

Gastroparesis

Gastroparesis is a partial paralysis of the stomach which causes delayed gastric emptying. This delayed emptying is often associated with poorly controlled diabetes mellitus. The effect of slowing the exit of carbohydrate from the stomach is especially dangerous for diabetics. Consider a situation in which a type I diabetic injects a calculated dose of short-acting insulin with a meal. If the carbohydrate absorption is delayed for up to 8-10 hours, life-threatening hypoglycemia is likely. Poor control of hyperglycemia, arterial complications, and diabetic neuropathy are all associated with gastroparesis.[10] It occurs in 55-75% of type I diabetics and 15-20% of type II diabetics. The incidence in the U.S is increasing and hospitalizations for gastroparesis as the primary diagnosis increased 158% to a total of 10,252 hospital stays in 2004. This is in contrast to a mere 53% increase in all hospitalizations for diabetes related problems that same year. Gastroparesis leads to the longest and most expensive hospital stays compared to the other five most common upper GI diagnoses.[11] Attaining long-term glycemic control improves gastric motility and improves upper abdominal symptoms in diabetic patients with gastroparesis.[12] It is thought that maintaining long term near normal glucose levels allows healing of vagal neuropathy with reversal of neuronal glycosylation.[13]

Other gastroparesis risk factors include medications, certain disease states and gluten intolerance.

TABLE 7.1 DRUGS THAT MAY INDUCE GASTROPARESIS	
Tobacco	Hyoscyamine
Tricyclic antidepressants	Bentyl
Calcium channel blockers	Levsin
L-dopa	Narcotics

TABLE 7.2 DISEASES THAT MAY INDUCE GASTROPARESIS	
Hypothyroidism	Parkinson's
Systemic lupus erythematosis	Stroke
Scleroderma	Traumatic brain injury

Diagnosis Of Gastroparesis

Symptoms and signs of gastroparesis include nausea or vomiting, bloating, early satiety, postprandial fullness and abdominal pain. A four hour gastric emptying study is the most common method of diagnosis. A one hour study may be fraught with false negatives, but a positive test is a reliable sign. The most accurate diagnostic method is antroduodenal manometry, but only a few centers in the U.S. currently perform this invasive test. Sometimes evidence of gastroparesis is seen on upper GI barium studies and small bowel follow-through series.

Upper GI barium studies of gastroparesis may reveal:

Gastric dilatation

Delayed emptying of barium

Retained gastric debris (bezoars)

Retained gastric fluid[14]

When reviewing lab results in diabetic patients, have a high index of suspicion of gastroparesis when you see the following trends:

- low blood sugar one to three hours postprandially
- high blood sugar five or more hours after meals with no other explanation
- difficulty controlling high morning blood glucose[15]

Treatment Of Gastroparesis

Table 7.3 Psychophysiology Of Digestion
Treatment and prevention of all digestive issues involves heeding the psychophysiology of digestion guidelines: **Savor the cephalic phase** • Eat in pleasant surroundings • Enjoy the sight and scent of food **Chew food until liquid before swallowing** **Eat slowly—unhurried** • Avoid eating while driving • Avoid watching television while eating • Practice mindfulness during meals **Use emotional clearing techniques for family of origin issues** **Avoid ice cold drinks during meals**

In addition, treatment of gastroparesis may include:

Dietary factors:

Adequate hydration

Smaller more frequent meals

Reduced intake of dietary fiber

Reduced portions of fat per meal

Avoidance of red meat

Reduced protein content of the evening meal

Smaller evening meal

Reduced alcohol consumption

Improved glucose regulation (discussed later)

Avoidance or limitation of cruciferous vegetables

Grain-free or gluten-free diet

Botanicals, etc.:

Aloe juice—up to 8 ounces 15-30 min ac

Iberogast (German prokinetic herbal tincture)—20 gtts ac or 60 gtts qhs

Papain (Super papaya enzyme plus) 3-5/meal

Antioxidants[16]

Atractylodes lancea (essential oil)[17]

Nervinum vagum (homeopathic vagus nerve) 10 gtts BID (children 3-5 gtts BID) for 3 weeks followed by one week off each month for three months

Other:

Normalize or replace HCl/pepsin output (see Chapter 13).

Normalize or replace pancreatic enzymes.[18] (see Chapter 14).

Have your patient chew gum for the first hour after meals to increase the production of saliva, stimulate smooth muscle contraction and relax the pylorus.

Therapeutic exercises:

Contract and relax the abdominal muscles with a regular rhythm immediately after meals. Work up to 100 repetitions per meal.

Flex and extend the abdomen (sitting or standing) twenty times after a meal.

Prescription Prokinetic agents

These medications increase the frequency (and possibly amplitude) of gastric contractions. These drugs should be taken 20-40 minutes before eating. Side effects include prolonged QT segment and other arrhythmias. Review all drug interactions and perform a cardiac exam prior to prescribing these agents:

Low dose erythromycin (motilin receptor agonist)—50-65 mg ac and qhs (either compounded or prescribe the commercial 250 mg tablets and have the patient divide them in quarters with a pill cutter. This is my first line prescription approach for gastroparesis. It increases the migrating motor complex which increases motility in the small intestine as well as gastric emptying. This dosage is too small to have a significant antibiotic effect.

Prucalopride (Resolor) a 5 HT_4 agonist—2 mg tablets. Dosage is 0.5 mg–2 mg ac and if needed qhs. Instruct the patient to divide these in quarters with a pill cutter. Start dosage trial with ¼ tablet and work up by an additional ¼ tablet ac until relief of symptoms is obtained. Note: 5 HT_4 agonists increase small and large bowel motility as well as gastric, so these are most appropriate for patients who tend toward constipation.

Metoclopramide (Reglan)—The dose is 10 mg taken 30 minutes ac and hs. (I have not prescribed this medicine.)

Domperidone—The dose is 10 mg with 8 ounces of water (or 10 mg in liquid form) one hour ac. (I have not prescribed this medicine.)

Autoimmune Gastritis And Achlorhydria

Autoimmune gastritis and pernicious anemia are diagnosed in 2% of the general population. The prevalence is 6-15% in patients with type 1 diabetes (15-20% of these patients produce anti-parietal cell antibodies.)[19] The same incidence of gastritis is seen in autoimmune thyroid disease.[20]

The clinical picture of autoimmune gastritis is:

1. Gastric mucosal atrophy
2. The presence of anti-parietal cell and anti-intrinsic factor antibodies
3. Achlorhydria
4. Iron deficiency anemia
5. Hypergastrinemia
6. Vitamin B_{12} deficiency (cognitive impairment, peripheral neuropathy, subacute combined degeneration of the cord or anemia)
7. Carcinoid tumors or gastric adenocarcinomas

Metformin And B_{12} Deficiency

Another important cause of B_{12} deficiency in type 2 diabetics is metformin and other biguanide medications. It has been known for over two decades that up to 30% of diabetics maintained on biguanides develop B_{12} deficiency.[21,22] An additional 18% may have borderline low B_{12} levels. Discontinuation of the medication reverses the deficiency in a majority of patients.[23] Up to 9% on long term biguanides develop B_{12} related megaloblastic anemia. The ileal cell membrane receptor for the B_{12} intrinsic factor complex is known to be calcium-dependent. Metformin affects calcium-dependent membrane action. The resulting B_{12} deficiency (determined by subnormal serum holotranscobalamin II) has been shown to be reversed by oral calcium supplementation.[24] Metformin also decreases enterohepatic recirculation of bile salts leading to more liquid stool and possibly malabsorption.[25]

Medication aside, diabetes is associated with neuropathy, cognitive impairment, and several causes of anemia. The following case is a good example of these phenomena:

Case presentation: 66 year old male with epigastic pain and peripheral paresthesias, occupation—CEO. Work history includes a high exposure to benzene.

Presenting complaints: Pt. PTC with a three month history of constipation, heartburn, epigastric pressure, and anorexia due to a metallic sensation on the tongue. Lifelong his bowel function has been very regular. Now he is using an herbal laxative in order to have one stool per day. He reports blood in the stool. He urinates more frequently in the last few years and has nocturia x2. There is hand and foot numbness, a "pins and needles" sensation bilaterally. His grip strength is reduced and he notices that he may drop his pen when writing. The patient complains of feeling chilly in the last few months. He has never used tobacco or alcohol and avoids medications. His job is stressful—he has worked 7 days a week for many years.

Examination findings: His weight is 232 pounds. He reports having lost 12 pounds over 3 months. Height 6'2", BP-120/78, P-54, T-97.1, RR-10, hands are warm with decreased grip strength on the right. The lower extremity reflexes are intact, but there is moderate loss of dull sensation bilaterally over the transverse arches (sharp is intact) and no ulcers or rashes. There is an erythematous perianal rash and proctoscopic exam reveals a ring of large painful internal hemorrhoids which bleed on exam.

Lab values: RBC-2.71K/mm3 (L), HCT-34.2% (L), HGB-12.3 (L), MCV-126.1 mc^3 (HH), MCH-45.4 PG (HH), RDW-14.6% (H), 79% hypersegmented neutrophils (HH), fasting insulin-26.8 mcU/ml (H), fasting glucose-110 mg/dl (H), gastric string test - pH-7, and zinc tally test reveals a low tissue zinc response.

Diagnosis: Prediabetes, megaloblastic anemia (probable pernicious anemia, but anti-parietal cell antibodies and serum B_{12} were not tested in favor of a clinical trial), B_{12} deficiency peripheral neuropathy, zinc deficiency and achlorhydria (chronic atrophic gastritis).

Management: Low glycemic index diet, daily 30 minute walks, betaine hydrochloride- 40 grains cc , zinc—15 mg. TID, B vitamin/Cr complex, cyanocobalamin (1000 mcg.) IM and folic acid (4 mg.) IM initially twice per week, hydroxycitric acid—1000 mg. TID, silymarin—80 mg. TID, Mg citrate—160 mg. BID, and referral for colonoscopy.

Outcomes: neuropathy and chilliness improved dramatically the first week and completely cleared within three months; the other sx of abdominal pain, reflux, metallic taste and anorexia all resolved within 2 weeks. The constipation gradually improved.

Discussion: This patient had all the signs/sx of atrophic gastritis and the associated B_{12} deficiency anemia and neuropathy. He was treated with replacement gastric acid, B_{12} and zinc. The zinc is needed to produce gastric acid and to cure the dysgeusia. Exercise, dietary changes, B vitamins, chromium, magnesium and hydroxycitric acid were aimed at improving his glucose metabolism and silymarin to prevent fatty liver and improve detoxification of solvents such as benzene. Although initially it appeared that he might have a GI malignancy or ulcer (anemia, GI bleeding, change in stool pattern, epigastric discomfort) a work-up proved negative. The patient was well at follow-up 8 years later. He no longer required B_{12} injections.

Small Intestine

In type 1 diabetic rats, duodenal, jejunal and ileal wall thickness was significantly increased.[26]

Bariatric Surgery And Insulin Resistance

Conventional gastrointestinal surgery for morbid obesity (Rouen-Y or biliopancreatic diversion) has been shown to dramatically improve type 2 diabetes, resulting in normal blood glucose and glycosylated hemoglobin levels, with discontinuation of all diabetes-related medications. The most radical of these procedures show reversal of diabetes in over 70% of patients.[73] At present, the improvement has been shown to continue for at least one year.[28] The same benefits of bariatric surgery are not found in obese patients diagnosed with type 1 diabetes mellitus.[74] These benefits are not dependant on the baseline BMI. According to Panaunzi et al:

> Diabetes resolution was 89% (95% CI, 83-94) after biliopancreatic diversion, 77% (95% CI, 72-82) after Roux-en-Y bypass, 62% (95% CI, 46-79) after gastric banding, and 60% (95% CI, 51-70) after sleeve gastrectomy.[75]

These impressive facts pertaining to type 2 diabetes are even more amazing because the euglycemia and normal insulin levels are observed within six days after surgery, before significant weight loss has occurred! A 2008 article in *Diabetes Care* asserts:

> Recent experimental studies point toward the rearrangement of gastrointestinal anatomy as a primary mediator of the surgical control of diabetes, suggesting a role of the small bowel in the pathophysiology of the disease. The significant mechanism is thought to involve the exclusion of the duodenum and proximal jejunum from the flow of nutrients.[78]

The surgical procedures producing the highest percentage of diabetes improvement both involve the re-routing of food so that it bypasses the distal stomach, duodenum, and at least several feet of jejunum. From a functional point of view, it is fascinating to entertain the idea that food is the trigger for insulin resistance via the mucosa of the upper intestinal tract (see Table 2.3 for GI hormones regulating insulin).

Liver

Non-Alcoholic Fatty Liver Disease And Non-Alcoholic Steatohepatitis

Non-alcoholic steatohepatitis (NASH) is a form of nonalcoholic fatty liver disease (NAFLD) which has the addition of a chronic inflammatory component. 30% of patients with NASH develop hepatic cirrhosis over 5–10 years. 10% of patients with NASH-induced cirrhosis develop hepatocellular carcinoma.

In the general population, the prevalence of NAFLD ranges from

3% to 24%, with most estimates in the 6% to 14% range. About half of diabetics have NAFLD.[29] The pathogenesis of NAFLD is attributed to a multi-hit process involving insulin resistance (regulated by the adipocytokines resistin, leptin and adiponectin), oxidative stress and apoptotic pathways.

Fatty liver is extremely common among patients undergoing bariatric surgery (84–96%). In these patients, 25–55% have NASH, 34–47% have fibrosis, and 2- 12% have bridging fibrosis or cirrhosis.[30]

NAFLD appears to be most strongly associated with obesity, insulin resistance, hyperlipidemia (high triglycerides, low HDL), increasing age (post-menopause), Mexican-American heritage, industrial toxins[31] (benzene, toluene, styrene, hexane, CCl^4, chloroform, methanol and vinyl chloride) and chemotherapy administration. Irinotecan is the most likely drug etiology and the resulting condition is known as chemotherapy associated steatohepatitis (CASH.)

A major dietary factor in the development of insulin resistance is the consumption of high fructose corn syrup.[32] Hepatic metabolism of fructose increases lipogenesis and ATP depletion. The fructose intake of the average American is 10.2% of total caloric intake.[33] Fructose consumption in patients with NAFLD was nearly 2- to 3-fold higher than controls.[34] In patients with NAFLD hepatic mRNA expression of fructokinase (an important enzyme for fructose metabolism) and fatty acid synthase (an important enzyme for lipogenesis) were increased.

Murine research shows intestinal hyperpermeability is associated with NASH.[35] Fructose consumption can lead to small intestinal bacterial overgrowth, which then leads to increased intestinal permeability, endotoxin absorption and the development of NAFLD.[36] When antibiotics were administered along with fructose feeding, mice were protected from steatosis[37] (see Figure 7.1).

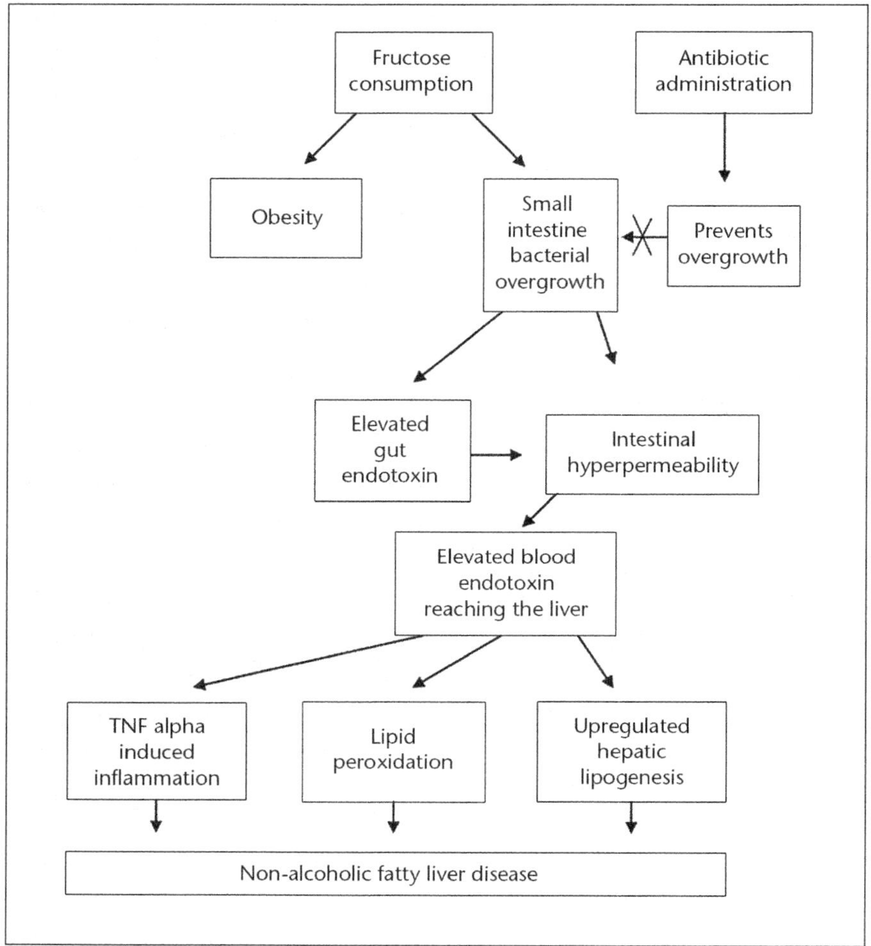

FIGURE 7.1 FACTORS IN THE ETIOLOGY AND PATHOGENESIS OF NAFLD

More advanced stages of NASH are associated with older age, higher body mass index, diabetes, hypertension and an AST/ALT ratio greater than one.[38] Less commonly, one may see NASH presenting in older female patients with normal transaminases and an isolated elevation of serum alkaline phosphatase.[39]

Celiac Disease And NASH

10-20% of celiac patients have Type 1 diabetes.[40] NASH may sometimes be the first sign of celiac disease. Many celiac patients are entirely asymptomatic for decades. A 2001 article in *Digestive and Liver Disease* states that 9% of patients with an unexplained elevation of transaminases have undiagnosed celiac disease.[41] Two studies found elevated transaminases in about half of new cases of celiac disease,[42] and in 18% of celiac patients on a strict gluten-free diet. In pediatric celiac patients (mean age 10) Lee et al found a 15.1% incidence of elevated transaminases.[76] Bardella et al reported that 3.4% of patients with NASH had hidden celiac disease.[44] The celiac diagnosis was based on elevated tissue transglutaminase antibody (tTG), anti-endomysial antibody (EMA) and duodenal biopsy. After six months on a gluten-free diet transaminase elevations decreased to normal values. Of note—another 10% of the study participants had elevated tTG levels, but normal EMA titers. These subjects were not biopsied or treated with a gluten free diet. tTG and EMA antibody assays have a similar sensitivity for celiac diagnosis. It seems to the author that they might also have had their NASH cured had they been given dietary intervention. In light of the new American College of Gastroenterology guidelines for evaluation of abnormal liver chemistries, the incidence of hepatic involvement in celiac disease may be significantly higher than that shown in current literature.[77] In the article announcing these new guidelines, Kwo et al state:

> Multiple studies have demonstrated that the presence of an elevated ALT has been associated with increased liver-related mortality. A true healthy normal ALT level ranges from 29 to 33 IU/l for males, 19 to 25 IU/l for females and levels above this should be assessed.

BARD Score

BMI equal or greater than 28 = 1 point

AST to ALT ratio equal or greater than 0.8 = 2 points

DM = 1 point

A score of 2-4 was associated with an odds ratio for advanced fibrosis of 17.

FIGURE 7.2 THE BARD SCORE FOR PREDICTING THE RISK OF FIBROSIS/CIRRHOSIS IN NAFLD

Elevated tTG in cirrhotic patients is an indicator of more advanced liver disease.[45]

Treatment Of NAFLD And NASH

- Weight loss
- Lipid, insulin and glucose normalization
- Exercise
- Diet
  - Higher protein
  - High fresh vegetables
  - Lower glycemic index/load
  - Complete abstention from alcohol
  - Frequent smaller meals
  - Grain-free or gluten-free
- Treat SIBO if present

Botanical and nutritional supplements

- Choleretics
- Betaine
- NAC[46, 47]
- Vitamin E
- Alpha lipoic acid
- B complex
- Cr, Zn, Mg, Mn, Va
- Balance cortisol/DHEA
- Probiotics

Glycogenic Hepatopathy

Distinct from NAFLD, glycogenic hepatopathy is an under-recognized complication of long-standing poorly controlled diabetes mellitus. Characterized by abnormal glycogen accumulation in hepatocytes, elevated transaminases and hepatomegaly, steatosis is not involved. Improved glycemic control has been shown to resolve this condition.[48]

Pancreas

Exocrine pancreas

Severe pancreatic insufficiency (fecal elastase <100/g) is seen in 10-40% of diabetics with steatorrhea that does not correlate with diabetes type, duration, or clinical symptoms.[49,50] Diabetes mellitus is associated with pancreatic atrophy and compromised digestion of carbohydrates due to reduction in α-amylase synthesis.[51] Obese patients have more severe pancreatitis than lean individuals. Obese leptin-deficient mice have more intra- and interlobular pancreatic fat and TNF-α compared to lean mice. Serum adiponectin levels are inversely correlated with the severity of pancreatitis. Analogous to the changes in the insulin resistant liver, nonalcoholic fatty pancreas disease (NAFPD) may lead to nonalcoholic steatopancreatitis (NASP.)

Twenty-five percent of celiac disease patients have *serum* elevations of pancreatic enzymes. Even if a patient has no digestive complaints, elevation of serum amylase or lipase should trigger screening for celiac disease.[52]

Both metabolic syndrome and diabetes are risk factors for pancreatic adenocarcinoma.[53,54]

Treatment options in pancreatic insufficiency (see Chapter 14)

Endocrine pancreas

A German study found that early life exposure to dietary gluten in the offspring of mothers with Type 1 diabetes is associated with an increased risk of developing anti-islet cell antibodies.[55]

Gall Bladder

Obesity, diabetes and hypertriglyceridemia are associated with an increased incidence of gallstones. Diets high in fat, cholesterol, and carbohydrates have been associated with gallstone formation as well in animals and humans. Consumption of fish oil and olive oil decreases the lithogenicity of bile.[56,57,58] Animal and human data suggest that insulin resistance is associated with increased gallbladder volume and/or impaired gallbladder emptying (stasis is a risk factor for stone formation). As a drug treatment for diabetes, pioglitazone, while improving insulin resistance, also increases gallbladder volume and may increase the propensity for gallstone formation. In addition, diabetic gall bladders are less responsive to acetylcholine, neuropeptide Y, and CCK.[59] It is believed that the hypertriglyceridemia of insulin resistance is the etiology of this lack of response.[60] One study of non-obese diabetics found impaired gallbladder emptying was associated with higher fasting glucose and insulin resistance. Curiously, this relationship was not seen in obese diabetics.[61] Gallstones and—with less certainty—obesity and diabetes are also risk factors for gallbladder cancer.[62,63]

Non-Alcoholic Fatty Gallbladder Disease (Cholecystosteatosis)

Patients with cholecystitis had more fat in the gallbladder wall (cholecystosteatosis) than non-diseased controls. High carbohydrate diet increases the fat deposition and presence of pro-inflammatory cytokines TNF-α, IL-6, and IL-1β in mice. These cytokines decrease gallbladder smooth muscle activity. The increase in toxic fats and pro-inflammatory cytokines may cause gallbladder pain even in the absence of gallstones.

Henry A. Pitt, a professor of surgery at Indiana University sums up these relationships in the digestive tract:

> The obesity epidemic has led to increased obesity research. Visceral fat is now considered to be an endocrine organ which produces multiple adipokines. The combination of high leptin and low adiponectin is associated with the metabolic syndrome, an insulin-resistant state in which steatosis and proinflammatory cytokines cause organ dysfunction. Over time and probably with a 'second hit', inflammation leads to fibrosis and, eventually, to cancer. This sequence of events has been most clearly elucidated in the liver where NAFLD → NASH → cirrhosis → HCC. However, a similar process most likely occurs in the pancreas where NAFPD → NASP → chronic pancreatitis → pancreatic cancer. Likewise, in the gallbladder NAFGBD (cholecystosteatosis) → steatocholecystitis → gallstones → gallbladder cancer. For the hepatopancreatobiliary surgeon, organ steatosis is significant because it increases the risk of liver resection, alters the function of the donor liver, increases the risk of pancreatic fistula following pancreatic resection, and increases the incidence of chronic acalculous cholecystitis and the need for cholecystectomy.[64]

NAFLD ⇨ NASH ⇨ cirrhosis ⇨ hepatocellular carcinoma

NAFPD ⇨ NASP ⇨ chronic pancreatitis ⇨ pancreatic adenocarcinoma

NAFGBD ⇨ steatocholecystitis ⇨ AC or gallstones ⇨ gallbladder cancer

NAFLD: non-alcoholic fatty liver disease, NASG: non-alchoholic steatohepatitis, NAFPD: non-alcoholic fatty pancreas disease, NASP: non-alcoholic steatopancreatitis, NAFGBD: non-alcoholic fatty gallbladder disease, (cholecystosteatosis), AC: acalculous cholecystitis

Figure 7.3 Fatty GI Changes Seen With Diabetes

Biliary Dyskinesia/Functional Gallbladder Disorder

This condition is not limited to metabolic syndrome or diabetes, yet it seems most appropriate to discuss it here. Often patients present in my office with typical symptoms of biliary pain, yet there are no abnormal findings on ultrasonic exam of the gallbladder. Symptoms include epigastric or right upper quadrant pain, nausea, and intolerance for fatty meals. A hepatobiliary iminodiacetic acid scan (HIDA scan) will allow for the diagnosis of this motility disorder of the gall bladder. Other terms for this diagnostic imaging study include cholescintigraphy or hepatobiliary scintigraphy. The results include estimation of the gallbladder ejection fraction (GBEF) in response to an intravenous injection of cholecystokinin. The GBEF should be at least 35-40%. Lower levels are found in biliary dyskinesia/functional gallbladder disorder.

Treatment Options For Biliary Sludge And Cholelithiasis

- improve insulin sensitivity (see NAFLD above) and serum lipids
- fish oil and olive oil use[65]
- improve digestive psychophysiology (see gastroparesis above)
- ox bile extract cc—2-6 grains per meal based on bowel tolerance
- Phosphatidylcholine (lecithin)—420 mg BID
- choleretics—menthol, Rosmarinus officinalis, Thymus vulgaris, Cynara scolymus

- cholegogues—Chelidonium, Chionanthus
- lipotropics—choline, inositol, methionine, betaine
- in addition for biliary dyskinesia/functional gallbladder disorder—add Fumaria amara to the cholegogues. A typical tincture formula includes 1 part each of Chelidonium majus and Chionanthus virginica and 2 parts of Fumaria amara. Dosage is 1 teaspoon QD or BID for 3-6 months.

Colon

Chronic constipation, diarrhea and fecal incontinence are all possible in diabetes, but slow transit constipation is the most typical.[66] Patient age, disease duration and poor control of diabetes mellitus all correlate positively with these changes.

Adenomatous colonic polyps are significantly associated with increased BMI levels. Korean males with even one component of the metabolic syndrome had a significantly higher risk for developing adenomatous polyps compared to those subjects without any component.[67] Elevated serum adiponectin is a risk factor and a possible diagnostic marker for obesity-related colon cancer. The same relationship may apply to adiponectin and cancers of the breast, endometrium, and prostate.[68] Comparing the risk factors of proximal and distal colorectal cancer reveals that Type 2 diabetes is associated with distal colorectal cancer in males whereas cholelithiasis is associated with proximal colon cancer in females.[69]

Recent data suggest that gut microbiota affect host nutritional metabolism with consequences regarding energy storage. A review discusses new findings that may explain how gut microbiota can be involved in the development of obesity and insulin resistance.[70]

Excess caloric intake in obese humans (and rodents) leads to greater numbers of the bacterial phylum Firmicutes which promotes enhanced absorption of nutrients and weight gain. Feeding cultures of Firmicutes flora to mice promotes obesity.[71] Inflammation induced by the systemically absorbed lipopolysaccharides of these bacteria is thought to be a factor in the pathophysiology of insulin resistance. Colonic transit was proven to be faster with obesity (BMI >30 kg/m.[72]

1 Siudikiene, J et al *Caries Res.* 2008;42(5):354-62.
2 Siudikeine, J et al *Eur J Oral Sci.* 2006 Feb;114(1):8-14.
3 Lopez, ME et al *Braz Dent J.* 2003;14(1):26-31.
4 Ship, JA, *J Am Dent Assoc.* 2003 Oct;134 Spec No:4S-10S.
5 Dodds, MW et al *Oral Surg Oral Med Oral Pathol Oral Radiol Endod.* 1997 Apr;83(4):465-70.
6 Yavuzyilmaz, E et al *Aust Dent J.* 1996 Jun;41(3):193-7.
7 Faraj, J et al *Diabet Med.* 2007 Nov;24(11):1235-9.
8 Beaumont H, Boeckxstaens G. *Curr Opin Gastroenterol.* 2007 Jul;23(4): 416-21.
9 Kinekawa, F et al *J Gastroenterol.* 2008;43(5):338-44. Epub 2008 Jul 1.
10 Moldovan C et al *Rom J Gastroenterol.* Mar 14(1):19-22, 2005.
11 Wang, YR *Am J Gastroenterol.* 2008 Feb;103(2):313-22.
12 Sogabe, M et al *J Gastroenterol.* Jun;40(6):583-90, 2005.
13 Bernstein, R *Dr. Bernstein's Diabetes Solution* 2007 Little, Brown and Company.
14 Levin, AA et al *Clin Radiol.* 2008 Apr;63(4):407-14.
15 Bernstein, R *Dr. Bernstein's Diabetes Solution* 2007 Little, Brown and Company.
16 Choy, KM et al *Gastroenterology.* 2008 Sep 11.
17 Zhang, H et al *Phytomedicine.* 2008 Aug;15(8):602-11.
18 Mizushima T, Ochi K, Ichimura M, Kiura K, Harada H, Koide N. Pancreatic enzyme supplement improves dysmotility in chronic pancreatitis patients. *J Gastroenterol Hepatol.* 2004 Sep;19(9):1005-9.
19 DE bock, CE et al *Diabetes Care.* 2003 Jan;26(1):82-8.
20 De Block, CE *J Clin Endocrinol Metab.* 2008 Feb;93(2):363-71.
21 Adams, JF et al *Diabetologia.* 1983 Jan;24(1):16-8.
22 Sparre Hermann, L et al *B J Diabetes Vasc Dis.* Nov 2004; 4(6): 401 - 406.
23 Tomkins, GH et al Br Med J. 1971 June 19; 2(5763): 685–687.
24 Bauman, WA et al *Diabetes Care* 2000; 23: 1227–31
25 Scarpello, JH et al *Diabet Med.* 1998 Aug;15(8):651-6.
26 Zhao, J et al *Diabetologia.* 2003 Dec;46(12):1688-97.
27 Rubino, F *Curr Opin Clin Nutr Metab Care.* 2006 Jul;9(4):497-507.
28 Wickremesekera, K et al *Obes Surg.* 2005 Apr;15(4):474-81.
29 Pit, HA *HPB (Oxford).* 2007;9(2):92-7.
30 Clark, JM *J Clin Gastroenterol.* 2006 Mar;40 Suppl 1:S5-10.
31 Cave, M et al *J Nutr Biochem.* 2007 Mar;18(3):184-95.
32 Tetri, LH et al *Am J Physiol Gastrointest Liver Physiol.* 2008 Sep 4.
33 Vos, MD et al *Medscape J Med.* 2008 Jul 9;10(7):160.
34 Ouyang, X et al *J Hepatol.* 2008 Jun;48(6):993-9.
35 Li, S et al *World J Gastroenterol.* 2008 May 28;14(20):3254-8.
36 Thuy, S et al *J Nutr.* 2008 Aug;138(8):1452-5.
37 Berfheim, I et al *J Hepatol.* 2008 Jun;48(6):983-92.
38 Rodriguez-Hernandez, H et al *Eur J Gastroenterol Hepatol.* 2008 May;20(5):399-403.
39 Pantsari MW, Harrison SA *J Clin Gastroenterol.* 2006 Aug;40(7):633-5.
40 Kanungo, A et al *Ann N Y Acad Sci.* 2002 Apr;958:232-4.
41 Volta, U et al *Dig Liver Dis.* 2001 Jun-Jul;33(5):420-5.
42 Selimoglu, MA et al *J Nutr.* 2008 Aug;138(8):1452-5.
43 Sabel'nikova, EA et al *Ter Arkh.* 2003;75(2):31-4
44 Bardella, MT et al *Dig Liver Dis.* 2004 May;36(5):333-6.
45 Vecci, M et al *Scand J Gastroenterol.* 2003 Jan;38(1):50-4

46 Thong-Ngam, D et al *World J Gastroenterol.* 2007 Oct 14;13(38):5127-32.
47 Ozarus, R et al *World J Gastroenterol.* 2003 Jan;9(1):125-8.
48 Hudacko, RM et al *J Diabetes Complications.* 2008 Sep-Oct;22(5):329-30.
49 Vsterhus, M et al *Diabetes Care.* 2008 Feb;31(2):306-10.
50 Hardt, PD et al *Dig Dis Sci.* 2003 Sep;48(9):1688-92.
51 Patel, R et al *Ann N Y Acad Sci.* 2006 Nov;1084:490-502.
52 Carroccio A, Di Prima L, Scalici C, Soresi M, Cefalù AB, Noto D, Averna MR, Montalto G, Iacono G. Unexplained elevated serum pancreatic enzymes: a reason to suspect celiac disease. *Clin Gastroenterol Hepatol.* 2006 Apr;4(4):455-9.
53 Russo, A et al *Eur J Cancer.* 2008 Jan;44(2):293-7.
54 Mesiterfield, R et al *Exp Clin Endocrinol Diabetes.* 2008 Sep;116 Suppl 1:S7-S12.
55 Füchtenbusch M, Ziegler AG, Hummel M. Elimination of dietary gluten and development of type 1 diabetes in high risk subjects. *Rev Diabet Stud.* 2004 Spring;1(1):39-41.
56 Jonkers, IJ et al *J Nutr.* 2006 Apr;136(4):987-91.
57 Mendez-Sanchez, M et al *J Nutr.* 2006 Apr;136(4):987-91.
58 Delgado-Aros, S et al *Am J Physiol Gastrointest Liver Physiol.* 2008 Aug;295(2): G382-8.
59 Al-Azzawi HH, et al *J Surg Res.* 2006 Dec;136(2):192-7.
60 Jonkers, IJ et al *Gut.* 2003 Jan;52(1):109-15.
61 *J Gastrointest Surg.* 2006 Jul-Aug;10(7):940-8; discussion 948-9.
62 Tavani A, Negri E, La Vecchia C. Biliary tract tumors *Ann Ist Super Sanita.* 1996;32(4):615
63 Fraumeni JF Jr. Cancers of the pancreas and biliary tract: epidemiological considerations. *Cancer Res.* 1975 Nov;35(11 Pt. 2):3437
64 Pitt, HA HPB (Oxford). 2007; 9(2): 92–97.
65 Alarcón de la Lastra C et al *Curr Pharm Des.* 2001 Jul;7(10):933-50
66 Rossol, S *MMW Fortschr Med.* 2007 Nov 1;149(44):39-42.
67 Lee, GE et al *Obesity (Silver Spring).* 2008 Jun;16(6):1434-9.
68 Barb, D et al *Am J Clin Nutr.* 2007 Sep;86(3):s858-66.
69 Oh, SW et al *Dis Colon Rectum.* 2008 Jan;51(1):56-61.
70 Yazigi, A et al *Presse Med.* 2008 Oct;37(10):1427-30.
71 He, ZQ et al *Med Hypotheses.* 2008;70(4):808-11.
72 Delgado-Aros, S et al *Am J Physiol Gastrointest Liver Physiol.* 2008 Aug;295(2): G382-8.
73 Brethauer, SA, Can diabetes be surgically cured? Long-term metabolic effects of bariatric surgery in obese patients with type 2 diabetes mellitus. . (4):628-36; discussion 636-7, s.l.: *Ann Surg.* 2013, Vol. 258.
74 Mahawar, KK, Bariatric Surgery in Type 1 Diabetes Mellitus: A Systematic Review. (1):196-204, s.l : *Obes Surg.* 2016, Vol. 26.
75 Panunzi, S. Predictors of remission of diabetes mellitus in severely obese individuals undergoing bariatric surgery: do BMI or procedure choice matter? A meta-analysis. (3):459-67, s.l.: *Ann Surg.* 2015, Vol. 261.
76 Lee, GJ, Hypertransaminasemia in Newly Diagnosed Pediatric Patients With Celiac Disease. (3):340-3, s.l.: *J Pediatr Gastroenterol Nutr.* 2016, Vol. 63.
77 Kwo, PY, 18-45 ACG Clinical Guideline: Evaluation of Abnormal Liver Chemistries. doi:10.1038/ajg.2016.517, s.l.: *Am J Gastroenterol.* 2017, Vol. 112 (Jan 2017).
78 Rubino F, Is type 2 diabetes an operable intestinal disease: A provative yet reasoable hypothesis. *Diabetes Care* 2008 Feb;31 Supp 2:S290-6.

Chapter 8

The Integrated Functional GI Physical Exam

Functional Gastroenterology Digestive Exam
Esophageal Transit Time
Lingual-neural Testing
Chapman's Digestive Reflexes
Tongue Reflex Markers
Hiatal Hernia Syndrome Point and Test
Ileocecal Valve Syndrome Test
Blood Sugar Imbalance Point
Adrenal Chapman Point

After completing standard inspection, auscultation, palpation and percussion of the abdominal organs to check for abnormalities and signs of disease, add the functional exam. The evaluation may include organ mobility, reflex point testing, muscle testing and therapy localization (having the patient contact specific areas while checking for changes in muscle strength) as well as lingual-neural testing which uses gustatory sensation as a measure of biochemical individuality.

Functional Gastroenterology Digestive Exam Outline

Note: bold type indicates the basics of a screening exam

Inspection
Auscultation
Palpation
Percussion

***Mouth:* inspection of lips ________________ tongue __________**
Mallampati score_________**Palatal rise and symmetry_________**
Ant. CR tongue (2nd ICS 3/4" lat. to sternum B) _______
Post. CR tongue (C2 mid SP/TP B) ________
Inspection of gums/buccal mucosa __________________________
Teeth: #root canals___ # of fillings ________ age of fillings ______
dental materials____

Esophagus
Esophageal transit time: _______ seconds (<10 secs.)
Ant. CR esophagus (2nd ICS at sternum B) _______
Post. CR esophagus (T2 mid SP/TP B) _______

Stomach
HCL point: 1 human inch (tsun) inferior to xyphoid on the left rib margin)
______
Ant. CR stomach (5th and 6th ICS mid-clavicular Left) _______
Post. CR stomach (T5 and T6 mid SP/TP Left) _______
Hiatal hernia syndrome point (immediately lateral to xyphoid Left) ______
Ant. CR pylorus (midline manubrium) ______
Post. CR pylorus (T10 lateral margin TP Left) ______
Hiatal hernia syndrome muscle test (patient pushes abdominal tissue superiorly)
Strong / weak
Associated muscles = **pectoralis major clavicular, biceps**

Pancreas
Pancreatic enzyme point: 1 human inch (tsun) inferior to xyphoid on the Right rib margin)_______
Pancreatic glycemic point (mid thenar pad B)_____
Ant. CR pancreas/spleen (7th ICS Left)______
Post. CR pancreas (T7 mid SP/TP Right) ______
Associated muscles = **latissimus dorsi**, triceps, mid and lower trapezius

Liver/gall bladder
DeJarnette Liver reflex (3rd rib costal junction Right): rigidity ____ tenderness _____
Ant. CR Sluggish Liver (5th ICS mid-clavicular Right) ______
Post. CR Sluggish Liver (T5 mid SP/TP Right) ———
Ant. CR Sluggish Liver/gall bladder (6th ICS mid-clavicular Right) ____
Post. CR Sluggish Liver/gall bladder (T6 mid SP/TP Right) ______
Gall bladder: Murphy's point ______
Associated muscles: liver = pectoralis major sternal, rhomboids
gall bladder = popliteus

Small Intestine
Bennett sm. intest. reflex (palpation in a 2" radius around umbilicus)
Ant. CR sm. intest. (8,9 and 10th ribs near the cartilage B) _____
Post. CR sm. intest. (T8,9, and10 mid SP/TP B) ________
Associated muscles = **quadriceps, abdominals**
Note: In newborns, umbilical erythema can be a sign of food intolerance, especially to cow's milk.[1]

Large Intestine
Tenderness to palpation over the colon
CR colon/spasm (iliotibial band tenderness) _____________
Post. CR colon/spasm (area from L2-4 paravertebral to iliac crest B) _____
ICV tenderness (McBurney point) ____________
"Open" ICV muscle test **iliacus**—strong / weak
"Closed" ICV muscle test **quadriceps group**— strong / weak
Ant. CR atonic constipation (between ASIS and femoral trochanter B)_____
Post. CR atonic constipation (T11 lateral margin TP B) _____
CR Appendix (upper aspect near the tip of the 12th rib Right) _____
Associated muscle = **tensor fascia lata** (entire colon), quadratus lumborum (appendix)

Rectum
Ant. CR rectum (adductor region) ______
Post. CR rectum (lower aspect of the SI joint B) _____
Rectum muscle test = hamstrings—strong / weak

Key
CR = Chapman reflex; **ICS** = intercostal space; **B** = bilateral;
SP = spinous process; **TP** = transverse process

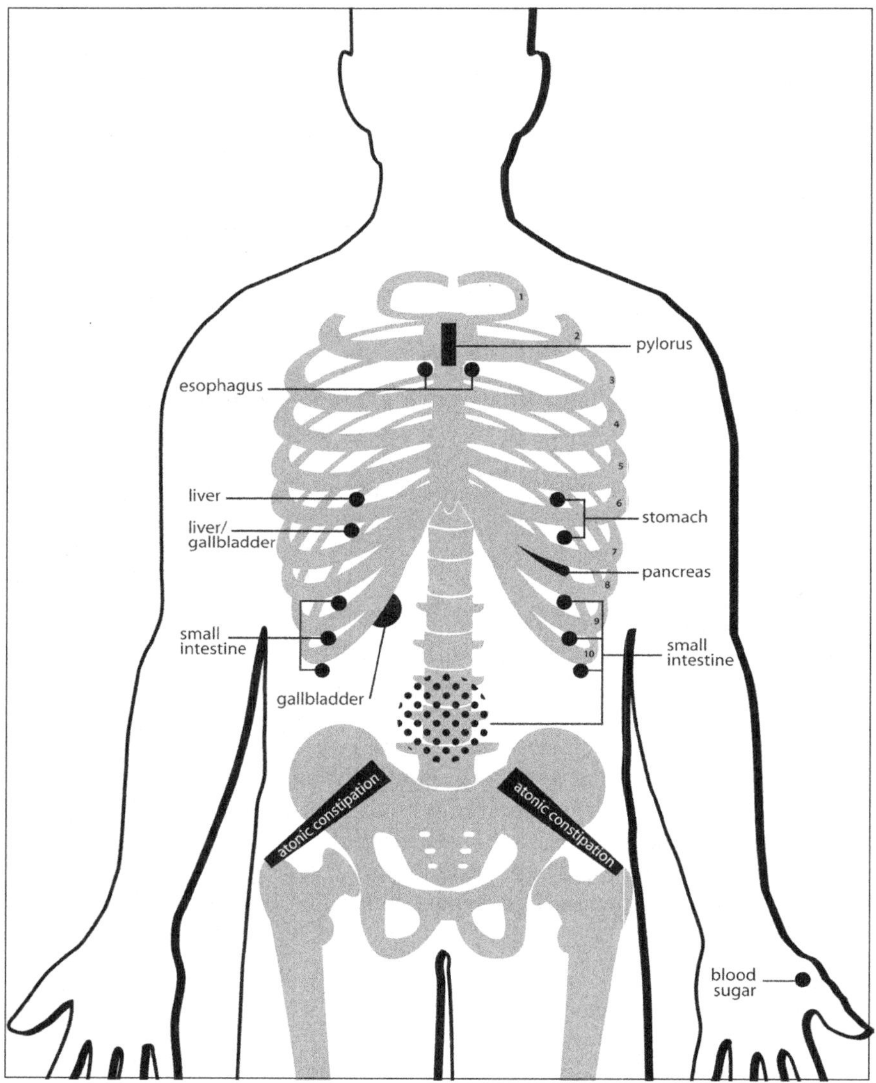

FIGURE 8.1 ANTERIOR CHAPMAN AND RELATED DIGESTIVE POINTS

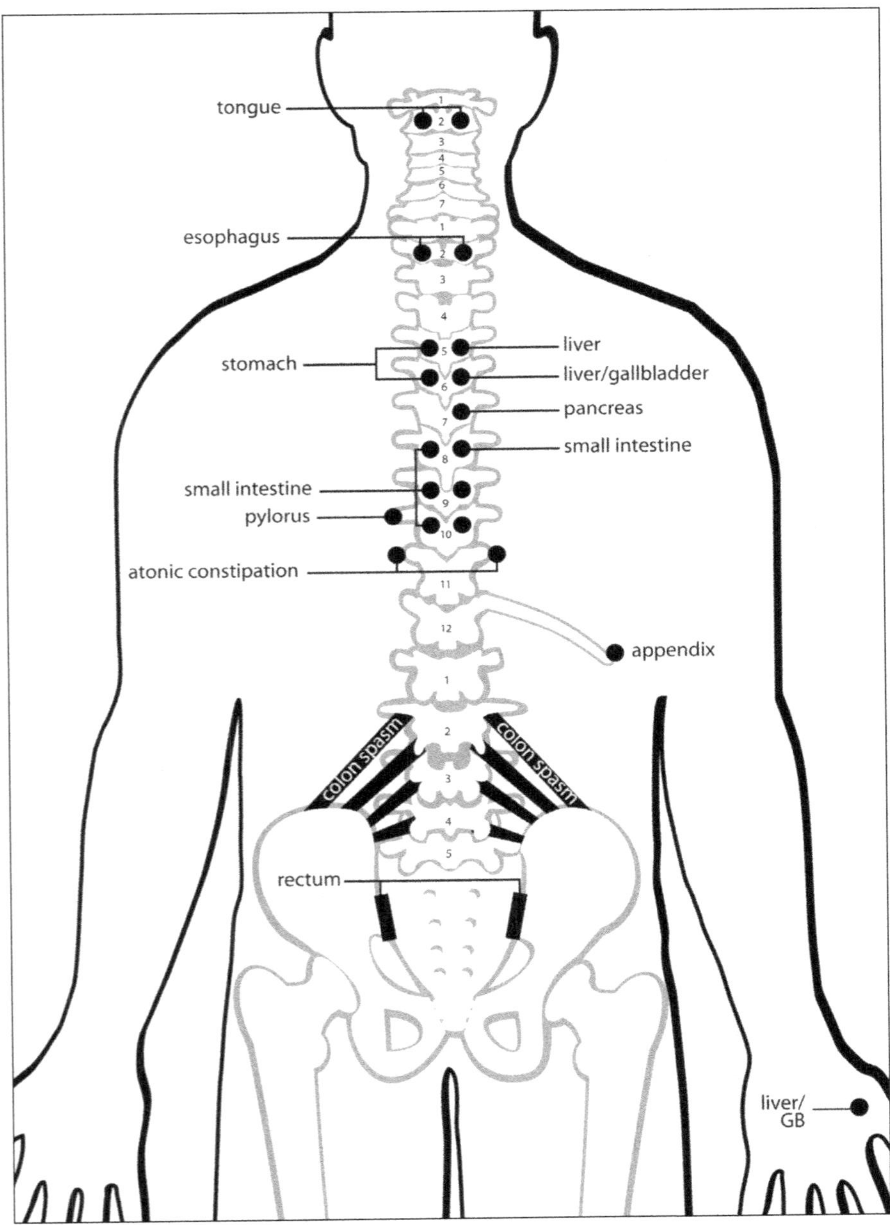

FIGURE 8.2 POSTERIOR CHAPMAN POINTS

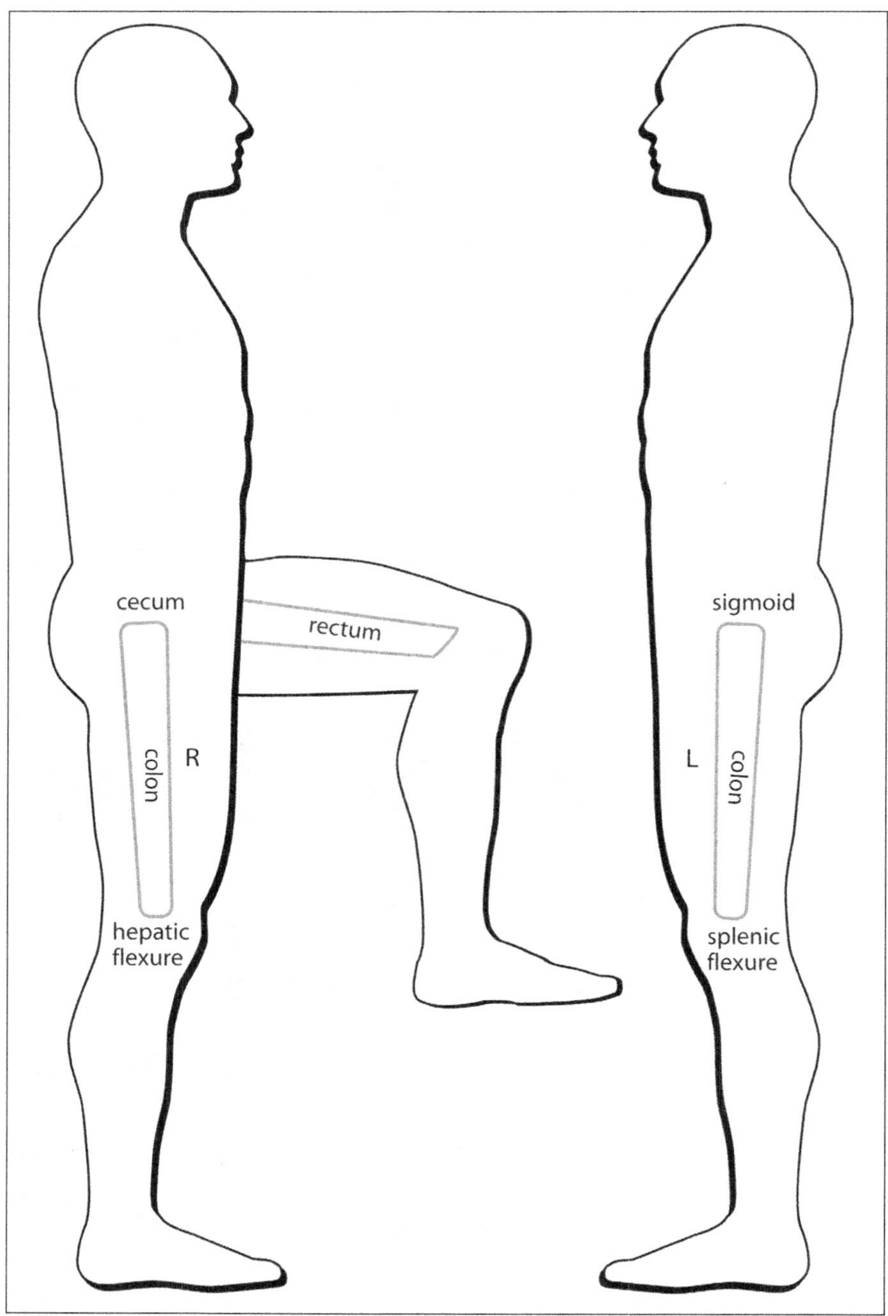

Figure 8.3 Lateral Chapman Areas

Esophageal Transit Time

This simple physical exam is a quick way to screen for an esophageal motility disorder. Place your stethoscope at the epigastrium and have a watch with a second hand available. Instruct the patient to swallow a liberal mouthful of water. Take note of the time it takes to audibly enter the stomach. An average swallow of water will take two or three seconds to enter the stomach. It will sound similar to bowel sounds on abdominal exam. A normal esophageal transit time is less than ten seconds.

Lingual-neural Testing

This is a rapid form of functional testing for the biochemical needs of your patient. Any substance which has a taste can be tested. Reflex point tenderness or muscle strength can be assessed before and after tasting a substance for 30 seconds or more. Chapman and Bennett reflexes will actually respond immediately—others take about 30 seconds. For example, the DeJarnette liver reflex is graded a 6 (0-10) by the patient. Put a lipotropic nutrient tablet on the patient's tongue and have her taste it (chew a bit if necessary) and then retest the reflex. If the tenderness drops (perhaps to a 3), that lipotropic formulation is indicated for that patient. If it does not decrease the tenderness, it is not well indicated for that individual. Additional substances can be added to test for a cumulative effect to the lipotropic (perhaps a choleretic such as artichoke) in order to further decrease the tenderness of the reflex. If successful (perhaps a drop to a tenderness of 1) both treatments are indicated.

Table 8.1 Indicators That Respond To Lingual-Neural Testing	
All Chapman reflexes	Bennett small intestine reflex
All muscle tests	DeJarnette liver reflex
Colon palpatory tenderness	Lowenberg's test

Four types of reflexes will be discussed: DeJarnette, Riddler, Bennett and Chapman. These are not diagnostic of disease states. They provide a good "hunch" and a quick method of getting an overview of GI function.

Only one DeJarnette reflex is included in the exam. It is on the right third rib and assesses the liver. Rub medially and laterally with three fingers over the mid clavicular line on the rib and ask for a rating of tenderness. This point will decrease in tenderness using lingual-neural testing.

Tenderness of the right dorsal base of the thumb is also used as a measure of chronic liver/gall bladder issues. The location is the area adjacent to the first metacarpal head. Have the patient rate the tenderness while the tissue is pinched between the examiner's thumb and index fingers.

There are two Riddler reflexes, which were discovered by Robert Riddler, ND. They are symmetrically placed one tsun (human inch = length of the distal phalanx of the patient's index finger) inferior to the tip of the xyphoid on the margin of the ribs. The left side is the gastric acid point; the one on the right is the pancreatic enzyme point. The examiner presses superolaterally against the inferior margin of the ribcage. The gastric acid point may be tender with acid hyposecretion or hypersecretion. The pancreatic enzyme point is a marker of hyposecretion.

Chapman's Digestive Reflexes

Catalogued in 1937 by osteopathic physician Charles Owens, these neurolymphatic points are the work of Frank Chapman, DO, who observed small, tender, palpable beads of fluid in the fascia over certain sites. The points are indicators of organ function, but massaging the points is also therapeutic. They may also be used to confirm organ dysfunction along with therapy localization in applied kinesiology. There are anterior points as well as corresponding points on the posterior aspect of the body. There are a large number of Chapman's points that can be used for most major organs and many conditions, but this chapter is limited to those directly related to GI function.

When testing Chapmans' points, use enough pressure to get to the muscle layer (external abdominals). Some authors rate this as 5 lbs of pressure. It is desirable to be consistent with the depth of pressure in order to get reliable information when retesting after treatment and when comparing tenderness among various patients. Have the patient rate the tenderness on a 0-4 or a 0-10 scale.

The anterior digestive Chapman's points are found by rubbing medially and laterally in the intercostal spaces (ICS). The anterior points include the liver reflex in the right 5th ICS in the mid-clavicular line; liver/

gallbladder reflex in the right 6th ICS in the mid-clavicular line; the stomach reflex in the left 5th and 6th ICS in the midclavicular line, the pancreas/spleen reflex in the left (sometimes right) 7th ICS, and the small intestine reflexes bilaterally at the 8th, 9th and 10th ribs near the cartilage. Additionally, the entire length of the bilateral tensor fascia lata is a colon reflex.

The posterior digestive Chapman's reflexes are found between the transverse processes either midway between the spinous and lateral border of the transverse process or at the lateral border of the transverse process.

The Bennett's point for the small intestine is included in the exam. It is a 2" radius circle around the umbilicus. Press in four quadrants to assess tenderness. This area responds well to lingual-neural testing.

Tongue Reflex Markers

The analysis of the coat and markings on the tongue is as ancient as medicine itself. The drawing (Figure 8.4) shows one system of tongue analysis based on the location of findings. In addition to coating, texture, lesions and fissures at the various reflex areas, liver/gallbladder indicators may include macroglossia (swelling of the tongue) which produces a scalloped appearance of the lateral border of the tongue.

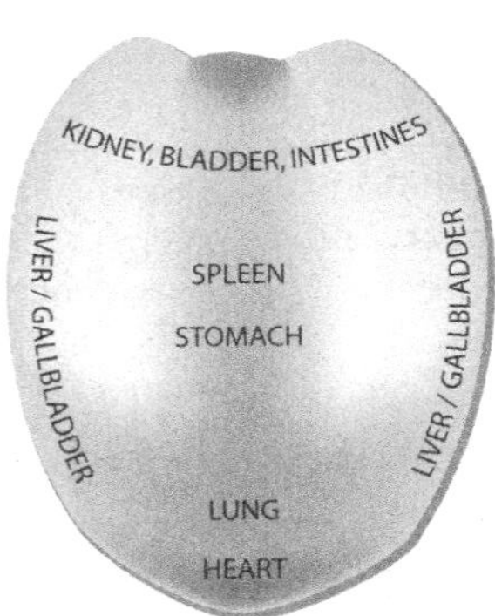

FIGURE 8.4
TONGUE REFLEX MARKERS

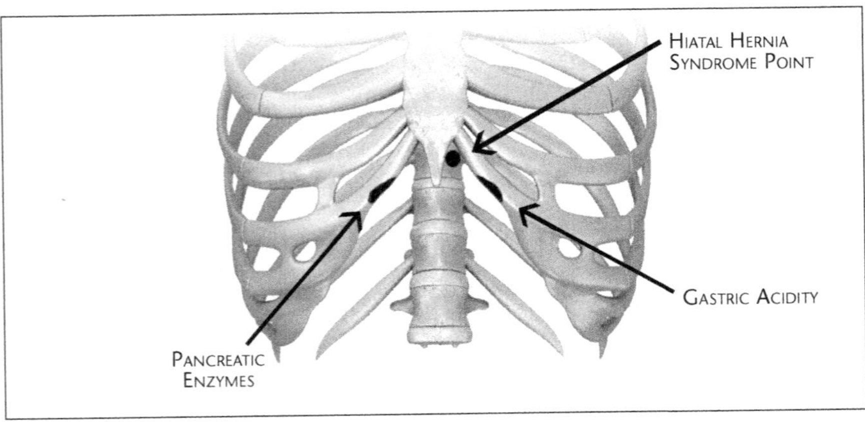

FIGURE 8.5 RIDDLER POINTS

Table 8.2 Riddler Gastric Acid

Point	Location	Muscles	Color	EFT Point	Emotion
Riddler gastric acid	1 tsun inferior to the xyphoid process on the left inferior rib margin	Pectoralis major clavicular	Golden	Under eye	**Worry**

Table 8.3 Riddler Pancreatic Enzyme

Point	Location	Muscles	Color	EFT Point	Emotion
Riddler pancreatic enzyme	1 tsun inferior to the xyphoid on the right inferior rib margin	Latissimus dorsi, Triceps, mid and lower trapezius	Golden	Under arm	**Worry**

Table 8.4 Acute Gallbladder

Point	Location	Muscles	Color	EFT Point	Emotion
Acute gallbladder	Murphy's point	Popliteus	Green	Lateral eyebrow	**Indecision**

Table 8.5 Bennett Small Intestine

Point	Location	Muscles	Color	EFT Point	Emotion
Bennett small intestine	A 2-inch radius around the umbilicus	Quadriceps, rectus femoris and external abdominals	Red	Hypothenar border	**Unclear thought process and expression of emotions**

Table 8.6 Chronic Liver/Gall Bladder

Point	Location	Muscles	Color	EFT Point	Emotion
Chronic liver/ gall bladder	In the web between the thumb and index finger	Pectoralis major sternal, Rhomboid, Popliteus	Green	Lateral eyebrow	**Indecision anger, depression**

Note: In infants, umbilical erythema can be a sign of food intolerance, especially to cow's milk protein. This food reaction may cause GI, respiratory or dermal symptoms. With dietary elimination of dairy, the erythema is reported to resolve within two weeks.[1]

Table 8.7 Colon

Point	Location	Muscles	Color	EFT Point	Emotion
Colon	Bilaterally along the tensor fascia lata	Tensor fascia lata, Hamstrings, Quadratus lumborum	White	Index finger	**Inflexibility (body and mind)**

Hiatal Hernia Syndrome Point And Test

This point—just to the left of the xyphoid process—can be checked for tenderness (0-4). It was introduced by Ralph Failor, DC, ND. An additional maneuver is to have the patient press anteroposterior and cephalad just below the costosternal angle while comparing the muscle strength against a previously strong muscle (for example rectus femoris). The hiatal hernia syndrome is often related to a finding at the occiput (see Chapter 12).

Ileocecal Valve Syndrome Test

Testing and treatment are explained in Chapter 15.

Related muscles:

Hypotonic ("open") = iliacus

Hypertonic ("closed") = quadriceps group

Related spinal levels:

Hypotonic ("open") = C5 and L1

Hypertonic ("closed") = C3 and L3

Blood Sugar Imbalance Point

This point is in the center of the thenar eminence on the adductor pollicis muscle. It may indicate low or high blood sugar imbalance. It is not specific for either, but may be followed up with a fasting blood sugar, a fasting insulin (3-4 mIU/L is ideal, >10 mIU/L is functional hyperinsulinemia[2], >22 mIU/L is pathological hyper-insulinemia), serum lactic dehydrogenase test (below 140 mg/dl is indicative reactive hypoglycemia[3] or hemoglobin A1c (normal is <5.7).

Adrenal Chapman Point

Although all organs have relationships to the GI tract, the adrenals —through blood sugar regulation and stress modulation—have a central role in governing the digestive tract. It may be part of what is found to be tender when checking the Bennett's small intestine area (discussed above.)

Table 8.8 Adrenal Chapman

Point	Location	Muscles	Color	Spinal Level	Emotion
Adrenal Chapman	Bilaterally 1 tsun lateral and 2 tsun superior to the umbilicus	Gracilis, Sartorius, Tibialis posterior, Gastrocnemius, Soleus	Yellow	T11 T12	**Worry**

Additional signs: +Orthostatic hypotension test and + hippus (pupillary light) test

1 Iacono G, Di Prima L, D'Amico D, Scalici C, Geraci G, Carroccio A. The "red umbilicus": a diagnostic sign of cow's milk protein intolerance. *J. Pediatr Gastroenterol Nutr. 2006 May;42(5):531-4.*

2 J. Mercola, MD

3 D. Kharazian, DC

Chapter 9
Laboratory Testing For FGID*

STOOL SPECIMENS

Culture for Yeast and Fungus

Culture for Bacteria

The Four "R" Program

Ova and Parasites (O&P)Microscopy

Blastocystis hominis

Dientamoeba fragilis

Entamoeba coli, dispar and hartmanni

Stool Antigens/Toxins

Giardia Specific Antigen

Cryptosporidium Antigen

Clostridium Difficile Toxins A & B

Occult Blood

Fecal Leukocytes

Inflammatory Markers

Lysozyme

Calprotectin

Alpha Anti-chymotrypsin

Fecal Lactoferrin

Digestive Enzyme Markers

Chymotrypsin and Pancreatic Elastase

Fecal Gluten Sensitivity Testing

Enterobius Vermicularis Tape Test

Stool Transit-retention Test

SALIVARY SPECIMENS

Entameoba Histolytica SIgA

Helicobacter Pylori IgG

Anti-gliadin Antibody SIgA

Total SigA

Other Food Specific SIgA Markers

Ascaris lumbricoides SIgA

Taenia solium SIgA

Trichinella spiralis SIgA

BREATH SPECIMENS

Helicobacter pylori Breath Test

Small Intestinal Bacterial Overgrowth Hydrogen/Methane Breath Test

BLOOD SPECIMENS

Neutrophilic Hypersegmentation Index

Fasting Glucose and Insulin

Transaminases, Alkaline Phosphatase and Gamma Glutamyl Transpeptidase

Complete Blood Count

Albumin, Globulin and Total Protein

Calcium, Magnesium

URINE SPECIMENS

Lactulose-mannitol Intestinal Permeability Test

Mast Cells and Permeability

GASTRIC SPECIMENS

Gastric String Test

Heidelberg Radiotelimetry Test

Esophagogastroduodenoscopy

COLONOSCOPY

* Many thanks to Dr. Jason Wysocki for his contributions to this chapter.

This section will discuss the use and analysis of the laboratory tests that I find most useful in the assessment, treatment and management of functional GI disorders. These have been chosen because they differentiate between pathology and dysfunction; uncover occult infections; determine nutrient levels or production of acid, enzymes and immune factors. I have not included dosages for prescription medicines in this section. Please use other reliable sources.

TABLE 9.1 INDICATIONS FOR STOOL/SALIVARY TESTING
• IBD/IBS • Traveler's diarrhea • Chronic loose stool or constipation • Multiple food intolerances • Bloating, belching, excess flatus, reflux • Chronic abdominal pain • Chronic fatigue • Behavioral disorders • Chronic skin problems • Sleep disorders • Arthritides • Autoimmune disorders • Osteoporosis • Chronic vitamin/mineral deficiency • Eating disorders

Stool Specimens

Culture For Yeast And Fungus

Candida is the most common GI fungal infection following antibiotic treatment. In a Japanese study, 110 patients with C. difficile toxin negative antibiotic associated diarrhea had stool samples cultured.[1] 28% of the cultures grew Candida species. The predominant isolates were C. tropicalis (n=16), C. albicans (n=14) and C. krusei (n=2). Smoking is highly associated with Candida overgrowth.[2] In humans, higher stool growth of Candida is associated with vaginitis, chronic fatigue,[3] food allergies and allergies in general. Post-antibiotic Candida overgrowth is associated with asthma in mice.[4] A small study in the *Annals of Allergy* showed that the presence of yeast overgrowth in the human intestinal tract (Candida albicans, Geotrichum candidum) can induce the typical symptoms of IBS.[5]

My experience is that the highest Candida growth you will see in most immuno-competent patients is 3+ (moderate growth.) This moderate growth is enough to cause a host of digestive and systemic symptoms. These may include excessive gas formation, abdominal bloating, sugar and complex carbohydrate cravings, fatigue, depression, muscle/joint pain, prostatitis, vaginitis, and rashes with a fungal or non-specific morphology.

There are relationships among excessive growth of yeast in the pharynx, vagina and colon, with a stronger correlation between pharynx and colon. Each year, millions of cases of vaginal Candidiasis occur in sexually active young women. *C. albicans* is regarded as a sexually transmitted infection (STI) because *C. albicans* gene sequences have been extracted from semen as well as vaginal secretions.[6] Oral-genital sexual contact may account for the presence of overgrowth in these two orifices. Sexual partners often grow identical yeast strains in the vagina, oral cavity, gastrointestinal tract and semen in cases of recurrent vulvovaginal Candidiasis.[7] Female risk factors for recurrence of vaginal Candidiasis include recent masturbation with saliva, cunnilingus and ingestion of two or more servings of bread per day. Male risk factors for recurrences in a female partner include history of the male masturbating with saliva in the previous month and younger age of first intercourse.[8] In immunocompromised patients and following major intestinal surgery, Candida may be blood borne and cause life-threatening systemic infections.

It is my experience that when present, hypochlorhydria decreases the success rate for treatment of yeast and bacterial overgrowth. Very little has been published on this relationship to fungal overgrowth,[9] but the relationship between bacterial overgrowth and hypochlorhydria is well documented.[10,11] Low levels of bifidobacteria are associated with intestinal fungal overgrowth.[12]

Natural therapy:

Antifungal—Any of the following: Caprylic acid (800-1200 mg TID cc), oregano extract (100 mg TID), garlic (whole herb) or allicin extract (180-450 mg QD to TID) or undecylenic acid (250 mg BID or TID)

Probiotics—5-20 billion BID cc

Treat hypo/achlorhydria if present (see Chapter 9)

Drug therapy: nystatin—a luminal agent, amphotericin B—a luminal agent, fluconazole (diflucan)—a systemic agent

Culture For Bacteria

This is an enormous topic. ***To simplify, we can divide the subject into two groups:***

1. bacterial gastroenteritis—infections such as Yersinia, Salmonella, Shigella, Vibrio cholera and the invasive, toxicogenic and pathogenic forms of E. coli.

This edition will not detail the treatment of these infections.

Note: No antibiotics should be used if E. coli O157:H7 is suspected or documented. Antibiotics increase the incidence of hemolytic uremic syndrome and toxicity especially in children.[13]

On a preventive note, in a study of 188 children in Mexico, vitamin A supplementation reduced the incidence of enteropathogenic E. coli (EPEC) diarrheal infections and the duration of both enteropathogenic E. coli and enterotoxigenic E. coli infections. The vitamin A group also had shorter durations of EPEC-associated diarrhea than did children who received placebo.[14]

2. dysbiosis (overgrowth of commensal and opportunistic bacteria)—moderate to heavy growth of organisms such as Klebsiella, Pseudomonas, Enterobacter, Citrobacter, α- and γ-Streptococcus. In the early 20th century, Eli Metchnikoff, Nobel laureate for his work on phagocytosis, coined the term "dysbiosis" and described it as the etiology of the majority of diseases. He found that yogurt could both prevent and treat gut bacterial infections.[15]

When dysbiosis occurs, the delicate balance of intestinal mucosal function may be lost. Overgrown commensals predispose to infections, putrefaction, nutrient depletion (B_{12}, iron, fat soluble vitamins, essential fatty acids), IBS and inactivation of digestive enzymes. The etiology of dysbiosis may be a result of antibiotic use, stress, high carbohydrate intake, maldigestion, toxic exposures, gut inflammation, lowered immunity and perhaps even obesity.[16]

The Four "R" Program

A general approach to dysbiosis (as well as for yeast, virus or parasitic infections) is to use the Four "R" program[17]—Remove, Replace, Reinoculate and Repair.

Remove: *diminish levels of bacterial overgrowth*

An elimination diet may be needed to lower the antigenic load and increase a depressed SIgA. Bacteria may be treated using Allium sativa, Origanum vulgare, probiotics, Cinnamomum cassia, Hydrastis canadensis, Berberis species and others (see Chapter 6 for SIBO treatment).

Garlic is bacteriocidal against Staph aureus, E. coli, Salmonella enteriditis, Pseudomonas aeruginosa, as well as Rotavirus, Candida albicans, Cryptosporidium and Giardia. Allicin is efficiently absorbed in the small intestine, so for colonic dysbiosis, a sustained release formulation might be more effective. Nigel Plummer, an international expert on intestinal flora, reports that Allicin—at doses many-fold more than are needed for an antibiotic effect—has no deleterious affect on the beneficial GI or GU flora.[18] Plummer also reports that oregano is especially active against H. pylori in vitro.[19,20]

An in vitro study found that cinnamon oil significantly reduced the intracellular pH of E. coli O157:H7 and damaged its cytoplasmic membrane.[21] A Chinese study revealed an equal effectiveness for cinnamon oil and the active fraction (cinnamaldehyde) in growth inhibition of bacterial isolates. These included Staphylococcus aureus, E. coli, Enterobacter aerogenes, Proteus vulgaris, Pseudomonas aeruginosa, Vibrio cholerae and Salmonella typhynurium. It also inhibited several Candida and Aspergillus species.[22]

Replace: *stimulate production of—or replenish—digestive factors*

The activity, quality and levels of hydrochloric acid and pepsin, bile salts, intrinsic factor, exocrine pancreatic factors and brush border enzymes are optimized in this phase of treatment (see Chapters 13 and 14 for details).

Increased numbers of colonic commensals such as Staphylococcus aureus, hemolytic Escherichia coli and nonfermenting gram negative bacteria are also found in hypochlorhydric patients. Overgrowth is also more common in patients with low SIgA.[23] SIgA is, in fact, the largest humoral immune system of the body.[24] Antibacterial and/or probiotic regimens are very helpful in these cases together with attempts to normalize the gut SIgA levels.

Reinoculate: *reintroduce probiotic flora*

A double-blind placebo-controlled study examined the effects of probiotic supplementation following antibiotic therapy. Growth of facultative anaerobes and enterobacteria increased significantly as well as the number of patients culture-positive for antibiotic-resistant enterococci post therapy in the placebo group. In contrast, there was no change in the number of facultative anaerobes or incidence of antibiotic resistance in the probiotic group[25] (See Chapter 3 for more details.)

Repair: *regenerate and heal the gastrointestinal mucosa*

Glutamine raises mucosal glutathione levels and reverses villous atrophy in malnourished rats.[26,27] In human studies, oral glutamine decreased intestinal injury, and intestinal hyperpermeability in patients with severe burns.[28] This amino acid prevents both changes in intestinal brush border absorption and increases in paracellular permeability in chemotherapy patients.[29] Aloe vera may improve intestinal bacterial short chain fatty acid production.[30] In murine research, Seacure—a whitefish protein concentrate—increased the phagocytic activity of peritoneal macrophages and the number of SIgA producing cells in the small intestine.[31]

Ova And Parasites (O&P) Microscopy

Intestinal parasitic infections are endemic worldwide and have been described as constituting the greatest single worldwide cause of illness and disease.[32] Parasites, their cysts or ova may be detected on microscopic exam, but may not be shed adequately with every bowel movement, therefore two or three samples are preferred.[33] In addition to three samples, care must be taken to use a lab that inspects all three samples for parasites rather than pooling the specimens and checking only once. Examining each of the three specimens individually allows for up to an additional 9% detection rate.

Blastocystis hominis (Blastocystis Species)

Epidemiology: Blastocystis is a protozoan flagellate. Morphological forms include avacuolar, vacuolar, multivacuolar, granular, cystic and ameboid. Fecal/oral transmission is thought to be the rule but a full understanding of the epidemiology is unclear.[168] According to Chandra et al:

> The baffling range of morphological forms of existence identified in *Blastocystis* species further mystifies the enigma surrounding the organism.
>
> At present, the most convincing yet unsatisfactory explanation to the pathogenicity of *Blastocystis* is the correlation of the subtype with virulence.

There are at least 6 subtypes but subtyping is not commercially available and would not allow you to determine pathogenicity. I decide whether to treat based on the symptom picture.

Clinical picture: Previously believed to be an asymptomatic infection, it can cause moderate to severe abdominal pain, distention, nausea/vomiting, fever and diarrhea.[34] Blastocystosis is quite common both in the developing world (30-50%) and the developed world (1.5-10%.)[35]

Natural therapy: I have seen Blastocystis eradicated by natural therapies only a couple of times. One was an adult using a broad-spectrum antiparasitic TID on alternating weeks for ten weeks (containing berberine sulfate, grapefruit seed extract, Gentian lutea, Allium sativa, Juglans nigra, Hydrastis canadensis, Ticrasma (Quassia) and Artemesia annua) plus a B. hominus 30X nosode (15 gtts TID daily for ten weeks) and a probiotic BID daily. Oregano oil has been shown to be effective in vivo.[36] Colloidal silver may be effective in eradicating up to 50% of cases.[37]

Drug therapy: Metronidazole is the standard but tinidazole, nitazoxanide, bactrim or iodoquinol are also used.

Dientamoeba fragilis

Epidemiology: Related to Trichomonas. The route of transmission is uncertain, but it is a cause of traveler's diarrhea.[38]

Clinical picture: Diarrhea is more commonly symptomatic in children. Other symptoms/signs include fatigue, nausea, abdominal pain, anorexia, malaise and eosinophilia. Cases may be misdiagnosed as IBS.[39]

Natural therapy: None confirmed.

Drug therapy: Iodoquinol (available in compounded formulation), nitazoxanide, tetracycline, metronidazole or paromomycin.[40]

Entamoeba coli, Entamoeba dispar And Entamoeba hartmanni

These protozoans are non-pathogenic but may be reported if seen on O&P. You may choose to treat these, but most agree that these organisms are benign.

Entamoeba histolytica, Giardia and other parasites may or may not be diagnosed by O&P, so they are discussed under alternate tests below.

Stool Antigens/Toxins

Giardia Specific Antigen (GSA) By Enzyme Immunoassay

Giardia lamblia is a flagellate detected by O&P or GSA. Giardia is considered to be the most common protozoal infection in humans.[41] Beavers, voles, muskrats and birds act as reservoirs and may be a source of Giardia in untreated water.[42] For either method multiple specimens are more accurate than single stool specimens.[43]

Epidemiology: Fecal-oral or food-waterborne transmission. The organism is usually ingested as a cyst with as few as 10-25 cysts being sufficient to cause infection. The cysts are the dormant stage. Digestion by stomach acid and proteases leads to excystation, leaving a replicative trophozoite which may attach to the small intestinal mucosa, but does not invade the bowel wall. Trophozoites may encyst and be shed in feces. Humans may be infected by dogs (who may be symptomatic or asymptomatic.)

Clinical picture: Giardiasis may be asymptomatic or present clinically as watery, frothy, foul smelling stool or diarrhea; weight loss; abdominal cramps; malodorous flatulence; fever/chills and nausea. There is an absence of blood, mucus or fecal leukocytes.

Natural therapy: I do not rely on natural therapies for Giardia, but the following research is included here. Probiotics, especially L. casei, prevent the adherence of Giardia trophozoites to the mucosal surface, promote IgA and mucin production and bind adhesion sites, perhaps offering an effective prevention and treatment.[44]

Ocimum basilicum (basil essential oil) was found highly effective in eradication of Giardia in a murine study.[45]

Allium sativa effectively treated twenty-six children infected with G. lamblia.[46] Either a 5 ml crude extract in 100 ml water was given in divided doses or a commercial preparation (0.6 mg capsules) 2 capsules twice/day was given for 3 days.

A study of 707 Mexican children found that prophylactic use of vitamin A plus zinc reduces G. lamblia incidence.[48] Please note that a related study found that vitamin A taken during infection *increased* the duration of illness.[49]

Drug therapy: Metronidazole or tinidazole. Nitazoxanide is FDA approved for treatment of this organism. In pregnancy, paromomycin is preferable.

Cryptosporidium Antigen

Epidemiology: This coccidian parasite (part of the Sporozoa—the same group as the malaria parasite) is detected by its antigen. Transmission is zoonotic, nosocomial, by person-to-person contact, waterborne, or ingestion of contaminated raw milk or meat. This infection can be life threatening especially in AIDS. It is likely to be asymptomatic in immunocompetent patients.

Clinical picture: *Immunocompromised patient*—nausea, fever, abdominal cramps, anorexia, 5-10 watery stools/day alternating with constipation. These symptoms can mimic Crohn's disease. Extra-intestinal effects may involve the respiratory tract, cholecystitis, hepatitis and pancreatitis.

Immune competent patient—It is often a self-limited disease but if it develops a chronic low grade course it responds well to natural therapy. The antigen should be retested in twenty-one days and again in 6 months.

Natural therapy: In the immune competent patient with symptoms, I have seen good results using chyawanprash, a variety of ayurvedic herbal formulas based on amla fruit paste (Emblica officianalis) which raises total SIgA. I give half a teaspoon twice a day for a month or more. In addition, I give Cryptosporidium 30X nosode—15 drops TID for a month.

Drug therapy: Nitazoxanide is FDA approved for treatment of this organism. In AIDS patients paromomycin, or azithromycin along with effective AIDS treatment.

Clostridium difficile Toxins A & B

Epidemiology: C. difficile is part of the normal intestinal flora, but when this anaerobic gram positive bacillus overgrows, it produces toxins A and B. 20-40% of cases are acquired in hospital patients. C. difficile has been isolated from sphygmomanometer cuffs[50] and hospital uniforms.[51] 60% of cases are asymptomatic carriers. Drugs with the highest risk of causing C. difficile overgrowth include clindamycin, cephalosporins, penicillins, and fluoroquinolones, but virtually any antibiotic may be implicated. Surgery, chemotherapy, proton pump inhibitors,[52] stool softeners and enemas may also encourage overgrowth of C. difficile. C. difficile toxins A and B have been shown to loosen the tight junctions of enterocytes.[53]

Clinical picture: Low to high grade fever, moderate to severe diarrhea, mild to severe abdominal cramps, pseudomembranous enterocolitis – severe cases are similar to the presentation of acute ulcerative colitis.

Natural therapy: Saccharomyces boulardii is useful in prevention and treatment.[54,55] I recommend a capsule containing 3-6 billion organisms TID for 14 days. A double-blind, placebo-controlled study tested the effect of antibiotics plus a probiotic containing both Lactobacillus and Bifidobacterium vs. placebo on the eradication of C. difficile. Trial probiotic or placebo was taken within 72 hours of commencing the prescription antibiotic. After treatment 2.9% of the probiotic treated group samples were positive for C. difficile toxins as compared with 7.25% in the placebo-control group.[56] A low dose of Cinnamonum zeylanicum bark extract (trans-cinnamaldehyde) was found to improve the antibiotic effect of clindamycin and decrease the dosage needed to treat C. difficile overgrowth by a factor of sixteen.[57]

Fecal microbiota transplantation by oral triple encapsulation method, enema or colonoscopic instillation has a near 99% cure rate. For insurance purposes, it is only considered after metronidazole and vancomycin treatment have failed to be successful.

Drug therapy: Metronidazole, vancomycin

Occult Blood

Blood in the stool—frank or occult—is one of the red flags for FGID.

The fecal occult blood test (FOBT or Hemoccult) is an older method of testing which may still be encountered. In order to avoid false positive stool occult blood, the following guidelines are given to the patient as printed on the *Hemoccult* home test sample envelope:

- For seven days before and during the stool collection period **avoid** non-steroidal and anti-inflammatory drugs such as ibuprofen, naproxen or aspirin (more than one adult aspirin a day).
- Acetaminophen (Tylenol) can be taken as needed.
- For three days before and during the stool collection period **avoid** citrus fruits and juices and supplements of vitamin C in excess of 250 mg a day.
- For three days before and during the stool collection period **avoid** red meats (beef, lamb and liver).
- Eat a well balanced diet including fiber (eg. bran cereals, fruits and vegetables.)[58]

A newer occult blood testing method is the fecal immune test (FIT). FIT has replaced FOBT and become the more mainstream screening test. It has improved sensitivity, specificity and low cost. There are fewer false positives because there are no confounding dietary factors. No preparatory diet is necessary for this type of testing. A single sample replaces the triple sample method used with FOBT.

Table 9.2 Causes For Positive Stool Occult Blood
Colorectal cancer
Adenoma
Diaphragmatic hernia
Gastric carcinoma
Peptic ulcer disease
Arteriovenous malformations
Inflammatory bowel disease
Gastritis
Vasculitis
Amyloidosis
Kaposi's sarcoma
Hemorrhoid or anal fissure

Fecal Leukocytes

The detection of leukocytes in a stool sample is a marker for several GI infections and inflammations.

Table 9.3 GI Conditions—Fecal Leukocyte Positive
Shigella
Campylobacter
Enterohemorrhagic E. coli 015:H7
Yersinia
Inflammatory bowel disease
Most bacterial infections of the colon

Table 9.4 GI Conditions—Fecal Leukocyte Negative
Vibrio cholera
Enterotoxigenic E. coli
Staph aureus
Clostridium botulinum and perfringens
Giardia
E. histolytica
Rotavirus
Norwalk virus
Cryptosporidium
Small intestinal bacterial overgrowth
Cyclospora
Isospora
Microsporidia

Table 9.5 GI Conditions—Fecal Leukocyte Variable
Salmonella
Yersinia
Clostridium difficile
Non-cholera Vibrios

Inflammatory Markers

Fecal Lysozyme: A Colon Specific Inflammation Marker

Several markers have been proposed to differentiate IBS from IBD. The fecal markers lactoferrin, calprotectin, and lysozyme are available and differentiate active IBD from inactive IBD as well as from IBS.[59,60,61] Fecal lysozyme has been shown to differentiate active UC or Crohn's colitis (Crohn's disease in the colon) from remission.[62,63] Fecal lysozyme concentrations in healthy controls and IBS tend to be in the normal range (0 to 6 mg/l.) In contrast, concentrations in patients with untreated IBD are increased (6 to 104 mg/l).[64] A Dutch study found that fecal lysozyme testing discriminates between normal individuals and patients with irritable bowel syndrome as well as between patients with inflammatory bowel disease and colonic cancer.[65] Fecal lysozyme levels can be used as a marker for relapse and to monitor therapeutic success in patients with inflammatory bowel disease. A consistently high level of fecal lysozyme excretion in adults over the age of forty may indicate the possibility of colorectal cancer and needs thorough investigation.[66] My experience with this marker is that modest elevations may be present in IBS. Calprotectin and lactoferrin are better tests to distinguish IBS from IBD.

Fecal Calprotectin

This protein is an antimicrobial factor in neutrophils, monocytes, macrophages and squamous epithelia. Calprotectin is thought to be stable in fecal specimens for up to seven days. However, fecal calprotectin sampling may be best acquired from first morning stool and if stored at room temperature, not for longer than 3 days.[169] It differentiates IBD from IBS and correlates with the severity of inflammation. A 2001 study found it to be a sensitive non-invasive marker of colorectal cancer and adenomatous polyps.[67] It is more sensitive than fecal occult blood tests for detection of colorectal neoplasia. A 2007 meta-analysis found calprotectin to be useful

Table 9.6 Calprotectin Levels In Health, Inflammation, Polyps, And Colorectal Carcinoma
normal/ insignificant inflammation = < 50 ug/g
a patient with positive Rome criteria for IBS and calprotectin <50 does not have IBD
mild/moderate inflammation (adenomatous polyps, neoplasia, NSAID use, IBD, or infection) = 50-100 ug/g
more significant inflammation = >100 ug/g
active disease, impending relapse of IBD = > 250 ug/g elevated fecal calprotectin (especially above 275 ug/g was significantly associated with SIBO in patients with systemic sclerosis

for IBD differentiation, but not for colon cancer screening.[68] Fecal calprotectin is lower when serum 25(OH) vitamin D levels were >75nmol/L, and higher when 25(OH)D was <25nmol/L.[170] Monoclonal fecal calprotectin assays have been shown to provide greater sensitivity when compared to polyclonal assays. [171]

Fecal calprotectin is more sensitive than *Hemoccult* in detecting colorectal neoplasia, but the specificity is lower.[69] It is reasonable to use calprotectin as a screening test when selecting high risk patients for colonoscopy. Calprotectin can be a marker of impending relapse for UC and CD.[70]

α-Anti-chymotrypsin

Elevation of α-anti-chymotrypsin in feces is a marker for intestinal inflammation.[71] In a study from the University of Melborne, levels above 360 mg% of dry weight positively predicted > 90% of patients with gastrointestinal inflammatory disease and 66% of patients with colorectal cancer.[72]

Table 9.7 Fecal α-Anti-chymotrypsin Assessment
Normal =< 60 mg% dry weight
Borderline elevation = 60-100 mg %
Mild or distal colitis = 100-180 mg %*
Colonic inflammation => 180 mg %*
* *The inflammation is small intestinal, unless fecal lysozyme is also elevated (see above)*

Fecal Lactoferrin

Lactoferrin is an iron binding glycoprotein that is present in various human body fluids such as colostrum, milk, saliva, tears, nasal and gastrointestinal secretions. It is a component of the innate immune system and neutrophilic secondary granules which are released during apoptosis.

It has been shown to have bactericidal, virucidal and fungicidal activity. It is a reliable biomarker of inflammation.[172] Similar to calprotectin, lactoferrin is detected in increased concentrations in stool in response to an active inflammatory process. It has similar specificity, sensitivity, and diagnostic accuracy to calprotectin for inflammatory bowel disease.[173]

TABLE 9.8 FECAL TOTAL LACTOFERRIN ASSESSMENT LEVELS
Normal= <7.25 µg/mL[174]
Elevated=>7.25 µg/mL
Note: Inaccurate tests are expected in breastfed infants as lactoferrin is a major component of human breastmilk.[175]

TABLE 9.9 FECAL LACTOFERRIN IBD SCREENING OBSERVATIONAL STUDY RESULTS

Group	#observations	µg/mL (x±SE)
Controls	55	1.6 (0.4)
IBS	31	1.3 (0.3)
Inactive UC	41	67 (24)
Active UC	31	815 (389)
Inactive CD	26	239 (83)
Active CD	51	672 (242)

Findings from observational study using fecal lactoferrin[176]

Digestive Enzyme Markers

Chymotrypsin And Pancreatic Elastase

Fecal chymotrypsin and pancreatic elastase are markers of total pancreatic exocrine output and are screening tests for pancreatic insufficiency. A patient who is supplementing most forms of plant pancreatic enzymes or pancreatin with meals will have a falsely elevated chymotrypsin level, but an accurate elastase level. The reason for this is that pancreatic supplements do not contain elastase which is unique to the human pancreas, but many contain chymotrypsin. A patient may continue these supplements while being tested for endogenous production of elastase.[73]

TABLE 9.10 CHYMOTRYPSIN LEVELS AND PANCREATIC EXOCRINE OUTPUT
*Very low output = <4 U/10 grams
*Low output = 4-9 U/10 grams
Adequate output = >9 U/10 grams
**Falsely low levels may occur with stool transit time >96 hours*

TABLE 9.11 PANCREATIC ELASTASE ASSESSMENT
Severe pancreatic insufficiency = <100 ug/g
Moderate pancreatic insufficiency = 100-200 ug/g
Indeterminate pancreatic exocrine function = 200-400 ug/g
Normal pancreatic exocrine function = >400 ug/g
Note: Falsely elevated levels of elastase may occur with liquid stool

See Chapter 14 for treatment of pancreatic insufficiency.

Fecal total secretory IgA

Total stool SIgA may be considered an evaluation of GI immune competence. This antibody is produced by mature Peyer's patches and isolated lymphoid follicles.

Natural therapy: Feeding of colostrum, prebiotics or probiotics raises the total SIgA level in children.[75,76,77] A diet high in pre-germinated brown rice (PGBR) significantly raises SIgA. This is a brown rice which is soaked to allow a small amount of sprouting to occur before cooking. PGBR also decreased depression, anger-hostility, and fatigue in lactating women[78] and was shown to lower blood-glucose levels and decrease serum homocysteine levels in mice.[79] Chyawanprash—an Ayurvedic herbal combination—is perported to raise SIgA.

A note on ordering Stool Testing:

Many labs offer stool testing available to practitioners with both culture and Polymerase Chain Reaction (PCR)-based methodology. To provide a brief discussion of a vast topic, PCR of stool is best reserved for acute-care situations. Based on current research, real-time PCR is the fastest method of determining the causative organism in diarrheal disease.[177,178] In sub-acute and chronic conditions, culture based technology remains the most sensitive and discriminating way to identify the greatest number of commensal and pathogenic gastrointestinal microorganisms.[179,180,181,182] DNA based testing currently available has not been shown to be specific and accurate in an independently conducted proficiency challenge.[183]

Table 9.12 Microorganism Detection Limits Of Various Stool Testing Methods [184]

Testing Method	Detection Limit	Linear Range
Culture	10 to 10^2 CFU/gm	10^2 to 10^9 CFU/gm
Real-time PCR	10^3 to 10^4 CFU/gm	10^6 to 10^8 CFU/gm
PCR ELISA	10^3 to 10^5 CFU/gm	10^3 to 10^9 CFU/gm
PCR	10^4 to 10^5 CFU/gm	10^5 to 10^7 CFU/gm

CFU=colony forming units, measured per gram of stool.

According to Gingras et al:

> Although there is a need to develop rapid molecular testing assays for characterization of the gut microbiome, physicians and patients need to be aware that all stool analysis assays may not be valid and users of these assays should demand to see verification study data in order to discern the claims of the commercial entity offering the lab developed assay. The claims made by the Subject Laboratory that their DNA assessment of stool samples is specific and accurate, could not be supported by this independently conducted proficiency challenge.[183]

Fecal Gluten Sensitivity Testing

It has always seemed logical to me to use a specimen from the GI tract, when looking for a measureable reaction in the GI tract. Standard celiac markers rely on serum samples—a less likely compartment for an accurate test. Stool measurement of antigliadin antibody IgA and anti-tissue transglutaminase antibody IgA are available and at least one article supports this."[186]

Enterobius Vermicularis—Anal Tape Test

A simple way to make the diagnosis is to have an appropriate family member use a flashlight to inspect the anal area early in the morning before washing or wiping. The worms are tiny, white, and threadlike. If none is seen, have the anal area viewed for one or two additional mornings. Even if a worm is not seen, a tape test specimen can be taken (see below).

The tape test sample is collected in the morning before bathing. The eggs are laid at night. The sticky side of a 1 inch strip of cellophane tape is pressed firmly against the anal area for a few seconds. If eggs are present they adhere to the tape. The tape is then affixed to a glass microscope slide, sticky side down. Ask the family to bring the slide to the office and microscopically examine for eggs.

Epidemiology: Pinworm is the most common intestinal worm infestation in the U.S. Transmission is fecal/oral. The organism lives in the colon, predominantly in the cecum. The females migrate to the perianal area during the night to lay eggs. Pruritis ani stimulates scratching—leading to reinfection and fecal oral spread, especially in children.

Clinical picture: Asymptomatic or pruritis ani, perioral discoloration, irritability, nightmares, sleeplessness and seizures. Some cases of diarrhea, abdominal pain and rectal bleeding in children have been diagnosed by colonoscopy to be due to E. vermicularis.[80] Rarely, obstruction of the appendix leads to acute appendicitis. Patients with symptomatic Enterobius vermicularis infections have lower vitamin B_{12} levels than asymptomatic patients.[81] An article in the journal Diabetologia points out that pinworms, by inducing immunomodulation, may prevent the development of diabetes in mice.[82]

Natural therapy: I have only used natural therapy in a few recurrent cases. Homeopathic potencies of sulphur or Cina (wormseed) have been effective in these unusual cases. Keeping the fingernails trimmed and using good handwashing practices are helpful.

Drug therapy: Mebendazole or albendazole for all household contacts.

Stool Transit-retention Test

This test is also done at home. Instruct the patient to swallow 6 charcoal capsules with breakfast. Have the patient take note of the number of hours elapsed before the first stool marked with grey or black. This is the transit time of food through the digestive tract. Have the patient continue to take note of the hours elapsed from the transit time until the last grey or black colored stool. This is the retention time. An ideal transit time plus the retention time should fall into the range of fourteen to thirty-six hours.

Salivary Specimens

Entamoeba Histolytica Antibody SIgA

Epidemiology: Transmission of this protozoan is fecal-oral. Onset of symptoms is gradual, over a week or more. The trophozoite stage exists in the host and in recently passed loose stools. In contrast, the cysts may be present in water, soil and food. Cysts are killed by heat or freezing. After ingestion, cysts become trophozoites in the intestines. E. histolytica may migrate to the liver.

Clinical picture: Asymptomatic or IBD-like symptoms (frequent bloody diarrhea); insidious onset of fatigue, diarrhea, bloody stool, colicky abdominal pain, tenesmus, weight loss (50% of cases) and fever (10% of cases.) It can cause perianal skin ulcers or condylloma-like lesions. Some extraintestinal manifestations such as cysts or abscesses in the liver may occur.

Testing: This protozoan may be detected on O & P (only detected by this method in <50% of cases) or, more predictably, by salivary antibody testing followed up by a stool antigen test. Stool antigen testing may be done to differentiate this organism from E. dispar and other non-invasive forms. *A positive stool antigen also indicates present infection rather than residual antibody levels from a previous infection.* No fecal leukocytes will be found in stool due to lysis of WBCs by the organism. Peripheral leukocytosis may be present with more severe cases and with liver abscesses.

Amoebic colitis should be ruled out before allopathic treatment of a presumed diagnosis of Crohn's disease because corticosteroids exacerbate amebiasis. Transaminases, alkaline phosphatase and possibly bilirubin may be elevated in hepatic cases.[83]

Natural therapy: I have seen a number of cases of E. histolytica symptomatically cleared with a broad spectrum parasidal agent (containing berberine sulfate, grapefruit seed extract, Gentian lutea, Allium sativa, Juglans nigra, Hydrastis canadensis, Ticrasma [Quassia] and Artemesia annua) 2 caps TID ic for 7 days every other week for 5-8 repetitions) and E. histolytica 30X bowel nosode (15 gtts TID for 1-2 months.) I have not been consistent about retesting, so my evidence is based on clinical picture only. Garlic has been shown to be effective against E histolytica.[84]

Drug therapy: Paromomycin or diloxanide furoate (asymptomatic pts.) Metronidazole or tinidazole or nitazoxanide if symptomatic. *I do not recommend drug therapy for Entamoeba without first obtaining a positive O & P or E. histolytica stool antigen.*

Helicobacter Pylori Antibody IgG

I use this only as a screening test and follow-up with an H. pylori breath test (see below) if the antibody is elevated.

Epidemiology: H. pylori is a gram negative spiral flagellated bacterium that produces urease. Transmission is fecal-oral, oral-oral or gastro-oral.

Clinical picture: Helicobacter may cause gastritis, hypochlorhydria, atrophic gastritis, vague or more severe epigastric pain, nausea, anorexia, fatigue, peptic ulcer, gastric cancer, and maltoma.[85] Treating H. pylori in ITP patients can cure their thrombocytopenia.[86] H. pylori is also a commensal organism essential for maturation of the immune system in infants and children. If typical peptic ulcer, gastric cancer or maltoma symptoms and signs are not present, treatment may not be warranted.[190]

Salivary IgG is a screening test which may be elevated due to past colonization. Duodenal sampling or the H. pylori breath test are indicative of current colonization and are more accurate for follow-up.

Natural therapy: Adding bovine lactoferrin (200 mg BID) and a probiotic (19 billion Lactobacillus, Bifidobacteria and Streptococcus organisms BID) to triple drug therapies—such as a proton pump inhibitor, clarithromycin and tinidazole—increases the eradication rate from 75% to 93% and decreases side effects of the antimicrobial therapy.[87] A study of 150 symptomatic H. pylori positive patients compared the use of a triple drug therapy alone against the triple therapy plus lactoferrin (no probiotic used in this study.) Eradication rate for the triple therapy alone was 72.5%. With the addition of lactoferrin, eradication was 95.9%.[88] It is presumed that these effects are due to the ability of lactoferrin to decrease bacterial adherence and also due to a direct antimicrobial effect.[89]

A seven day course of curcumin (30 mg b.i.d.), bovine lactoferrin (100 mg b.i.d.), N-acetylcysteine (600 mg b.i.d.), and pantoprazole (20 mg BID) did not eradicate the organism but conferred significant symptomatic improvement and reduced signs of gastric inflammation both at the end of treatment and at two months follow up.[90]

Lactoferrin as a single agent (200 mg BID x twelve weeks) produced a 33% eradication of H. pylori.[91] Administration of lactoferrin during pregnancy may be contraindicated due to evidence that it inhibits metalloproteinases and may prevent cervical maturation/effacement.[92] Pistacia lentiscus (Mastic gum) is partially effective in vitro and in vivo (murine) against H. pylori.[93] Of note: No solitary pharmaceutical is considered effective against H. pylori and none has been studied individually.

Oregano oil is effective in vitro against H. pylori.[94]

Drug therapy: Triple therapies such as clarithromycin, ampicillin and a proton pump inhibitor or tetracycline, metronidazole (or tinidazole) and a proton pump inhibitor are standard. I add 900-1000 mg of lactoferrin qhs and a probiotic BID cc to either of the above protocols as discussed above under natural therapy.

Clarithromycin resistant H. pylori is becoming common in many areas of the U.S. so alternate regimens are recommended in these areas and 14 day courses of treatment are becoming standard (7-10 day courses were standard in the past).

Total secretory IgA

Total secretory IgA may be measured in saliva, stool or serum. The most common reason for depressed levels is excessive endogenous or exogenous cortisol. Salivary levels may be decreased and risk of respiratory infection may be increased in elite high performance swimmers and others exercising to exhaustion.[95]

Food antigen specific antibodies (SIgA)

Individuals with genetic or acquired food intolerances may experience intestinal inflammation after consumption of the offending foods. Subsequently, the intestinal mucosa releases SIgA which can be measured in saliva. Anti-gliadin antibodies may be detected in this way. If total intestinal SIgA is decreased, there will be false negative food specific antibody levels.

Table 9.13 Salivary Anti-Gliadin Antibody SIgA Assessment
Negative = <13 correct for depressed total SIgA if necessary (see Table 9.14 below)
Borderline = 13-15 Elevated = >15

TABLE 9.14 CORRECTING FOR A DEPRESSED TOTAL SIGA
If total stool or salivary SIgA levels are depressed, determine a multiplier that brings the IgA into the low normal range. Multiply the food antigen specific IgA by the same number to correct.
Example: A patient has a total stool IgA level of 40 (low). Multiplying by a factor of 10 brings the IgA to 400 (normal range). If the uncorrected anti-gliadin SIgA level is 3 (negative), multiplying by 10 gives a corrected level of 30 (positive.)
Salivary anti-gliadin antibody SIgA (salivary AGA SIgA) is not a valid test for celiac disease. It is a marker for immune reactivity against gliadin and gluten, and indicates that a gluten-free diet (GFD) is indicated. Offer the patient serum testing for celiac markers before commencing the GFD in order to insure an accurate result. Serum anti-tissue transglutaminase (anti-tTG) IgA and IgG and deamidated gliadin peptide IgA and IgG are available for this purpose. Should the patient decide to have serum testing after avoiding gluten for weeks to months, the results will likely be falsely negative. Similarly, salivary AGA SIgA will drop into the negative range within weeks to months on a GFD. It can therefore be used as a test of compliance and/or unwitting gluten contamination in the diet. I recommend running the salivary AGA SIgA follow-up test three months after commencing the GFD.

TABLE 9.15 DISEASE STATES ASSOCIATED WITH GLUTEN INTOLERANCE	
Diabetes mellitus	Fibrosing alveolitis
Thyroiditis	Idiopathic pulmonary hemosiderosis
Osteopenia/porosis	Recurrent pericarditis
Sjogrens dz	Myocarditis
Primary biliary cirrhosis	Dilated cardiomyopathy
Adrenocortical deficiency	Splenic atrophy
IgA nephrosis	Dementia/schizophrenia
Rheumatoid arthritis	Dermatitis herpetiformis
Down syndrome	Maltoma
Seizure disorders	

Table 9.16 Lab Findings Suggestive Of Gluten Intolerance	
Hypocalcemia	Thrombocytosis
Vitamin D deficiency	Prolonged prothrombin time
Hypoproteinemia	Elevated transaminases or alk phos
Iron deficiency anemia	Elevated serum amylase
Folate/B_{12} deficiency anemia	

Table 9.17 History Findings Suggestive Of Gluten Intolerance	
Short stature	Delayed menarche/puberty
Anxiety, irritability	Amenorrhea
Chronic fatigue	Infertility
Muscle cramping	Recurrent spontaneous abortion
Tetany	Night blindness
Bone/joint/muscle pain	Chronic anemia
Ataxia	Chronic bruising
Neuropathy	Recurrent oral apthae
Paraesthesia	Dental enamel defects
Migraine/headpain	Skin pigment changes
Generalized itching	Follicular hyperkeratosis
	Vesicular pruritic rash

Ascaris lumbricoides SIgA

Epidemiology: Ascaris lumbricoides ("roundworm") is the most common worm infection worldwide. A 1989 Lancet editorial suggested that if all the Ascaris on the globe were placed head to tail, they would encircle the world 50 times.[96] It is more concentrated in warm, moist climates (southeastern U.S.) and on swine farms or where pig feces are used as fertilizer. Humans acquire it by swallowing eggs from contaminated soil, water, fruits or vegetables and through the fecal-oral route. Larvae penetrate the wall of the duodenum and travel to the liver via blood or lymph. Microscopic egg detection is elusive because the time required from egg ingestion to shedding in stool is 2-3 months. Detection may be by either salivary SIgA or the O & P, but the O & P is less reliable.

Clinical picture: Patients are often asymptomatic. Initial coughing and difficulty breathing (possibly pneumonia-like) subside only to be followed by abdominal discomfort or pain, nausea/vomiting, and diarrhea. Less often, intestinal, biliary or pancreatic obstruction may occur as well as peritonitis.[97] A Romanian study found a relationship between angioedema or chronic rash and Ascariasis.[98] A common finding is anemia and malnutrition, especially in children. Palmar pallor may be used as a screening test in children.[99]

A study at Memorial Sloan-Kettering noted the clearing of Ascaris worms in the emesis of a patient who had received whole-body irradiation in preparation for a bone marrow biopsy.[100]

With respect to nutrition, children with Ascariasis may experience a reduced growth rate; protein deficit; vitamin A and fat malabsorption; lactose intolerance and a decreased intestinal transit time.[101]

Natural therapy: A Harvard study found that zinc supplementation *increased* the incidence of A. lumbricoides infecton in Mexican children.[102] Carica papaya (dried papaya seed) may be effective against Ascariasis.[103] In a study of 26 Nigerian children with Ascariasis, a single 20 ml dose of C. papaya air dried seed blended in honey cleared 86% of the cases. Extracts prepared from heat-treated seeds had no anthelmintic activity and benzyl isothiocyanate is presumed to be the essential factor.[104] An Egyptian study found a 1% solution of Artemesia santonica to be effective in killing both the infective larvae in approximately forty days and ova in twenty days.[105]

Drug therapy: Mebendazole, albendazole or pyrantel pamoate for all household contacts

Taenia Solium SIgA

Epidemiology: Taenia ("pork tapeworm") infections are worldwide and concentrated in countries where pork is consumed and sanitation is poor. The human harbors the adult worm which is 6-20 feet long and inhabits the small intestine. The head is armed with about 22-32 hooks and the worm sheds 250,000 or more eggs a day.

Transmission: Pigs consume the eggs from human feces (sewage or fertilizer), the eggs partially mature into the intermediate form, the cysticercus, which infects the muscle and brains of swine. Humans consuming infected undercooked pork, or eating food contaminated with infested human feces can develop intestinal tapeworm and/or tissue migrating tapeworm larvae (cysticercosis).

Clinical picture: Muscles and the brain are sites of larval hatching. Myositis, headache, fibromyalgia-like symptoms and CNS related problems such as seizures, and headaches are the most common symptoms. Other CNS signs include confusion, lack of attention to people and surroundings, difficulty with balance, and hydrocephalus. According to the CDC, "although rare, cysticerci may float in the eye and cause blurry or disturbed vision. Infection in the eyes may cause swelling or detachment of the retina."[106]

Calcified CNS lesions may be present. Salivary SIgA and/or O&P are used for detection.

Natural therapy: Cucurbita maxima (pumpkin seed)—One handful daily for two weeks. In albino rats, tapeworm was killed by administering pumpkin seed at a dose equivalent to 73 seeds for an adult human.[107]

Drug therapy: Albendazole or praziquantel

Trichinella Spiralis SIgA

Epidemiology: Trichinella spiralis "pork worm" is a tissue worm of swine.

Transmission: Humans acquire the infection by ingesting the larvae from undercooked pork.

Clinical picture: After days to weeks of nausea, vomiting and diarrhea, the parasite resides mainly in skeletal muscle causing long standing inflammation and fibromyalgia-like symptoms (myositis and dyspnea due to involvement of respiratory muscles). Respiratory muscle involvement leads to dyspnea and infection in cardiac muscle may cause myocarditis, CHF and arrhythmias. The larvae can migrate through CNS leading to meningitis, hemorrhages, seizures, or psychiatric disturbances. There may be leukocytosis and eosinophilia (may continue for years after treatment).

Natural therapy: Podophyllum mother tincture, Cina 30 C and Santoninum 30C reduced the larval population of T. spiralis in mice by 68%, 84% and 81%, respectively, as compared to an untreated control group.[108] In a 2008 study, Artemesia vulgaris and A. absinthium reduced the larval load in rat muscle by 75% and 63% respectively.[109] A combination of Echinacea purpurea extract, Allium sativum extract and cocoa significantly decreased adult T. spiralis in the GI tract and muscular larvae in mice.[110]

Drug therapy: Albendazole or mebendazole. Cook meat thoroughly.

Breath Specimens

Helicobacter Pylori Breath Test

I prefer this test over serological testing because, if positive, it indicates a current infection and within 4 weeks after treatment, it can be used to determine if eradication has been achieved. The finding of antibodies to H. pylori does not distinguish between a present infection and past exposure. Serological tests cannot be used for post-therapy testing.

Method: After obtaining a baseline breath sample, the patient drinks a 3 gram dose of Pranactin-Citric, a solution of a synthetic non-radioactive 13C-urea (also contains citric acid, aspartame and mannitol). If H. pylori is present in the stomach, urease splits the 13C-urea into 13CO2 + 2NH4 13C-urea. The 13CO2 is absorbed into the blood and eventually becomes exhaled in the breath. The change in 13CO2 is measured in the post-dose breath sample by an infrared spectrophotometer.

Patient preparation: Let the patient know that the test drink contains aspartame and therefore phenylalanine (in case they have phenylketonuria). The patient should not eat or drink for an hour prior to the test. No antimicrobials, proton pump inhibitors or bismuth preparations should be taken for at least two weeks prior to the test.

False positive results may occur in achlorhydric patients and with H. heilmannii infection. This organism is rare in humans, but if transmitted from a dog, cat or pig to a human, it may cause peptic ulcer. As with any H. pylori test method, rare false negatives may occur. Repeat testing or an alternate method may be used.

Follow-up testing post treatment should be done at least four weeks after completion of therapy. Treatment was discussed above under salivary anti-helicobacter IgG.

Small Intestinal Bacterial Overgrowth (SIBO) Breath Hydrogen/Methane Test

The overgrowth of flora in any portion of the small intestine can lead to severe digestive consequences. This condition is discussed in every major reference on GI disease, but is often forgotten as part of the differential for abdominal pain, maldigestion, malabsorption, diarrhea, weight loss and anemia. This elegant test for SIBO is underutilized. SIBO is especially likely to occur after gastroduodenal or intestinal surgery and with the presence of achlorhydria, small intestinal diverticulosis, GI motility disorders, Crohn's disease and fistulas.[111] SIBO often causes lactose intolerance which normalizes when the overgrowth is corrected.[112] A recent Italian study found that 45% of IBS patients had SIBO.[113] Overgrowth was found to be even more prevalent among rosacea patients (51%).[114] After bacterial eradication with rifaximin, rosacea cleared in twenty of twenty-eight and greatly improved in six of the remaining eight. Subjects treated with placebo had no improvement in cutaneous lesions. A study of IBS and restless leg syndrome (RLS) in patients with SIBO found dramatic lasting improvement (>80%) in RLS symptoms after treatment of SIBO.[115] A French study found that morbid obesity and severe hepatic steatosis was associated with SIBO.[116] Italian research on celiac patients who failed to improve after a gluten-free diet found a high incidence of SIBO. Rifaximin treatment was effective in removing the residual symptoms in these celiac patients.[117]

Table 9.18 Clinical Picture Of Small Intestinal Bacterial Overgrowth	
Steatorrhea Bloating Cramping Abdominal pain Weight loss	**Malabsorption of fat soluble vitamins, iron and B_{12}:** Neuropathy Anemia Osteomalacia Coagulopathy Night blindness Tetany

When bacteria overgrow in any part of the small intestine, the following can be the result: Inactivation/destruction of pancreatic and brush border enzymes, flavonoids, vitamin B_{12}; deconjugation of bile salts; hydrogenation of fatty acids and production of nitrosamines.

Table 9.19 Risk Factors For Small Intestinal Bacterial Overgrowth	
Hypochlorhydria, achlorhydria, atrophic gastritis Proton pump inhibitors High dose H2 receptor blockers	**Reduced motility:** Obstruction (strictures, adhesions) Small bowel diverticuli Surgical blind loops Intestinal resection Diabetes Scleroderma Fistulas

The basis of the SIBO test is the ability of intestinal organisms to ferment lactulose to hydrogen and methane. Lactulose is virtually unabsorbable, so it is an ideal substance to assess overgrowth in any part of the small bowel. Breath samples are collected prior to lactulose ingestion and again every 20 minutes for a total of three hours. Hydrogen and methane are measured in each specimen and are presented as a graph for analysis.[118]

See page 114 for test interpretation guidelines.[119]

Table 9.20 Decreasing The Risk Of False Positive Results In SIBO Testing
Avoid high fiber foods for 24 hours before testing (eat no starches except rice the evening before—ie. rice and a protein) For constipated patients, a 48 hour avoidance should be considered.
Avoid tobacco smoke in the area of the test
Avoid allowing the patient to fall asleep during the test

Table 9.21 Decreasing The Risk Of False Negative Results In SIBO Testing
If the patient has had recent severe diarrhea postpone the test for at least 7 days
If the patient has used antibiotics, laxatives or enemas postpone the test for at least 7 days
R/O the presence of heavy concentrations of sulfate-reducing bacteria (the patient's intestinal gas will have a rotten egg odor)
If bacterial overgrowth is present only in the distal ileum the test may be incorrect, but this situation is not common

Spot Breath Testing

(Only available with on-site breath testing capabilities)

Before Full Lactulose Breath Test: Due to the cost/time constraints of the full lactulose breath test at initial evaluation, an alternative method has emerged in SIBO gas testing evaluation. If methane symptoms are clinically present, a single "spot" test (single breath sample with no lactulose or glucose administration) can be used prior to performing a full breath test to evaluate methane gas levels. A recent study has suggested that methane readings equal to or greater than 5 PPM on a spot test, preceded by an overnight fast, is highly accurate in detecting methane. [185] A full breath test should normally follow a spot test to validate expected results and provide additional information on methane gas levels throughout the GI tract as well as hydrogen levels.

After Full Lactulose Breath Test / Methane Treatment Evaluation: The spot test can also be used to ascertain response to treatment. It can be used before a full lactulose breath test is repeated. Further study is required as to whether this requires fasting in order to provide useful clinical information. Random repeat spot tests, in the same visit for confirmation, further validate accuracy of single breath sample results.

Natural therapy: Research on a probiotic called Yakult® and IBS has been reported. This Lactobacillus casei strain Shirota (6.5 billion bacteria) was taken by SIBO positive IBS patients each morning prior to breakfast for 6 weeks. 64% had a normalization of the breath test and cases with at least moderate symptoms had an average improvement in symptoms of 55%.[120] Enteric coated peppermint oil (25 mg. TID) may be effective in lowering breath hydrogen and IBS symptoms in patients with SIBO.[121,122] The specific carbohydrate diet, SIBO Specific Foodguide, low FODMAPs diet, and Cedars-Sinai diet are used for primary treatment or to follow antibiotic treatment to prevent recurrence. [123, 124, 125]

Drug therapy: Rifaximin, a luminal antibiotic, is specific for hydrogen dominant SIBO. Up to 43% of patients treated with antibiotics have recurrence by 9 months. The rate of recurrence is increased in advancing age, status post-appendectomy, and chronic use of proton pump inhibitors.[126]

See Chapter 6 for an expanded discussion of SIBO treatment/evaluation

Blood Specimens

Neutrophilic Hypersegmentation Index (NHI)

The NHI is an inexpensive early diagnostic indicator of folic acid deficiency. In folate deficiency, the nuclei of polymorphonuclear cells are altered from an average of 3 lobes to an average of 5 lobes.[127] This is perhaps the earliest folate deficiency sign, before changes in MCV or serum folate. I use this test to determine the folate status of my patients and in my IBD patients, in order to prevent a heightened risk of colonic adenocarcinoma. A 2008 study shows a 7-fold increase in colon cancer risk in IBD patients with folate deficiency. An isolated hyperhomocysteinemia increases the risk 2.5 fold.[128] Sulfasalazine in its various forms is the standard baseline allopathic treatment for IBD, and a competitive inhibitor of folate absorption. A study published in *Gastroenterology* found that folate supplementation was associated with a 62% lower incidence of colorectal carcinoma in ulcerative colitis patients.[129]

Fasting Glucose And Insulin

See Chapter 7 for the details of insulin resistance on the GI tract.

Table 9.22 Fasting Glucose Ranges	
Normal range	70-99 mg/dl
Ideal range	80-99 mg/dl
Prediabetes	100-125 mg/dl
Diabetes	126 and above on more than one reading

Table 9.23 Fasting Insulin Ranges	
Normal range	3-22 mIU/L
Ideal range	3-4 mIU/L
Early intervention range hyperinsulinemia	>10 mIU/L
Pathological range hyperinsulinemia	>22 mIU/L

Transaminases, Alkaline Phosphatase And Gamma Glutamyl Transpeptidase

Transaminases are elevated in inflammatory states while alkaline phosphatase and GGT are generally signs of biliary stasis. I find that average healthy transaminase levels range from the high teens to the mid twenties. Transaminases do not need to be elevated in the pathological ranges to be indicators of liver disease. A 2004 study of 94,533 men and 47,522 women researched the predictive value of normal range liver function tests. The article, which was published in the *British Medical Journal,* showed people with slightly increased transaminase levels, but still within the normal range, had higher risk for mortality from liver diseases over an eight year follow-up.[130]

Table 9.24 Slightly Elevated (Normal Range) Transaminases Compared To Levels Less Than 20 IU/L And Adjusted Relative Risk Of Death From Liver Disease

	AST 20-29 IU/L	AST 30-39 IU/L	ALT 20-29 IU/L	ALT 30-39 IU/L
Men	2.5	8.0	2.9	9.5
Women	3.3	18.2	3.8	6.6

Based on these findings and others, the American College of Gastroenterology published new guidelines for transaminase normal ranges. They state that a true healthy normal ALT level ranges from 29 to 33 IU/l for males and 19 to 25 IU/l for females. They recommend that levels above this should be assessed.[187]

Chronic unexplained "transaminitis" has been reported in about 40% of adult and 60% of pediatric celiac patients compared to 0.5% of the general population.[131,132] Elimination of gluten from the diet will usually normalize transaminase levels in these individuals. Always order screening serum tests for celiac disease (anti-gliadin antibody IgA and IgG, and/or anti-tissue transglutaminase IgA and IgG) when other causes of hepatic disease are not found in patients with elevated transaminases.

Some authorities consider a GGT below 15 to be a possible indicator of hypothyroidism, hypothalamic malfunction and/or very low levels of magnesium.[133,189]

Complete Blood Count (CBC)

The CBC is a good screening test for anemia due to GI blood loss, malabsorption, dietary deficiencies (iron, B_{12}, folate) etc. I follow-up a low MCV with a ferritin level. Chronic iron deficiency anemia is a common presenting sign of upper GI malabsorption such as celiac disease and other gluten reactivity states. I consider vitamin B_{12} and folate problems when the MCV reaches 93 um^3 and follow-up with a NHI (discussed above.)

Albumin, Globulin, Total Protein

I find that low or low-normal protein levels are often found in hypo/achlorhydria (especially when the anion gap is high) as well as in pancreatic insufficiency. These test values may also be low in other malabsorptive states or in cases of low dietary intake of protein.

Serum Calcium And Magnesium

In my experience, these minerals will test low or low-normal when malabsorption is present, especially with low gastric HCl output which may be secondary to H. pylori induced gastritis or proton pump inhibitor use. A low serum albumin, as in hepatic or renal disease, will decrease the serum calcium value.

Urine Specimens

Lactulose-mannitol intestinal permeability test (test for "leaky gut syndrome")

As discussed in Chapter 4, optimal control of paracellular and transcellular permeability is essential to mucosal and systemic health. These epithelial barriers are in place to prevent absorption of bacterial and dietary antigens which induce antibody production, cytokine release and resultant inflammation, autoimmunity and even multiple organ failure.[134,135,136] Infants have a hyperpermeable intestinal mucosa, perhaps to allow for intact absorption of the immunoglobulins in colostrum.[137] Seventy-two full-term, healthy neonates were divided into two dietary categories—exclusively breast-fed or formula fed. Intestinal permeability decreased faster in breast-fed babies than in those fed bovine formulas.[138] Children with functional abdominal pain syndrome and IBS have evidence of low-grade GI inflammation and increased intestinal permeability.[139] A serious pathological effect of this altered permeability, according to the *Annals of the New York Academy of Science*, is that early dietary intake of bovine insulin (formula feeding of infants) may break down neonatal tolerance to self-insulin—leading to anti-insulin antibody production. In fact, intestinal immune activation and increased gut permeability are associated with type 1 diabetes.[140]

HIV positive persons suffer from intestinal hyperpermeability and villous atrophy which becomes normalized with highly active antiretroviral therapy (HAART).[141] Intestinal hyperpermeability is also induced by food allergy and in turn increases the formation of food-immune reactions.[142]

IBS and IBD patients have more mast cells in the intestine than controls.[143] Mast cells produce and release inflammatory mediators upon activation and are in proximity to intestinal neurons.

Mast cells are key modulators of intestinal motility and intestinal hyperpermeability.[144] Patients with postinfectious IBS have chronic mucosal immunologic dysregulation, altered intestinal permeability and motility.[145]

Acute pancreatitis,[146] bacterial overgrowths and viral infections, medications, alcohol abuse and stress can all induce intestinal hyperpermeability.[147]

Chronic psychological stress elevates CRH and mast cell activity, impairing host defense mechanisms and increasing intestinal permeability.[148]

Description of the test: The test requires an overnight fast. No food, drink or water should be taken after 11 PM on the night before testing. The next morning, after a baseline urine test, mannitol and lactulose – two non-metabolized sugars – are taken as a drink. Urine is then collected over a six hour period. Mannitol is well absorbed by the brush border and—in the post-drink urine sample—serves as a marker of the transcellular route of absorption. Lactulose is poorly absorbed which—in the post-drink urine sample—gives it value as a marker of paracellular absorption. A higher lactulose to mannitol ratio indicates hyperpermeability. A low level of mannitol recovery is an indicator of brush border malabsorption.

Natural therapy: Polyunsaturated fatty acids (GLA, AA, EPA and DHA) are effective in supporting barrier integrity and reducing IL-4 mediated hyperpermeability.[149]

Bifidobacter infantis culture has been found to normalize or prevent changes in the intestinal permeability of mice.[150,151] In IBS-D patients, probiotic treatment decreased small bowel hyperpermeability and mean global IBS scores significantly.[152] Saccharomyces boulardii partially corrected hyperpermeability in Crohn's disease patients in remission, despite the fact that they were taking mesalamine, azathioprine, or prednisone—all potent inducers of hyperpermeability.[153]

The expected rise in small intestinal permeability after administration of indomethacin (an NSAID) was significantly prevented by the addition of 5 g of recombinant human lactoferrin, compared to indomethacin and placebo.[154] A partially hydrolysed and dried product of Pacific white fish had a similar significant protective affect.[155] Lactoferrin also normalized permeability due to the bacterial endotoxin lipopolysaccharide.[156] Ingested lactoferrin is absorbed in the small bowel.[157]

Glutamine is effective in both the prevention and treatment of intestinal hyperpermeabiilty.[158,159]

The fermentable carbohydrate in common beans (black bean, navy bean) is a source for butyric acid production in the colon.[160] Butyrate has a rapid normalizing effect on intestinal permeability in rats.[161] The

TABLE 9.25 SELECTED MAST-CELL MEDIATORS AND THEIR ACTIONS	
Mediator	**Action**
Histamine	Vasodilation, angiogenesis, mitogenesis, pain
Serotonin	Vasoconstriction, pain
Chemokines	Chemoattraction and tissue infiltration of leukocytes
Metalloproteinases	Tissue damage
Phospholipases	Generation of arachidonic acid
Corticotropin-releasing factor	Inflammation, vasodilation
Bradykinin	Inflammation, pain, vasodilation
Endorphins	Analgesia
Endothelin and renin	Vasoconstriction
Somatostatin	Suppresses secretion of GI peptides
Substance P	Inflammation, pain
VIP and Nitric oxide	Vasodilation
IL-1, 2, 3, 4, 5, 6, 8,10,13,16,17 32	Inflammation, leukocyte migration, pain
IFN-g; TNF-a, TGF-b	Inflammation, leukocyte proliferation, activation
Leukotriene B4	Leukocyte chemotaxis

mechanism may be modulation of lipoxygenase and cyclo-oxygenase (COX).[162] Curcumin acts by a similar mechanism.[163] In contrast, typical NSAIDS inhibit COX and the production of gastroprotective prostaglandins, leading to increased intestinal permeability.[164]

Drug therapy: Enteragam is a bovine serum immunoglobulin containing prescription product designed to bind bacterial pathogens and allow for healing of intestinal hyperpermeability. It has been shown to improve symptoms in patients with HIV or diarrhea-predominant irritable bowel syndrome. [166]

Gastric Specimens

Gastric String Test: Rapid, Inexpensive, Gastric pH Screening

Description of the test capsule: This low tech, in office device is a weighted gelatin capsule containing a seventy cm coil of cotton floss. One end of the floss extends through a small hole in the capsule. A separate pH reagent-coated wand and color chart are included in the test kit. Periodically this test becomes unavailable due to FDA related issues.

See Chapter 13 for treatment of hypochlorhydria.

Heidelberg Radiotelemetry Test: Definitive Gastric pH Testing

This test employs a radiotelemetry capsule which communicates with a computer to provide a continuous gastric pH analysis. A limited number of clinics do this testing, but equipment is available (Heidelberg International, Inc., Norcross, GA.) After being carefully calibrated, the capsule is typically tied to a length of floss and tethered to the patient's cheek by a piece of dermal tape. The capsule can also be "untethered," but this requires extra post-procedure monitoring for complete evacuation of the capsule. Once swallowed, the capsule reads the pH over a period of 60-90 minutes. Immediate information is provided to assess frank hyperchlorhydria, hypochlorhydria, or achlorhydria. Longer tests, with multiple challenges of super-saturated bicarbonate solution, are required for hidden hypochlorhydria, pyloric insufficiency, etc. Other substances can be tested (such as bitters, hydrochloric acid, herbs) to ascertain effects on gastric re-acidification.

Procedure: An overnight water-only fast of ten hours duration precedes the test. No water should be consumed for one hour previous to testing. If possible the patient should also have discontinued use of proton pump inhibitors, H2-blockers, antibiotics, or antihistamine agents at least a week preceding testing. The patient is screened about dysphagia as above (gastric string test). The capsule is either swallowed untethered or it is first tied to floss, then swallowed and the proximal end affixed to the patient's cheek, with micropore tape. A device worn around the patient's neck allows the capsule to interface with the computer. An initial reading higher than pH 3 indicates hypochlorhydria. A reading above 6 indicates achlorhydria. As with the gastric string test, the test may be concluded or a 200-400 mg tablet of caffeine may be given to see if re-acidification occurs within 30 minutes (a sign of some parietal cell reserve.) Should the ambient pH be determined to be below pH 3, a series of up to five bicarbonate challenges (5cc of super saturated H2CO3) is administered. The amount of time and the resultant pH after re-acidification are seen on an ongoing graphic readout. Progressively longer re-acidification times or failure of gastric re-acidification indicates "hidden hypochlorhydria" and various other graphed patterns give the suggestion of pyloric insufficiency, or other gastric dysfunction, for further workup.

Esophagogastroduodenoscopy (EGD)

EGD or "upper endoscopy" allows for gross visualization and biopsy of the esophagus, stomach and the first two portions of the duodenum. Biopsy of the duodenum provides the "gold standard" of diagnosis for celiac disease (employing the revised Marsh criteria.) Interventions such as banding of esophageal varices, dilation of stenotic areas and destruction of webs and rings are also possible with this technology.

Colonoscopy

Colonoscopy provides gross visualization and biopsy of the entire colon, ileocecal valve and the terminal ileum. Interventions such as polypectomy are performed via colonoscopy or flexible sigmoidoscopy. Colonoscopic biopsy is the only current method for diagnosing microscopic colitis, a cause of copious, non-bloody diarrhea.

According to Charapata and Mertz, physicians order endoscopic procedures in 67% of IBS patients with diarrhea and in 46% with constipation. This may be excessive.[167] Using non-invasive testing, such as calprotectin, may decrease the necessity of endoscopic procedures in these cases.

---

1 Vaishnavi, C et al *Jpn J Infect Dis.* 2008 Jan;61(1):1-4.
2 Jobst D, Kraft, K. *Mycoses.* 2006 Sep;49(5):415-20.
3 Evengard, B et al *Scan J Gastroent.* 2007;42:1514-1515.
4 Liu, CH et al *Zhonghua Er Ke Za Zhi.* 2007 Jun;45(6):450-4.
5 Petitpierre, M et al *Ann Allergy.* 1985 Jun;54(6):538-40.
6 Southern, P et al *PLoS ONE.* 2008; 3(4): e2067.
7 Mendling, W et al *Mycoses.* 1998;41 Suppl 2:23-5.
8 Reed, BD et al *J Womens Health (Larchmt).* 2003 Dec;12(10):979-89.
9 Veselov AIa, Ruchkin EI, *Antibiot Med Biotekhnol.* 1987 Oct;32(10):785-9.
10 Husebye, E *Chemotherapy.* 2005;51 Suppl 1:1-22.
11 Williams, C et al *Best Pract Res Clin Gastroenterol.* 2001 Jun;15(3):511-21.
12 Bukharin, OV et al *Zh Mikrobiol Epidemiol Immunobiol.* 2002 Sep-Oct;(5):45-8.
13 http://prod.hopkins-abxguide.org/pathogens/bacteria/escherichia_coli.
14 Long, KZ et al *J Infect Dis.* 2006 Nov 1;194(9):1217-25.
15 Lipski, E (2004) *Digestive Wellness :McGraw-Hill Professional*
16 Saputo, L (1999) *Optimal Digestion* (N. Fass and T.W. Nichols, Ed). New York, NY: Harper Collins.
17 Galland, L (2008) *Gastrointestinal Dysregulation: Connections to Chronic Dis*eases, Gig Harbor, WA, Institute for Functional Medicine
18 Plummer, NT *Plant Antimicrobials*—Pharmax Technical Monograph: Bellevue, Washington:2002.
19 Plummer, NT *Plant Antimicrobials*—Pharmax Technical Monograph: Bellevue, Washington:2002.
20 Mahady GB, Pendland SL, Stoia A, Hamill FA, Fabricant D, Dietz BM, Chadwick LR. In vitro susceptibility of Helicobacter pylori to botanical extracts used traditionally for the treatment of gastrointestinal disorders. *Phytother Res.* 2005 Nov;19(11):988-91.
21 Oussalah, M; Caillet, S; Lacroix,M Mechanism of action of Spanish oregano, Chinese cinnamon, and savory essential oils against cell membranes and walls of Escherichia coli O157:H7 and Listeria monocytogenes. *Journal-of-food-protection.* 2006 May; 69(5): 1046-1055.
22 Ooi, LSM; Li-YaoLan; Kam-SheungLau; Wang-Hua; Wong, EYL; Ooi, VEC Antimicrobial activities of cinnamon oil and cinnamaldehyde from the Chinese medicinal herb Cinnamomum cassia Blume. *American-Journal-of-Chinese-Medicine.* 2006; 34(3): 511-522
23 Bollinger, RR et al *Immunology.* 2003 Aug;109(4):580-7.
24 Brandtzaeg, P et al *Vaccine.* 2007 Jul 26;25(30):5467-84.
25 Madden, JA; Plummer, SF; Tang, J; Garaiova, I; Plummer, NT; Herbison, M; Hunter, J O; Shimada, T; Cheng, L; Shirakawa,T Effect of probiotics on preventing disruption of the intestinal microflora following antibiotic therapy: a double-blind, placebo-controlled pilot study. *Int-Immunopharmacol.* 2005 Jun; 5(6): 1091-7.

26 Belmonte,L; Coeffier, M; Le-Pessot, F; Miralles Barrachina, O; Hiron, M; Leplingard, A; Lemeland, JF; Hecketsweiler, B; Daveau, M; Ducrotte, P; Dechelotte, P Effects of glutamine supplementation on gut barrier, glutathione content and acute phase response in malnourished rats during inflammatory shock. *World-J-Gastroenterol*. 2007 May 28; 13(20): 2833-40.

27 Sukhotnik, I; Khateeb, K; Mogilner, JG; Helou, H; Lurie, M; Coran, AG; Shiloni, E Dietary glutamine supplementation prevents mucosal injury and modulates intestinal epithelial restitution following ischemia-reperfusion injury in the rat. *Dig-Dis-Sci*. 2007 Jun; 52(6): 1497-504.

28 Peng, X; Yan, H; You, Z; Wang, P; Wang,S Effects of enteral supplementation with glutamine granules on intestinal mucosal barrier function in severe burned patients. *Burns*. 2004 Mar; 30(2): 135-9.

29 Daniele, B: Perrone, F: Gallo, C: Pignata, S: De Martino, S: De Vivo, R: Barletta, E: Tambaro, R: Abbiati, R: D'Agostino, L Oral glutamine in the prevention of fluorouracil induced intestinal toxicity: a double blind, placebo controlled, randomised trial. *Gut*. 2001 Jan; 48(1): 28-33.

30 Pogribna, M; Freeman, JP; Paine, D; Boudreau, MD Effect of Aloe vera whole leaf extract on short chain fatty acids production by Bacteroides fragilis, Bifidobacterium infantis and Eubacterium limosum. *Lett-Appl-Microbiol*. 2008 May; 46(5): 575-80.

31 Duarte, J; Vinderola, G; Ritz, B; Perdigon, G; Matar, C Immunomodulating capacity of commercial fish protein hydrolysate for diet supplementation *Immunobiology*. 2006; 211(5): 341-50.

32 Mehraj, V et al *PLoS ONE*. 2008;3(11):e3680.

33 Garcia, LS; Bruckner, DA. (1997) *Diagnostic medical parasitology. 3rd ed.* Wash, D.C.:Am. Soc. Micro.

34 Kaya, S et al *Turkiye Parazitol Derg*. 2007;31(3):184-7.

35 Al FD, Hokelek M, *Turkiye Parazitol Derg*. 2007;31(1):28-36

36 Force M, Sparks WS, Ronzio RA. Inhibition of enteric parasites by emulsified oil of oregano in vivo. *Phytother Res*. 2000 May;14(3):213-4.

37 Personal conversation with Dr. Rami at Diagnostechs lab.

38 Stark, D et al *J Travel Med*. 2007 Jan-Feb;14(1):72-3.

39 Stark, D et al *Int J Parasitol*. 2007 Jan;37(1):11-20.

40 Vandenberg, O et al *Pediatr Infect Dis J*. 2007 Jan;26(1):88-90.

41 Hawrelak, J *Alt Med Rev* 2003 May;8(2):129-142.

42 Fayer, R et al *J Zoo Wildl Med*. 2006 Dec;37(4):492-7.

43 Hanson KL, Cartwirght CE, *J Clin Microbiol*. 2001 Feb;39(2):474-7.

44 Shukla, G et al *Dig Dis Sci*. 2008 Oct;53(10):2671-9.

45 Di Almeida, I et al *Parasitol Res*. 2007 Jul;101(2):443-52.

46 Soffar SA, Mokhtar GM *J Egypt Soc Parasitol*. 1991 Aug;21(2):497-502.

47 Agarwal, AK et al *J Ethnopharmacol*. 1997 May;56(3):233-6.

48 Long, KZ et al *Pediatrics*. 2007 Oct;120(4):e846-55.

49 Long, KZ et al *J Infect Dis*. 2006 Nov 1;194(9):1217-25.

50 Walker, N et al *J Hosp Infect*. 2006 Jun;63(2):167-9.

51 Perry C. et al *J Hosp Infect*. 2001 Jul;48(3):238-41.

52 Dial, S et al *CMAJ*. 2006 Sep 26;175(7):745-8.

53 Fasano, A , *Ann N Y Acad Sci*. 2000;915:214-22.

54 Surawicz, CM , *Best Pract Res Clin Gastroenterol*. 2003 Oct;17(5):775-83.

55 McFarland, LV, *Am J Gastroenterol*. 2006 Apr;101(4):812-22.

56 Plummer, S; Weaver, MA; Harris, JC; Dee, P; Hunter, J Clostridium difficile pilot study:effects of probiotic supplementation on the incidence of C. difficile diarrhoea. *Int-Microbiol.* 2004 Mar; 7(1): 59-62

57 Shahverdi, AR; Monsef Esfahani, HR; Tavasoli, F; Zaheri, A; Mirjani, R Trans-Cinnamaldehyde from Cinnamomum zeylanicum Bark Essential Oil Reduces the Clindamycin Resistance of Clostridium difficile in vitro. *Journal-of-food-science.* 2007 Jan-Feb; 72(1): S055-S058

58 Hemoccult brand fecal occult blood screening test 2001 Aug: Beckman Coulter, Inc

59 Langhorst, J et al *Am J Gastroenterol.* 2008 Jan;103(1):162-9.

60 Langhorst, J et al *Inflamm Bowel Dis.* 2005 Dec;11(12):1085-91.

61 Schoepfer, AM et al *Inflamm Bowel Dis.* 2008 Jan;14(1):32-9.

62 Hidaka, M et al *Nippon Shokakibyo Gakkai Zasshi.* 2000 Feb;97(2):161-9.

63 Van der sluys Veer, A et al *Dig Dis Sci.* 1998 Mar;43(3):590-5.

64 Hemrika, MH et al *Neth J Med.* 1989 Apr;34(3-4):174-81.

65 Costongs, GM et al *Clin Chim Acta.* 1987 Aug 14;167(2):125-34.

66 Dick, W, *Fortschr Med.* 1982 Jul 8;100(26):1230-4.

67 Tibble, J et al *Gut* 2001 Sept;49:402-8.

68 Bret A Lashner How useful is fecal calprotectin for the diagnosis of IBD and colorectal cancer? *Nature Clinical Practice Gastroenterology & Hepatology* (2008) 5, 16-17

69 Kristinsson J, Nygaard K, Aadland E, Barstad S, Sauar J, Hofstad B, Stray N, Stallemo A, Haug B, Ugstad M, Tøn H, Fuglerud P. Screening of first degree relatives of patients operated for colorectal cancer: evaluation of fecal calprotectin vs. hemoccult II. *Digestion.* 2001;64(2):104-10.

70 D'Inca, R et al *Am J Gastroenterol* 2008;103:2007-2014

71 Van der sluys Veer, A et al *Scand J Gastroenterol Suppl.* 1999;230:106-10.

72 Choudhary, S et al *J Gastroenterol Hepatol.* 1996 Apr;11(4):311-8.

73 Kampanis, P et al *Ann Clin Biochem.* 2008 Nov 13.

74 Lenander-Lumikari, M et al *Arch Oral Biol.* 2000 May;45(5):347-54.

75 Fukushima, Y et al *Int J Food Microbiol.* 1998 Jun 30;42(1-2):39-44.

76 Scholtens, PA et al *J Nutr.* 2008 Jun;138(6):1141-7.

77 Arau'jo, ED et al *Acta Cir Bras.* 2005;20 Suppl 1:178-84.

78 Sakamoto, S et al *Eur J Nutr.* 2007 Oct;46(7):391-6

79 Usuki, S et al *Nutrition & Metabolism* 2007, 4:25

80 Jardine, M, et al *J Pediatr Gastroenterol Nutr.* 2006 Nov;43(5):610-2

81 Olivares, JL et al *J Am Coll Nutr.* 2002 Apr;21(2):109-13.

82 Gale, EA, *Diabetologia.* 2002 Apr;45(4):588-94.

83 Vinetz, J http://prod.hopkins-abxguide.org/pathogens/parasitesentamoeba_histolytica

84 Ankri S, Mirelman, D, *Microbes Infect.* 1999 Feb;1(2):125-9.

85 Richter, J et al *Cas Lek Cesk.* 2003;142(11):665-9.

86 Inaba T et al. Eur J Clin Invest. 2005 Mar;35(3):214-9.Also on the topic of 86: CinesDB, Liebman H, Stasi R. *Semin Hematol.* 2009 Jan;46(1 Suppl 2):S2-14.

87 de Bortoli, N et al *Am J Gastroenterol.* 2007 May;102(5):951-6.

88 Di Mario, F et al *Dig Liver Dis.* 2003 Oct;35(10):706-10.

89 Wada,T et al *Scand J Gastroenterol.* 1999 Mar;34(3):238-43.

90 Di Mariao, F et al *Helicobacter.* 2007 Jun;12(3):238-43.

91 Okuda, M et al *J Infect Chemother.* 2005 Dec;11(6):265-9.

92 Nakayama K, Otsuki K, Yakuwa K et al, *J Obstet Gynaecol Res.* 2008 Dec;34(6):931-4.

93 Paraschos, S et al *Antimicrob Agents Chemother.* 2007 Feb;51(2):551-9.
94 Stamatis G, Kyriazopoulos P, Golegou S, Basayiannis A, Skaltsas S, Skaltsa H. In vitro anti-Helicobacter pylori activity of Greek herbal medicines. *J Ethnopharmacol.* 2003 Oct;88(2-3):175-9.
95 Maree Gleeson, Sharron T Hall, Warren A McDonald, Adrian J Flanagan and Robert L Clancy Salivary IgA subclasses and infection risk in elite swimmers *Immunology and Cell Biology* 1999 77, 351–355.
96 Markell, EK Medical Parasitology 1999;Saunders, Phil. PA: 270-276.
97 Mello, CM et al *J Pediatr Surg.* 1992 Sep;27(9):1229-30.
98 Varga, M et al *Roum Arch Microbiol Immunol.* 2001 Oct-Dec;60(4):359-69.
99 CDC *MMWR Morb Mortal Wkly Rep.* 2000 Apr 7;49(13):278-81.
100 Jurcic, JG et al *Bone Marrow Transplant.* 1994 Apr;13(4):491-3.
101 Crompton, DW, *Soc Trop Med Hyg.* 1986;80(5):697-705.
102 Long, KZ et al *Pediatrics.* 2007 Oct;120(4):e846-55.
103 Okeniyi, JA et al *J Med Food.* 2007 Mar;10(1):194-6.
104 Kermanshai R, *Phytochemistry.* 2001 Jun;57(3):427-35.
105 El Garhy MF, Mahmoud L, *J Egypt Soc Parasitol.* 2002 Dec;32(3):893-900.
106 www.cdc.gov/ncidoc/dpd/parasites/cysticercosis/factsht
107 Díaz Obregón D et al *Rev Gastroenterol Peru.* 2004 Oct-Dec;24(4):323-7.
108 Sukul, NC et al *Forsch Komplementarmed Klass Naturheilkd.* 2005 Aug;12(4):202-5.
109 Caner, A et al *Exp Parasitol.* 2008 May;119(1):173-9.
110 Bany, J et al *Pol J Vet Sci.* 2003;6(3 Suppl):6-8.
111 McNally, P *GI/Liver Secrets* 1996 Hanley and Belfus, Inc. Phila, PA.
112 Tursi, A et al *Dig Dis Sci.* 2006 Mar;51(3):461-5.
113 Carrara, M et al *Eur Rev Med Pharmacol Sci.* 2008 May-Jun;12(3):197-202.
114 Parodi, A et al *Clin Gastroenterol Hepatol.* 2008 Jul;6(7):759-64.
115 Weinstock, LB et al *Dig Dis Sci.* 2008 May;53(5):1252-6.
116 Sabate, JM et al *Obes Surg.* 2008 Apr;18(4):371-7.
117 Tursi, A et al *Am J Gastroentero.* 2003 Apr;98(4):839-43.
118 Application guide: Genova Diagnostics 2006 www.genovadiagnostics.com
119 Application guide: Genova Diagnostics 2006 www.genovadiagnostics.com
120 Barrett, JS et al *World J Gastroentero.* 2008 Aug 28;14(32):5020-4.
121 Kline, RM et al *J Pediatr.* 2001 Jan;138(1):125-8.
122 Logan AC, Beaulne TM.. *Altern Med Rev.* 2002 Oct;7(5):410-7.
123 Elaine Gottschall, *Breaking the Vicious Cycle: Intestinal Health Through Diet,* 1994, Kirkton Press Ltd, Ontario, Canada.
124 Campbell-Mcbride N, *Gut and Psychology Syndrome*, 2004, International Nutrition, Inc., Middle River, MD.
125 Pimentel M, *A New IBS Solution*, 2006, Health Point Press, Sherman Oaks, CA.
126 Lauritano, EC et al *Am J Gastroenterol.* 2008 Aug;103(8):2031-5.
127 Bills T, Spatz L, *Am J Clin Pathol.* 1977 Aug;68(2):263-7.
128 Phelip, JM et al *Inflamm Bowel Dis.* 2008 Feb;14(2):242-8.
129 Lashner, BA et al *Gastroenterology.* 1989 Aug;97(2):255-9.
130 Kim, HC et al *BMJ* 2004 Apr 24;328(7446):983.
131 Bardella MT et al *Hepatology.* 1999 Mar;29(3):654-7.
132 Rubio Tapia A, Murray JA. *Minerva Med.* 2008 Dec;99(6):595-604.
133 Ray Sahelian, M.D. http://www.raysahelian.com/ggt.html

134 Swank GM, Deitch EA, *World J Surg.* 1996 May;20(4):411-7.
135 Fasano, A *Am J Pathol.* 2008 Nov;173(5):1243-52.
136 Fasano, A *Am J Pathol.* 2008 Nov;173(5):1243-52.
137 Westerbeek, EA et al *Clin Nutr.* 2006 Jun;25(3):361-8.
138 Catassi, C et al *J Pediatr Gastroenterol Nutr.* 1995 Nov;21(4):383-6.
139 Schulman, RJ et al *J Pediatr.* 2008 Nov;153(5):646-50.
140 Vaarala, O, *Ann N Y Acad Sci.* 2006 Oct;1079:350-9.
141 Eppel, HJ et al *Gut.* 2008 Nov 4.
142 Farhadi, A et al *J Gastroenterol Hepatol.* 2003 May;18(5):479-97.
143 Rijnierse A, et al *Pharmacol Ther.* 2007 Nov;116(2):207-35.
144 Farhadi, A et al *World J Gastroenterol.* 2007 Jun 14;13(22):3027-30.
145 Dupont, AW *Clin Infect Dis.* 2008 Feb 15;46(4):594-9.
146 Liu, H et al *Pancreas.* 2008 Mar;36(2):192-6.
147 Galland L, Lafferty H, *Gastrointestinal Dysregulation,* 2008 p. 39 Inst for Func Med, Gig Harbor, WA.
148 Teitelbaum, AA et al *Am J Physiol Gastrointest Liver Physiol.* 2008 Sep;295(3): G452-9.
149 Willemsen, LE et al *Eur J Nutr.* 2008 Jun;47(4):183-91.
150 Ewaschuk, JB et al *Am J Physiol Gastrointest Liver Physiol.* 2008 Nov;295(5): G1025-34.
151 Southcott, E et al *Dig Dis Sci.* 2008 Jul;53(7):1837-41.
152 Zeng, J et al *Alimen Pharmacol Ther.* 2008 Oct 15;28(8):994-1002.
153 Garcia Vilela, E. et al *Scand J Gastroenterol.* 2008;43(7):842-8.
154 Troost, F et al *Eur J Clin Nutr.* 2003 Dec; 57(12): 1579-85.
155 Marchbank, T et al *Aliment Pharmacol Ther`.* 2008 Jun 26.
156 Hirotani, Y et al *Yakugaku Zashi.* 2008 Sep;128(9):1363-8.
157 Troost, F et al *J Nutr.* 2002 Sep; 132(9): 2597-600.
158 Kouznetsova, L et al *J Parenter Enteral Nutr.* 1999 May-Jun; 23(3): 136-9
159 Li, N et al *J. Nutr. Biochem.* 2003 Jul;14(7):401-8.
160 Hangen L, Bennink M, *Nutr Cancer.* 2002;44(1):60-5.
161 Suzuki, T et al *Br J Nutr.* 2008 Aug;100(2):297-305.
162 Ohata, A et al *Nutrition.* 2005 Jul-Aug;21(7-8):838-47.
163 Rao. CV, *Adv Exp Med Biol.* 2007;595:213-26.
164 Leone, S et al *Curr Top Med Chem.* 2007;7(3):265-75.
165 Banan, A et al *Free Radic Biol Med.* 2001 Feb 1; 30(3): 287-98.
166 Petschow BW, 2014 May 24;7:181-90
167 Charapata C, Mertz H,, *Neurogastroenterol Motil.* 2006 Mar;18(3):211-6.
168 Branda J et al *Clin Infect Dis* (2006) April; 42(7): 972-978
169 Lasson A et al *J Crohns Colitis.* 2015 Jan;9(1):26-32.
170 Raftery, Tet al *Dig Dis Sci.* 2015 Aug;60(8):2427-35.
171 Burri, E et al *Clinica Chimica Acta* 2013 Feb; (416): 41-47.
172 Kpoylov, U et al *Inflamm Bowel Dis.* 2014 20 (4):742-756.
173 Lehmann, FS et al *Ther Adv Gastroenterol.* 2015; 8(1) 23-36.
174 Lamb, CA et al *Frontline Gastroenterol.* 2011 Jan; 2(1):13-18.
175 Fan, K et al *J. Clin Microbiol.* 1993; (31):2233-2235.
176 Sunanda, V et al *Am J Gastroenterol.* 2003; (98):1309-14.
177 Eigner, U et al *Diagn Microbiol Infect Dis.* 2017 Feb; (17)30035-4. [Epub ahead of print]

178 Chen, O L et al *Ann Clin Microbiol Antimicrob.* 2014 Jul 15;13:30.
179 Croxatto, A et al *FEMS Microbiol.* 2012 (36):380-407
180 Ikryannikova, et al *Clin Microbiol Infect.* 2013 19(11):1066-71
181 Mellman, A et al, *J Clin Microbiol.* 2009 (47):3732-34
182 Castanheira, M et al, *J Clin Microbiol.* 2013 (51):117-24
183 Gingras, B et al, *Intr Journal of Hum Nutr & Funct Med.* 2014:2(1);1
184 Pirnay, JP et al, *Crit. Care* 2000;4(4):255-61.
185 Klaus, G et al, *Gastroenterol Rept.*2017 Jan 27; 1–7.
186 Halblaub, JM et al, *Clin. Lab.* 2004;50(9-10):551-7.
187 Kwo, PY et al, *Am J Gastroenterol.* 18-45 doi:10.1038/ajg.2016.517, s.l.:, 2017, Vol.112 (Jan 2017).
188 Whalen MB, Massidda O, *J Infect Dev Ctries.* 2015 Jul 4;9(6):674-8.
189 Kwo Y et al, *Am J Gastroenterol.* 2017; 112:18–35; doi:10.1038/ajg.2016.517; published online 20 December 2016
190 Whalen M, Massidda O, *J Infect Dev Ctries* 2015; 9(6):674-678.

Chapter 10

Diets For The Treatment Of Gastrointestinal Conditions

The Essential Role Of Diet And Nutrition For Gastrointestinal Disorders

I have found that diet and nutrition are key features in symptom reduction and/or resolution of functional gastrointestinal disorders. In previous years, many patients would tell me that their gastroenterologist had said "diet has nothing to do with Crohn's disease" or that the same was said about irritable bowel syndrome. Nearly 2/3 of patients with IBS believe their symptoms are food-related.[4]

Until the late 1980s, even classic conditions known to be associated with diet were virtually ignored by conventional specialists. Celiac serology and Marsh criteria based biopsies were rarely considered to be part of a differential for GI symptoms. Celiac was considered rare with an estimated prevalence of 0.03% of the U.S. population.[15] Because of this skewed belief, the diagnosis typically was made only after an average of 10 years of medical visits. Now we know that celiac disease affects about 1% of the population. A work-up for celiac disease is now part of any standard GI workup.[14]

Much has changed with respect to diet in mainstream medicine. The low FODMAP diet is well researched for IBS and most physicians recognize its value. Even the Specific Carbohydrate Diet has now had some initial studies which have been published in respected peer reviewed journals.

Although inflammatory bowel disease (IBD) and irritable bowel syndrome (IBS) are distinct diseases, there is considerable overlap in many patients. These two conditions can coexist in patients and may be opposite ends of a spectrum.[12,13] This may be the reason I find that in the majority of cases, diets such as the Specific Carbohydrate Diet and the low FODMAP are central in the effective treatment for both diseases.

The Specific Carbohydrate Diet (SCD)

The specific carbohydrate diet was developed by Sidney Haas (a pediatric gastroenterologist) in the 1930s and published in 1951.[1] It became more popular in the 1980s when Elaine Gottschall (biochemist) wrote about an expanded version of the diet in her book *Breaking the Vicious Cycle: Intestinal Health Through Diet.* The diet allows monosaccharides while excluding disaccharides and all but certain polysaccharides. Yogurt fermented for 24 hours is an important component of the diet when tolerated. Commercial yogurt is fermented for 6–8 hours which allows exposure to traces of lactose (a disaccharide not permitted on SCD). Full 24 hour fermentation converts all the lactose to lactic acid.

The SCD is designed to promote restoration of a healthy microbiome.

Included ("legal" foods):[1,2,3]

- Vegetables—especially those that have more amylose (linear-chain polysaccharide) than amylopectin (branched-chain polysaccharide)
- Fruits
- Nut flours
- Certain soaked beans/lentils
- Dry curd cottage cheese
- Firm cheeses (aged at least 30 days)
- Meat
- Poultry
- Fish

- Eggs
- Honey
- Butter
- Oils

Excluded ("illegal" foods)

- Sucrose
- Maltose
- Isomaltose
- Lactose
- Grains
- Potatoes
- Okra
- Corn
- Fluid milk
- Soy
- High lactose soft cheese fermented less than 30 days
- Processed meats
- Dietary additives/preservatives

When beginning this diet, patients with more sensitive digestive tracts may need to cook, peel, and deseed fruits and vegetables as well as avoid legumes. This diet is not designed to be low-carbohydrate and this should be kept in mind especially when working with underweight patients. Winter squash, white jasmine rice and higher intake of medium chain triglycerides as well as long chain and saturated fats may be needed to supply adequate calories to prevent weight loss. Alternatively, I have found that some patients with malabsorption may gain weight when starting the SCD, likely due to improved absorption.

The working hypotheses behind the mechanism of the SCD is that those with IBD and some forms of IBS have brush border destruction (villous and/or microvillous) which prevents proper digestion of disaccharides and foods with a high amylose to amylopectin ratio.[1] Another proposed mechanism suggests that excessive mucus production prevents brush border disaccharidases from reacting with disaccharides and amylopectin leading to carbohydrate malabsorption. As in lactose intolerance and other malabsorption syndromes, this leads to hyperosmolar diarrhea and increased substrate for small intestine bacterial overgrowth. The undigested sugars lead to gas production, bloating and pain secondary to distention of the bowel. Bacterial overgrowth increases glycosidase levels which damage the enterocyte brush border. The microvilli are the site of disaccharidase production and the glycocalyx the site of disaccaridase storage. It is believed that the SCD benefits diversity and/or volume of the GI microbiome and helps to shift it from a pro-inflammatory mode to a more balanced state with decreased intestinal inflammation.[3] The lipopolysaccharide excess underlying this proinflammatory mode was discussed in Chapter 5.

Research studies on the SCD predominantly focus on populations diagnosed with inflammatory bowel disease (IBD). A 2015 case series studied the details of remission induced by the SCD in 50 individuals diagnosed with IBD. 36 were diagnosed with Crohn's disease (CD), 9 with ulcerative colitis (UC), and 5 with indeterminate colitis (IC). Subjects were all diagnosed by a U.S. physician and the diagnosis re-confirmed by a board-certified gastroenterologist specializing in IBD at Rush University. Remission was defined as a Harvey-Bradshaw Index <5 for CD and St Mark's Index <4 for UC and both for IC. Subjects followed the diet for an average of 35.4 months with an average adherence rate of 95%. Sixteen subjects reported occasionally eating some "forbidden foods." Initial improvement occurred within 30 days and complete symptom resolution was experienced by two-thirds of the subjects within 10 months.

A 2016 study took the format of a retrospective chart review for the evaluation of the clinical response to the SCD in 11 pediatric Crohn's patients. Results from strict versus liberalized versions of the SCD were compared.[2] The definition of "liberalized" was "any significant variance from the SCD including one illegal meal more than once every month or the addition of an illegal ingredient on a regular basis."

Results:

- 90% moved up in weight percentile following strict SCD
- 82% had stable or increased height percentiles following strict SCD
- In patients who were less strict, weight loss occurred in 50%

A study at Seattle Children's Hospital also relied on a retrospective chart review. Subjects were 36 children who used SCD as treatment for ulcerative colitis (UC) and Crohn's disease (CD).[3] The mean duration of SCD adherence was 10 months. 46% of those who remained on the diet experienced significant improvements in clinical & inflammatory markers (C reactive protein, erythrocyte sedimentation rate, calprotectin and Crohn's quality of life questionnaire). Improvements in a UC quality of life questionnaire did not reach statistical significance perhaps due to a smaller number of UC subjects in the study compared to CD subjects.

In the CD group, only one patient experienced a flare. C reactive protein (CRP) normalized in 10 of the 14 (71%) and erythrocyte sedimentation rate (ESR) improved in 5 out of 9 (56%) who experienced elevated levels before SCD. Serum albumin increased from a mean of 4.1g/dL to 4.3 g/dL at 4 weeks and also at 6 months. Calprotectin decreased for 6 of 13 (46%) who had their levels checked. Some patients succeeded in discontinuing medications, using the SCD alone for maintenance of remission. Some subjects followed a moderately liberalized version of the diet by including rice, oatmeal, potatoes, or cocoa powder.

A single case report of a 73-yr-old Asian female with ulcerative pancolitis was published in 2015.[4] Prior to the dietary intervention, this subject's condition followed a course of continuous decline in spite of a variety of standard treatments. After 3 months, improvement was noted and by 12 months there was an improved general state; abdominal pain and diarrhea had ceased. Follow-up colonoscopy showed resolution of pancolitis.

The Low FODMAP Diet

The term FODMAP was originally coined by Monash University in Melbourne, Australia.[5] The mnemonic stands for:

- F—fermentable
- O—oligosaccharides
- D—disaccharides
- M—monosaccharides
- A—and
- P—polyols

FODMAPs are poorly absorbed short-chain fermentable carbohydrates (prebiotics) that, in excess, exert osmotic pressure, drawing water into the lumen of the distal small intestine and proximal colon. These prebiotics may also feed small intestine commensals, increasing gas production and symptoms in small intestine bacterial overgrowth (SIBO). This diet has been shown to be effective in as many as 74% of patients with IBS[6] reducing the symptoms of bloating, nausea, abdominal pain and diarrhea. This diet has also been used to reduce symptoms of IBD. A retrospective pilot study produced improvement in approximately half of patients.[5] Oligosaccharides include fructo-oligosaccharides, fructans (such as inulin) and galacto-oligosaccharides. Humans have no digestive mechanism for absorbing fructans. Examples of sources include wheat and onion.

Galacto-oligosaccharides are fermented in the colon because humans do not have α-galactosidase. Examples include:

- Legumes
- Nuts
- Seeds
- Some grains
- Dairy products
- Human milk
- Some commercial infant formulas

Disaccharides include lactose, sucrose, maltose and trehalose. Lactose is poorly absorbed in lactase deficiency and, as discussed under SCD, feeds small intestine commensals in patients with SIBO. Up to 70% of the world's inhabitants have primary lactose deficiency. Typical age of onset is between 2 and 6.[6]

Lactose sources include:

- Dairy products
- Possible additives in breads, cakes, diet products

The major source of monosaccharide is fructose. It is absorbed in the small bowel via GLUT-5 and GLUT-2 transporters. GLUT-2 is more efficient, but requires the presence of glucose for activation. Fructose is more likely to be malabsorbed when consumed in excess of glucose.

Fructose sources include:

- Fruit
- Fruit products
- Honey
- High-fructose sweeteners

Both sucrose and honey are cleaved into fructose and glucose during digestion. Many patients with IBD, IBS and SIBO tolerate honey unless they have a distinct fructose malabsorption syndrome. A breath test is commercially available for diagnosis of fructose malabsorption. This test may be useful for patients who do not improve on the SCD, the SIBO Specific Foodguide or a FODMAP diet that has been liberalized with the use of honey.

Polyols are sugar-alcohols which include mannitol, xylitol, erythritol and sorbitol. These are absorbed by slow passive diffusion since they do not have an active intestinal transport system.

Polyol sources include:

- Certain fruits & vegetables
- Sugar-free chewing gum & other "sugar-free" or "diet" foods

FODMAP are rapidly fermented by colonic bacteria, leading to symptoms of gas, distention, altered motility and abdominal pain.[5,6] Because of increased fructose consumption in the form of fruit juice and high fructose corn syrup, intake of FODMAP has increased in Western diets. A Monash University smart phone application is a useful source of up to date information on the FODMAP content of various foods. FODMAP intake has an additive effect, therefore, considering the total per meal is important for symptom reduction.

The diet is implemented in two phases: an elimination phase for 6-8 weeks followed by gradual reintroduction once symptoms are controlled. Transition to a less restrictive version of the diet is the goal because prebiotics are necessary for the health of the colonic microbiota. Adding foods slowly while monitoring for an increase in symptoms is key to individualizing the diet during this latter phase. Because of the inclusion of grains, I find that this diet, or the Cedars-Sinai diet, is the best choice for strict vegetarians or vegans. Websites for vegan-friendly FODMAP diet guidelines may be useful for these patients. The SCD and the SIBO Specific Foodguide are generally not suitable for these patients.

Possible drawbacks of the low FODMAP diet include difficulties with adherence, reduction in bifidobacteria concentration or absolute abundance of colonic bacteria, reduced total fiber intake and deficient calcium intake. If tolerated, the addition of lactose-free dairy products (discussed above in the SCD section) provides a good source of calcium for these patients.

Research On Low FODMAP Diet And IBS

A meta-analysis of low FODMAP diet treatment for IBS strongly supports efficacy of this approach. Six randomized clinical trials and 16 non-randomized studies were included. Assessment instruments employed were the IBS Symptoms Severity Score (SSS) and the IBS quality of life (QOL) score. There was a significant decrease in SSS scores for those individuals on a low FODMAP diet and a significant improvement in the QOL score. The low FODMAP diet significantly reduced symptom severity for abdominal pain (OR 1.81), bloating (OR 1.75) and overall symptoms (OR 1.81).[7] A systematic review of 6 studies concluded that "a FODMAP-restricted diet may be effective in short-term management of selected patients with IBS".[8]

SIBO Specific Food Guide (SSFG)

I rely on this diet plan to:

1) reduce symptoms in most functional GI disorders
2) induce remission in IBD (Crohn's, ulcerative colitis and microscopic colitis)
3) treat celiac disease or non-celiac gluten intolerance that is non-responsive to a standard gluten-free diet
4) prevent recurrence of SIBO after effective treatment

I believe that handing a patient two different diet guides to follow is never a good idea because it leads to confusion and excessive restriction of foods. Allison Siebecker, ND MSOM has done a great service to the world by synthesizing into one chart the details of the low FODMAP diet, the SCD, some aspects of the Cedars-Sinai diet and her own clinical experience with thousands of SIBO/IBS patients. It is an excellent first choice for treatment of IBD, IBS, celiac disease and SIBO or for those who have not had sufficient symptomatic relief from trials of other diets.[9] A colorful chart of this guide is available at no charge at www.siboinfo.com under the treatment/diet menu. The SSFG encourages the use of carbohydrates that are easily absorbed in the upper small intestine which are less likely to become substrate for overgrown small bowel flora. It is low in starch, fiber, and fermentable fruits and vegetables.

Guidelines include:

- Begin with no beans or raw foods for sensitive patients (these can be added later).
- Begin with peeled, de-seeded vegetables and fruits for sensitive patients.
- Allow at least 4 hours between meals and a 12 hour fast overnight to allow the migrating motor complex (MMC) to function optimally. These guidelines should be overlooked if contraindicated for those who are underweight or have unstable blood sugar levels.
- A handout of a 5 phase introductory SSFG is available for especially sensitive or highly inflamed digestive tracts.

Foods avoided:

- Grains
- Sugars other than honey or liquid stevia extract
- Corn, soy, tubers
- Thickeners—carrageenan, guar gum, xanthan gum
- Mucilaginous foods—flax, chia, seaweed, okra and demulcent herbs
- Beans (lentils, navy and lima beans may be added progressively)

Foods permitted:

Unlimited

- Meat
- Fat
- Lactose-free dairy (if casein is tolerated)
    —Ghee
    —Aged cheeses
    —24 hour yogurt

        To provide a higher calorie content for underweight patients, a base of 50:50 milk/cream may be used.

        For casein sensitivity, a base of coconut milk without added gum thickeners may be use in place of mammalian milk.

Per FODMAP quantity restrictions or Dr. Siebecker's clinical experience

- Vegetables (Although garlic and onion are high FODMAP and therefore not part of this diet, the green portion of a green onion stalk is often well tolerated. Garlic infused oil may be used in cooking as the problematic fructans in garlic remain in the solids of the garlic clove after cooking garlic in oil. Garlic powder cannot be used on this diet.)
- Fruit
- Nuts/seeds
- Winter squash
- Sweeteners

Foods with special explanations:

- Honey
  - —Typically excluded on a low FODMAP diet, but permitted on SIBO Specific Food Guide
  - —Certain varieties (for example, clover honey) have been permitted on the premise that they have a favorable glucose to fructose ratio and therefore are low FODMAP
- Bone broth
  - —Bone broth made from whole bones containing cartilage is not permitted due to glycosaminoglycans content
  - —Bone broth made from marrow bones is permitted

Consider individualizing the diet. The following 5 categories may be problematic for some even though they are included for most patients. I call these the "high five":*

- Dairy
- Eggs
- Raw fruits and vegetables
- Too much fruit or honey
- Nuts and seeds

After several months of remission, patients may carefully, one at a time, reintroduce moderate and eventually high FODMAP items back into the diet—with a careful eye for aggravation of symptoms. Working with a knowledgeable SSFG physician or nutritionist is highly advised for best results during all phases of the diet.

Cedars-Sinai/Low Fermentation Diet

Dr. Mark Pimentel and his team at Cedars-Sinai medical center have developed a dietary protocol for prevention of relapse after successful treatment of SIBO.[10] Of the four diets described in this chapter, this is the simplest to follow and supports the broadest choice of foods. It is a good choice for vegetarians, vegans and patients who do not want many nutritional restrictions.

---

*This is a slight expansion of a concept from scdlifestyle.com originally and colorfully called "the four horsemen of the apocalypse".

Key features are:

Food timing to promote motility

The recommendation is to space meals at least 4 hours apart to allow migrating motor complex production of "cleansing waves/housekeeping waves" in the small intestine. Snacking between meals and at bedtime[10] is discouraged.

Low carbohydrate:

- This approach limits the quantity of starches but allows most grains, potato, etc.
- Permitted sugars= sucrose, glucose, aspartame (Nutrasweet)
- Total sugar intake is limited to less than 40 grams per day
- It eliminates most hard-to-digest sugars [11]
    - Fructose (such as high fructose corn syrup), lactose, sucralose (Splenda), sugar alcohols such as sorbitol, xylitol, mannitol, erythritol, lactulose, and lactitol

Other permitted foods:

- Lactase treated milk products
- Almond milk
- Rice milk
- Carbohydrates: limit to ½-1 cup serving per meal
    - White rice
    - Potatoes
    - Sweet Potatoes
    - White bread (sourdough, Italian, French, potato)
    - Rice Krispies cereal
    - White pasta
    - Cream of wheat hot breakfast cereal
- Nuts
- Chocolate
- Meat/seafood/eggs- chicken, pork, beef, fish, eggs
- Whey protein powder (and other protein powders not sweetened with prohibited sugars)

- Fats
- Vegetables
    - Moderate use of raw vegetables/small salads
    - Peppers, tomatoes, cucumber, zucchini, squash, eggplant, peas (but not the edible pod). These vegetables are considered more "fruit-like vegetables" due to their botanical type (prominent seeds; grow above ground)
    - Vegetables that grow underground: onions, garlic, beets, carrots, turnips, etc.
    - Recommended intake of 3-5 cups of cooked vegetables daily
- Fruits—limited to 2 servings/day
    - Apples, pears, and bananas are only allowed in small amounts on rare occasions.
    - Fresh fruits rather than dried fruit
- Coffee
    - 1-2 cups daily

Foods excluded:[10,11]

- Probiotic-rich foods (such as yogurt)
- Dairy products—cheese, non-lactase treated milk, butter, yogurt
- Chewing gum or other products containing sugar alcohols
- High fiber foods and supplements-
- Metamucil
- Oatmeal
- Wild rice
- Whole wheat or multigrain breads
- Beans/legumes—hummus, lentils, peas, soy products (tofu, soymilk) etc.
- Cabbage, brussel sprouts, broccoli, cauliflower, leafy vegetables
- Eat, but limit apples, pears, bananas
- Fruit juice

1 Kakodkar S, Farooqui AJ, Mikolaitis SL, Mutlu EA. The Specific Carbohydrate Diet for Inflammatory Bowel Disease: A Case Series. *J Acad Nutr Diet.* 2015;115(8): 1226-32.
2 Burgis JC, Nguyen K, Park KT, Cox K. Response to strict and liberalized specific carbohydrate diet in pediatric Crohn's disease. *World J Gastroenterol.* 2016;22(6): 2111-7.
3 Obih C, Wahbeh G, Lee D, et al. Specific carbohydrate diet for pediatric inflammatory bowel disease in clinical practice within an academic IBD center. *Nutrition.* 2016;32(4):418-25.
4 Khandalavala BN, Nirmalraj MC. Resolution of Severe Ulcerative Colitis with the Specific Carbohydrate Diet. *Case Rep Gastroenterol.* 2015;9(2):291-5.
5 Dugum M, Barco K, Garg S. Managing irritable bowel syndrome: The low-FODMAP diet. *Cleve Clin J Med.* 2016;83(9):655-62.
6 Nanayakkara WS, Skidmore PM, O'brien L, Wilkinson TJ, Gearry RB. Efficacy of the low FODMAP diet for treating irritable bowel syndrome: the evidence to date. *Clin Exp Gastroenterol.* 2016;9:131-42.
7 Marsh A, Eslick EM, Eslick G, Does a diet low in FODMAPs reduce symptoms associated with functional gastrointestinal disorders? A comprehensive systematic review and meta-analysis Eur J Nutr. 2016 Apr;55(3):897-906.
8 Rao SS, Yu S, Fedewa A Systematic review: dietary fibre and FODMAP-restricted diet in the management of constipation and irritable bowel syndrome
9 Johnson S. The SIBO Specific Diet. www.sibodietrecipes.com
10 Cedars-Sinai Medical Center. Low Fermentation Diet/SIBO Diet. Handout.
11 Cedars-Sinai Medical Center. Low Fermentation Diet/SIBO Diet. Handout [13] Pimentel M, Pimentel MA. A New IBS Solution, Bacteria-the Missing Link in Treating Irritable Bowel Syndrome. Sherman Oaks, CA : Health Point Press, c2006.
12 Abdul Rani, R. (2016). Irritable bowel syndrome and inflammatory bowel disease overlap syndrome: pieces of the puzzle are falling into place. *Intest Res*, (4):297-304.
13 Burgell , R. (2015). Irritable bowel syndrome in quiescent inflammatory bowel disease: a review. *Minerva Gastroenterol Dietol.*, (4):201-13.
14 Dubé C, R. A. (2005). The prevalence of celiac disease in average-risk and at-risk Western European populations: a systematic review. *Gastroenterology*, 128: S57–S67.
15 Lohi S, M. K. (2007). Increasing prevalence of coeliac disease over time. *Aliment Pharmacol Ther*, 26: 1217–1225.

Chapter 11

Homeotherapeutics For Gastrointestinal Conditions

Stomatitis	*Hepatitis*
Heartburn	*Acute Appendicitis**
Vomiting	*Diarrhea*
Indigestion (functional dyspepsia)	*Abdominal Bloating*
Peptic ulcer disease	*Constipation*
Abdominal pain	*Hemorrhoids*
Biliary system pain	*Pruritis ani*

This information comes from an original lecture by Bernardo Vijnovsky, MD which was translated from Spanish by Ian Mussman, ND, CHM. I have added additional differentials and indicators gleaned from my clinical practice. In this chapter, the numbers 1-3 are indicators of the strength of the symptom in relationship to the remedy (as is standard in the homeopathic literature) or for the strength of the remedy with regards to the condition being discussed, rather than references to journal citations. An added asterisk means, according to Vijnovsky, that the remedy is the leader for the topic being discussed.

Stomatitis

Arsenicum album (2)

Aphthous ulcers with burning pain (3)
Burning pain (3), better from hot drinks (2)
Ulcers are whitish (2) or bluish (3)
Gangrenous ulcers (2)
Geographic tongue (2) or thick white coating appearing as if painted (2)

---

* The author does not recommend using homeopathic treatment in lieu of surgical consultation in acute appendicitis.

Thirst for small sips frequently (3)
Anxiety (3) and restlessness (3)
Desire for company (3)
Aggravation after midnight until 3 AM (3)

Borax (3)

The main remedy for stomatitis followed by Mercurius and Sulfuric acid
Very painful ulcers on the buccal and lingual mucosa (3) which bleed easily (3) when rubbed or while eating
Excess salivation (3) and heat in the mouth (3)
Aphthae in nursing infants (3)
Infants start nursing but stop sucking and start crying (2) due to the pain
The nursing mother feels the infant's mouth is very hot (3)
The child is upset and cries a lot (2)
The patient is easily startled (3)
Intense fear of downward motion (3) especially when infants are lowered onto the mattress (2)

Hepar sulph (2)

Diffuse ulcerations in the mouth with a lard-like base
Very painful ulcers (2)
Tendency to suppuration (2)
Splinter-like pain (2)
The gums are bloody and painful
Extreme irritability (3)

Kali muriaticum (2)

White stomatitis in babies or nursing mothers
Bad breath with whitish-grayish tongue (2), dry, geographic tongue
Cervical lymphadenopathy
Edematous, erythematous and friable gingiva

Mercurius solubilis (3)

Stomatitis especially in children (3)
Mouth, tongue and pharynx are very painful (2)
Intense thirst (3) for cold drinks; patient has excessive salivation (3)
Flaccid (3) and swollen tongue with indented edges (3)
Breath described as smelling horrid or putrid (3)
Metallic taste (3)
Pain on opening the mouth or swallowing (2)

Mercurius corrosivus (2)

Stomatitis with burning pain (2)

Salty taste (2) with excessive (3) salivation (3)

Intense thirst (2)

Putrid odor to breath (2)

Cervical adenopathy (2)

Associated with bloody diarrhea (2), scanty (3) volume of stool passed frequently (2)

Constant painful tenesmus (2)

Mercurius cyanathus (2)

Whitish-grayish (2) aphthae, mouth filled with ulcers

A specific remedy for diphtheria (2)

Necrotic destruction of soft palate and fauces (2)

Rapid profound prostration (3) cannot stand up (2)

Vincent's angina, syphilitic ulcers (2)

Putrid odor to breath (2)

Muriatic acid (2)

Stomatitis especially in children (2) on the tongue (2)

Fetid odor to breath

Cracked painful lips (2) with dry leathery tongue (2)

Great prostration keeps them in bed (3)

Eyelids half closed (2)

Mandible hangs open (2)

Nitric acid (2)

Splinter-like pain with the ulcers (3)

Yellow color of tongue (2); burning pain in small vesicles on the tongue (2)

Edematous, bleeding gingiva with fetid breath

Urine has the strong odor like that of a horse's urine (3)

Sulphuric acid (3)

Bloody (3) offensive exudate from aphthous ulcers

Plaques especially on the tongue (2), gums and diffusely in the mouth

Stomatitis especially in neonates and children (3) [see Borax, Merc-sol]

Babies have a sour body odor despite being bathed (2)

The child is weak and feeble (2)

Heartburn

Arsenicum album (2)

Burning pain (2) better hot drinks (2)

Nausea from smelling, thinking about or looking at food (2)

Thirst for small quantities frequently (2)

Anxiety (3) and desire for company (3)

Agitation (3) and physical restlessness (3)

Carbo veg (2)

Acid eructations (2)

Worse after eating greasy food (3), lard (3), rich foods (3)

Burning gastralgia: better eructations

Great distention after eating

Better eructations (3)

Great flatulence (3); worse after eating, especially in hypochondriacal patients

Conium maculatum (2)

Heartburn in the elderly

Acid eructation (2)

Worse in bed (2)

Pyrosis in elderly celibate patients (2)

Crocus sativa (2)

Heartburn after eating (1)

Sensation that something is alive in the abdomen (2) which is moving

Frequent change of mood (2)

Hysterical behavior followed by quick repentance

Sudden changes from hilarity to melancholy

Iris versicolor (3)

Intense heartburn (2)

Everything that is eaten feels as if it turns to vinegar

The entire GI tract burns from mouth to anus (3)

Acrid diarrhea (2) and acid vomiting

Lycopodium clavatum (3)

Burning eructations (2)

Intolerable burning sensation (3) in the pharynx

Burning sensation persists after eructations (2)

Worse after eating (2)
Worse 4-8 PM
Easy satiety (3)
Worse after eating to satiety (3)
Worse from onions (2), seafood (2), cabbage (2), legumes (2)
Fullness in the abdomen from excess gas (3)
Intolerance of tight clothing around the waist (3)
Irritability (3)

Magnesium carbonicum (2)

Acid eructations and regurgitation (3)
Constant acid taste in the mouth (2)
All secretions and excretions smell sour (3)
Nervous exhaustion (2)

Nux vomica (3)

Heartburn in people who eat and drink excessively (2)
Worse in the morning (2), before breakfast (2), after eating (2)
Sour eructations (2)
Sensation of hardness in the abdomen (3)
Distention is worse one hour after eating (2)
Needs to loosen tight clothing (2)
Desire to vomit to relieve the discomfort (2); may induce vomiting (3)
Relief after vomiting (3)
Sour vomiting (2)
Vomiting tastes like food (2)
Aggressive behavior (3); irritable (3)

Robinia (3)

Profuse acid vomiting (3)
Sour eructations; worse evening (3), worse at bedtime (3)
Hyperchlorhydria (2)
Everything eaten feels as if it turns to acid
Constant acid taste in mouth (2)

Sulphuric acid (3)

Violent heartburn (3)
Very acidic regurgitation (3)
Heartburn in alcoholics (3); heartburn after drinking alcohol (3)
Craving for alcohol (3)

Non-alcoholic beverages cause a cold sensation in the stomach (3)
Constant acidic taste in the mouth and esophagus (2)
Vomitus is very acidic (2)

Vomiting

Aethusa cynapium (3)

Violent sudden projectile vomiting (3)
Vomiting in newborns and children (2)
Total intolerance to any form of milk
Vomiting of large greenish or yellowish curds
Sleepy (3) with clammy (2) sweat after vomiting

Apomorphinum (3)

Violent sudden vomiting (3) without previous nausea (2)
Vomiting until the stomach is completely empty (2)
Vomiting from motion sickness (2) during pregnancy
Sweating, salivation and prostration may accompany the bouts

Arsenicum album (2)

Simultaneous vomiting and diarrhea (3)
Associated with anxiety (3) and fear of death (3)
Desire for company (3)
Paroxysmal violent vomiting (2)
Worse from eating or drinking even the smallest quantity (2)

*Ipecac (3)**

Vomiting with constant persistent nausea (3)
Nausea is not ameliorated after vomiting (3)
Nausea both before and after vomiting (3)
Vomiting followed by sleepiness (2)
Feels as if the stomach is hanging (2)
Tongue is clean (3) with intense salivation (2) and absence of thirst (2)
Vomiting while coughing (2), after eating (2), during headache (2)
Vomiting after stooping

Iris versicolor (2)

Vomitus is viscous and ropy (2)
Bilious vomiting (3)
Hematemesis (3)

Intense burning throughout the GI tract (3) from mouth to anus

Vomiting associated with hemicrania (3) or other headache (3)

Vomiting associated with watery diarrhea (2)

Nux vomica (3)

Vomiting after anger (2)

Vomiting in sedentary people or big eaters (3)

Vomiting after alcoholic intoxication (2)

Sense of heaviness or swelling in the epigastrium (3)

Symptoms worse one hour after eating (2)

Sense that they would feel better if they could make themselves vomit (2)

Induces vomiting; relief afterwards (2)

Desire to loosen their clothing after eating

Vomiting triggers palpitations (2)

Phosphorus (3)

Intense thirst for cold water which is vomited as soon as it warms in the stomach (2)

Hematemesis of bright red blood or coffee ground emesis (2)

Post surgical vomiting (2)

Intense sensation of emptiness in the epigastrium (3)

Burning fever (2)

Burning heat sensation in the palms of the hands

Intense heat in the abdomen

Chills radiating to the spine in the interscapular region

Pulsatilla (3)

Vomiting after eating greasy rich food (3)

Sense of a heavy stone in the stomach (2) on awakening

Greasy, rancid tasting eructations (2)

Nausea with heartburn leading to vomiting of undigested food which was ingested long before

Dry mouth without thirst (3)

Symphoricarpos (3)

One of the leading remedies for vomiting of pregnancy (3)

Continuous (2), persistent (2), violent (2) vomiting

Vomiting preceded by intense nausea

Vomiting associated with aversion to food (2)

Intense nausea worse from any motion (2), looking at food, smelling food
Better lying on back (2)

Tabacum (2)

Persistent nausea and vomiting (3)
Vomiting with a pale face (3), cold sweats (3) and vertigo (3)
Worse from least movement (2)
The vertigo (3) and faintness (2) are better from fresh air (3) and uncovering the abdomen (3)
Vomiting from seasickness (2)
Vomiting of pregnancy
Vomiting better with the eyes closed (2)
Nausea and vomiting with icy cold extremities (2)
Nausea and vomiting with prostration (2)
Nausea and vomiting with sensation of fatigue (2)
Nausea and vomiting with sensation of emptiness in the stomach (2)

Indigestion

Antimonium crudum (3)

Indigestion from:
- overeating (3)
- eating specific foods (2)—acidic food (3)
  - vinegar (3)
  - unripe fruit (3)
  - sour wine (3)
- taking a cold bath (2)
- exposure to heat (2)

eructations smell and taste like food (2)
nausea (2) and vomiting (2)
retching (2)
thick, milky-white coating on tongue (3)
constant nausea (2)

Carbo vegetabilis (2)

Indigestion from eating fatty foods (3), greasy foods (3), lard (3), ice cream (2)
Marked epigastric distention (2)

Sensation of fullness (2), better eructations (3), better after loosening clothing (2)

Acid regurgitations (2)

Chelidonium majus (3)

Hepatic insufficiency (3)

Headache over the right eye (3)

Bitter taste in the mouth (3)

Halitosis (2)

Stomach can't tolerate anything but warm drinks (2)

Hepatic pain extending to the inferior angle of the right scapula (2)

China (Cinchona officinalis) (3)

Indigestion from fruits (3), excess tea (2) or milk (2)

Gastric fermentation (3) with acidic eructations (3)

Great flatulence (3) associated with lienteric diarrhea (2)

Sensation of fullness (2) and heaviness (2) after eating even though they eat very little

Easy satiety (2)

Marked distention of the stomach after meals (3); not better from eructation (3)

Eructation tastes bitter (2) or like food (2)

Regurgitation tastes like food (2)

Food eaten tastes bitter (2)

Hydrastis Canadensis (2)

Intense sensation of emptiness in the epigastrium (3) associated with fainting sensation (3)

Indigestion especially from legumes (2)

Sensation of emptiness and fainting not improved by eating (2)

Ipecac (2)

Cannot tolerate greasy food (2), lard (2), ham (2), fruit (2)

Indigestion with violent nausea (3) with unproductive vomiting (3) OR

Persistent violent nausea (3) with vomiting which does not bring any relief (3)

Vomiting with a clean tongue (3)

Sensation that the stomach is hanging (2) and dilated (2)

Lycopodium (3)

Indigestion from legumes (3), cabbage (3), seafood (2), cold food (3)

Great sensation of fullness after eating (3)

Sensation of fullness after only a mouthful of food (2)

Persistent laryngeal burning (3) from acrid eructations (2)

Great abdominal distention (3): better passing flatulence (2)

*Nux vomica (3)**

Main remedy for the effects of overeating (3)

Indigestion from excess coffee (3), excess alcohol (3), excess mental activity (3)

Dull heaviness in the epigastrium (3)

Sensation of a stone in the stomach (3)

Worse one hour after eating (2)

Compelled to induce vomiting (3) which ameliorates (3)

Sleepiness after meals (3)

Irritability (3) and impatience (3)

Abdomen very sensitive to pressure (2) and distended (2)

Need to loosen clothing over the abdomen (2)

Pulsatilla (3)

Indigestion from greasy (3), rich food (3); cream (2), lard (3), sausage (3), butter (3), ice cream (3), cake (2), pancakes (2)

The main keynote is absence of thirst (3)

Heaviness in the epigastrium (2); worse one hour after eating

Sulphur (2)

Indigestion from milk (3), greasy food (2), farinaceous food (grains) (2), bread (2)

Great thirst with no appetite (3)

Worse 11 AM (3)

Stomach feels empty : worse 11 AM (3)

Putrid eructations (2)

Sensation that the stomach is hanging (2)

Peptic Ulcer Disease

Anacardium orientale (2)

Gastralgia when the stomach is empty (2); one to two hours after eating and lasts until the next meal (opposite of Nux vomica)

Painful hunger relieved by eating (3)

Nausea, heartburn, sensation of emptiness in stomach relieved by eating (2)

Patient eats and drinks very rapidly and nervously (2)
Irritable (2)
Patient is malicious and insulting to others (2)
Absentminded (2)
Mental symptoms are relieved by eating (2)

Argentum nitricum (3)

Gnawing ulcer pain (2)
Piercing pain (3) which radiates (2)
Radiating pains (2)
Pain worse from a deep breath (2), palpation, after eating, especially eating sweets (3)
Craving for sweets (3)
Sharp circumscribed pain in epigastrium radiating to the left hypochondrial area (2)
Ulcer pain under the left lower ribs
Retching (2)
Hematemesis (2)
Greenish diarrhea (3)
Belching difficult (3), loud (2) associated with enormous painful abdominal distention
Painful gastric distention; worse after meals (2)
Violent loud eructations (2), following many unsuccessful attempts,which greatly relieve (2) the painful distention
Painful episodes from eating sweets (3) or from anticipation (3) of important events

Arsenicum album (2)

Burning stomach pain (2) like a fire; worse midnight to 3 AM (3), after eating, cold drinks, ice cream and cold food
Better from hot drinks, locally applied heat
Nausea from smelling (2) seeing (2) or thinking (2) about food
Frequent thirst for small quantities (2)
Simultaneous vomiting and diarrhea (3) from taking in the least amount of food or drink (2)
Vomiting is followed by prostration (3)
A mix of black and bright red hematemesis
Pains are associated with fear of death (2)

Great anxiety (3) and fear which makes them get out of bed and pace (2)
Desire for company (3)

Atropinium (2) (an alkaloid of Belladonna)

Paroxysmal and intense pains (2)
Vomiting of digested food (2)
Pain is better after vomiting
Pyloric region is very sensitive to touch (2)
Great dryness of throat (2); so dry that it is difficult to swallow
Bruxism (2)
Objects appear enlarged with a red halo (2) or double (2) or visual hallucinations (2)
Dry mouth (2)

Bismuth (2)

Burning (2) or pressing pain (2)
Pressing pain feels like a stone in the stomach (2)
Better bending backwards (3) [see also dioscorea]
Vomits liquids immediately after they are consumed (3); even just a sip
Vomits undigested food from several days previous (3) from pyloric stasis (3)
Mental state similar to Arsenicum: anxiety (3) and anguish (3) with the pain
Restlessness (3): makes the patient get up and pace
Anxiety (3) with great desire for company (3)

Kali bichromicum (3) *

Burning pain (2)
Pain is worse after eating (2), worse at 2 AM (3)
Pain is very localized (2)—pain in small spots (2) [see also benzoic acid]
Pain in small spots that comes and goes suddenly
Sensation of heaviness and swelling in stomach especially after eating meat (2)
Sudden nausea with acid vomiting (2)
Vomitus is viscous (2) and ropy (2), may contain mucus (2) and blood (2)
Great desire for beer (3) which causes diarrhea and vomiting
Peptic ulcers in beer drinkers and excessive beer drinkers
Stomach pains alternate with joint pains (2)
Intense thirst

Lycopodium (3)

Burning stomach pain (2)

Sensation that the stomach is enlarged and distended (2)
Great flatulence especially in the hypogastrium (2)
Worse from 4-8 PM (3)
Voracious hunger (2) even at night, but feels full after a few bites of food (3)
A few bites of food leads to an intense sensation of fullness and distention (3)
Sensation of abdominal distention (3) which forces them to loosen clothing around the waist (3) which ameliorates the pain (2)
Burning eructations (2) associated with intolerable burning in the pharynx (3)
The pain increases emotional irritability (3); sensitive to the least contradiction (3)

Nux vomica (2)

Gastralgia soon after eating
Pain; better from warm drinks (2) and warmth of the bed
Nausea in bed in the morning (2)
Nausea after meals (2)
Sensation of a dull heaviness in the stomach (3); worse one hour after eating (3)
Desire to vomit for relief (3); self-induced vomiting relieves the pain (2)
Relief after vomiting (2)
Violent vomiting (2) of black, acrid, acidic food
Most of their symptoms are provoked by worry (2) or aggravation over business (2) which increases their natural state of irritability (3) and aggressiveness (3)
Patient feels better after a short nap (3)

Ornithogalum (2)

Gastragia extending to the chest (2) to lower extremities (2); preceded by chills

- worse at night (2), from cold drink or food
- better from warm drinks or food (2), loosening clothing around the abdomen (2)

Frequent forceful fetid tasting eructations (2)
Vomitus is acrid (2), bloody (2); coffee ground appearance or frothy
Vomiting ameliorates the pain
Pain worse when food passes through the pylorus
Sensation that the stomach is a bag filled with water that is rolling around

Uranium nit (2)

Boring pain in the pyloric area (3) better after eating (2)

Associated with coffee ground vomitus, intense thirst (2) and polyuria

Voracious appetite (3); despite appetite they become emaciated (2) and weak

Epigastrium very tender to palpation

Abdominal pain

Belladonna (3)

Abdominal pain (2) all types

Pain comes and goes suddenly (3)

Worse coughing (3), morning (3), pressure (3), jar (3), breathing (2), any abdominal movement

Better lying prone (3); doubling up with legs flexed (2)

Face is red and hot (3)

Mydriasis (3) with bright eyes (3); pulsating arteries (3)

Bryonia alba (3)

Abdominal pain (2) especially sharp pains (3)

Needs to double up (2)

Worse from motion (3), coughing (3), inspiration (2), during bowel movement (2) waking (2)

Better lying prone (2), better flexing legs on abdomen (2)

Chamomilla (3)

Pain especially during diarrhea (3)

Worse after a fit of anger (2), after drinking coffee (2), after chilling drinks (3), during heat (2)

Pain is gripping (3)

Pain forces patient to double up (2)

Better local heat (3)

Irritability (3), intolerance to everything (3), hypersensitivity to pain (3)

Colicky baby (2); better being carried (3)

Worse from emotional excitement (2), during or after anger (2)

*Colocynth (3)**

Colicky pain (3), violent abdominal pain (2), paroxysmal pain (3)

Cutting pain (3) especially after eating, cramping pain (3), pinching pain (3)

Feels as if the intestines were crushed between rocks (2)

Pain in the umbilical region (3)
Patient is forced to double up (3) and flex the knees (3)
Better from doubling up (3), better from pressure on the abdomen (3)
Worse after a fit of anger (3) or indignation (3), after consuming fruit (3) or cold drinks (3)
Better sitting (2), local heat (2), drinking coffee (3), after bowel movement (3)
Often associated with diarrhea, associated with gas (2)
Better after passing flatulence (2), passing a bowel movement (2), vomiting (2)
Pain radiates to the pubis (3)
Electric-like pain (3) radiates to the anus (3)
Colic in babies ameliorated lying prone (2)
Nash writes, "No substance produces such severe colic and no remedy cures it so promptly."

Dioscorea villosa (3)

Cramping pain (3), radiating to distant parts (3)
Violent colicky pain (3), worse morning (3)
Comes in regular paroxysms (2) followed by remission
Feels as if a powerful hand was squeezing the intestines (2)
Worse lying (2), stooping (2)
Better standing erect (3), arching the back (3), motion (1)
Periumbilical pain (3) radiating to the extremities (2), radiating to distant parts (3)

Magnesium phosphate (3)

Cramping pain (3) which makes them double up (3)
Better doubling up (2), pressure (3), local heat (3), friction (2), hot drinks (2)
Radiating pains (3)

Nux vomica (2)

Worse in the morning in bed (3), getting chilled (3), motion (3), pressure (2)
Better local heat (3), after a bowel movement (3)
Pain radiates to the anus (2), and chest (2)

Phosphorus (2)

Burning pain (2)
Worse from getting chilled (2), after eating (2)
Better lying prone (2), motion (1), doubling up (1)
Intense burning thirst (3) for cold drinks; vomits cold fluids as soon as they become warmed in the stomach (2)

Plumbum metallicum (2)

Violent colicky pain (3)

Hard abdomen (3)

Looks as if the umbilicus were drawn towards the spine by a wire (3)

Retracted abdomen (3)

Pain radiates all over the body (3) forcing the patient to stretch in various positions

Better from pressure (2)

Associated with constipation (2) with hard black balls of feces (3)

Pulsatilla (3)

Cramping pain (2)

Tearing pain (2)

Pain radiating to genitals (3)

Worse in the evening (3)

Pain makes the patient double up (3)

Worse during menses (3) before a bowel movement (2), before urinating (2)

Better doubling up (3), local heat (2), open air (2)

Biliary System Pain

Belladonna (3)

Paroxysmal pain (3)

Worse from least jar (3), breathing (3). Lying on the right side (3)

Hot head and cold extremities (2)

Red (3) and bright face (3)

Mydriasis (2)

High fever (3)

Hyperexcitability (3)

Berberis vulgaris (3)

Sticking pain (2)

Pain comes on suddenly with great intensity

Paroxysmal pain (2)

Worse motion (2), pressure (2)

Pain causes shallow breathing (2)

Pain localized to left side, radiating to left lower ribs (3) and lumbar region (3)

Icterus (3) associated with clay colored stools (2)

Bryonia alba (3)*

Better from total immobility (3)

Worse from any type of motion (3), breathing (3), coughing (3), jar (3), diaphragmatic motion

Better pressure (3), lying on the painful side

Dry mouth (2) with thirst for large quantities of water infrequently (opposite of Arsenicum)

Carduus marianus (3)

Sticking pain (2)

Tearing pain (2)]

Worse pressure (2), lying on the left side

Intense nausea (2), worse palpating the liver or epigastrium (2)

Bilious vomiting

Chelidonium (2)

Sticking pain (2), paroxysmal pain (2)

Radiates to the inferior angle of the right scapula (3)

Worse 4-9 PM (2)

Better eating (2), drinking (2), warmth (2), milk (2)

China (Cinchona officinalis) (3)

Worse touch (3), light pressure (3), doubling up (2), least jar (1)

Better from deep pressure (3)

Pain associated with enormous distention and flatulence (3) not ameliorated by eructations or passing flatus (3) [opposite of lycopodium]

Colocynthis (2)

Pain appears suddenly (2), paroxysmal pain (3)

Pain forces the patient to (3) in knee-chest position (2)

Can't tolerate any other position (2)

Pain radiates to the periumbilical region (2)

Dioscorea villosa (2)

Cutting pain (3), worse in the evening (2)

Pain radiates to thorax and upper extremity (2)

Better from extending the trunk (3)

Lycopodium clavatum (2)

Worse 4-8 PM (3), eating to satiety (3), tight clothing (3), touch (3), any constriction

Worse lying on the right side (2)
Associated with excessive flatulence
Right sided pain or begins on the right, radiates to the spine (3)

Natrum sulphuricum (2)

Worse lying on the left side (3) [see also Carduus, Phosphorus]
Worse breathing (2), touch (2), jar (2)
Better stepping
Associated with flatulence (2)

Hepatitis

Bryonia (3)

Sticking hepatic pain (3)
Worse from coughing (3), deep breathing (3), any jar (3), least motion (3)
Better from lying on the painful side (3)
Thirst for great quantities of cold water at long intervals (3)
Dry mouth (1) and white tongue, bitter taste (3)
Nausea while sitting up in bed (3)
Weakness from least effort (2, worse when waking (3), before noon (3)
Constipation (2) with hard dry stools (2), stool dry as if burnt (2), dark urine (2)
Burning pruritis (2)
Fever in the evening (2) or around 9 PM (2)
Chills which start at the tips of finger and toes (2)

Chelidonium (3)

Marked icterus (3); dirty yellow appearance (2)
Especially of sclera (2), face (2), palms (2), tongue and palate (2),
Tongue indented on margins by the teeth (3)
Bilious vomiting (2), bitter taste (2) and fetid breath, fecaloid odor of entire body (2)
Violent pruritis (2)
Dark brown urine (2) with hard white feces (2) or pasty light yellow stool (2)
Sharp pain extending from liver to right inferior angle of the scapula (3) and to spine (3)
Pain better from eating (2) or cannot tolerate anything but very warm drinks (3)
Desire for warm drinks (3) especially milk (3) which ameliorates (2)

Better at noon (3), after lunch (3)
Enlarged liver especially of right lobe

Lycopodium (3)

Hepatic pain worse from: lying on right side (2) palpitation (2). touch (2), eating to satiety (2)
Feels full after a mouthful of food (2)
Hepatic pain extending to the back (2)
Great abdominal flatulence (2), worse in the hypogastrium (2)
Intolerance to tight clothing around the abdomen (3)
Constipation (1), stools hard at first followed by liquid (2)
Irritability (3), worse in the morning when waking (3), intolerant to contradiction
Worse from 4-8 PM (3)

Magnesium muriaticum (2)

Liver indurated (2), enlarged (2), burning pain (2), pressing pain (3)
Better lying on the right side (3), extending to the back (3), worse touch (1), worse stepping (2)
Yellow tongue (2), painful tongue (2)
Nausea from milk (2), constipation (2), hard (3), dry (3), crumbling (3), sheep-like feces (3)

Mercurius solubilis (2)

Hepatic pain, worse: touch (2), right lobe (3) lying on the right side (2) constipation (2), ineffectual urge (2)
Pruritis (2), worse from heat of the bed (2)
Profuse sweat which does not ameliorate (3)
Excess salivation (3): metallic taste (3), great thirst (2), flaccid tongue with indentations (3)

Natrum sulphuricum (3)

Hepatic pain worse from: stepping (2), diaphragmatic motion (2), lying on the left side (3)
Feels as if the liver is pulled to the right side , better lying on the right side (1)
Icterus (2)
Diarrhea, worse before rising or in morning (3)
Bilious stool (3), clay colored stool (3), associated with noisy flatus which ameliorates (3)

Great amelioration after bowel movements (2)
Coated tongue; greenish gray or brownish (3), dirty coating of posterior half of tongue (3)

Phosphorus (3)*

Hypertrophied liver (2)
Pain prevents patient from lying on the right side (2)
Severe icterus (2)
Intense thirst for cold drinks (3) which are vomited as soon as they warm up in the stomach (3)
Tendency to hemorrhage (3)
Prostration (3)
Indifference (3) or desire for company (3)
Fear of death (3)
Involuntary stool (2), sensation that the anus is open (2)

Ptelea (2)

Hepatic pain worse:
- lying on right side (2)
- lying on the left side (2), as if the liver were pulled to the left side
- after eating (2)

Hepatic pain better lying on the right side (2)
Sensation of heaviness in the liver (2), sensation of a stone in epigastrium (2)
Frontal headache (2)
Bitter taste in mouth (2)

Acute Appendicitis

Belladonna (3)*

Paroxysmal pain which comes and goes suddenly (3)
Pain worse from:
motion (3)
jar (3)
stepping (3)
Pain better from:
lying prone (3)
flexing legs on trunk (2)
Dry burning fever (3) with red hot face (3), fever increases at night,

Pulsating carotids (3) and other major arteries
Tachycardia with a full hard pulse (2), mydriasis (3)

Bryonia alba (3)*

Pain in iliac fossa (3)
Pain is worse from:
- least motion (3)
- breathing (3)
- any diaphragmatic movement (3)
- passing stool (3)

Pain is better from:
- flexing the legs on the trunk (2)
- lying on the right side
- lying on the painful side

Sticking pain in right lower quadrant when breathing deeply (3)
Constipation (3) with dry (2) and hard (2) feces as if burnt (3)
Nausea when sitting up in bed (3), vomiting after drinking (3)
thirst for large quantities at infrequent intervals (3)

Crotalus horridus (2)

Septic appendicitis (3)
Septic fever (2) associated with loquacious delirium (2)
Delirium with desire to escape from the bed (2)
Delerium with hallucinations (2)
Sudden profound prostration of vital energy (3)
Tendency to hemorrhage (2), ecchymosis, purpura
Vomiting from:
- the least motion (2)
- lying on the right side (2)
- lying supine (2)

Positive psoas sign and RLQ very tender to palpation

Echinacea (2)

Septic appendicitis (2) or appendicular abscess (2)
Nausea (2) and chills down the spine (2)
Fever (2) and exhaustion (2)

Hepar sulph (2)

Appendicitis in the abscess stage

Psychological and physical hypersensitivity (3) especially to pain (3)
Cannot tolerate the least touch over painful areas (3)
Cannot tolerate the contact of a bedsheet or clothing
Patient becomes violent from the pain (3), great irritability (3)
Sweats without relief (3), fever alternates with chills (2)
Nausea (3), tense abdomen (2)
Pulsating (2), cutting (2), drawing pains (2)

Iris tenax (3)

One of the main remedies for appendicitis
Cutting (2) ulcerative pains (2)
Sensation of heavy dullness in the epigastrium with palpation of the RLQ (3)
Constipation (2),
greenish vomiting, dry mouth (2)
intense chills around 2 PM (3) followed by fever

Lachesis (2)

Acute appendicitis with rigid abdomen
Intolerance to the least constriction around the abdomen (3)
Intolerance to the least contact or touch in the RLQ (3)
Aggravation after sleeping (3)
Sensation of rising heat (3) with profuse sweating (3)

Mercurius corrosivus (2)

Bruised sensation in the RLQ (3), worse from the least pressure (2)
Abdomen rigid and contracted
persistent vomiting (2)
diarrhea with blood and mucus (2), scanty (3) but with constant urge (3) and tenesmus (3)
frequent burning dysuria (3), passes drop by drop (3)
patient desires to lay supine with the legs flexed on the trunk (2)

Phosphorus (3)

Pain which is burning (2) cutting or stinging
Empty sensation in the abdomen (3)
Pain is better from lying prone (2) or flexing the legs on the trunk
Abdomen rigid and contracted
Intense thirst for cold drinks (3) which are vomited as soon as they warm in the stomach (3)

Apathy (3)
Great desire for company (3)

Pyrogenum (2)

Septic appendicitis (2)
Main remedy for septicemia
Putrid, cadaverous odor of the whole body (3), of all secretions (3) and excretions (3)
Glossy red tongue (3)
Prostration with agitation (2), intense restlessness (2)
Very rapid pulse which is out of proportion to the fever (moderate fever)
Sensation that the bed is very hard, parts in contact with the bed feel bruised (2)

Diarrhea

Aethusa (3)—this remedy is mostly used for infants*

Greenish diarrhea (2) with violent tenesmus (2)
Intolerance to milk (3), violent vomiting of milk (3), vomits curds (3), yellow or green (2)
Sleepy (2) and sweaty (2), falls asleep immediately after vomiting or diarrhea (2)
Cannot hold up head, exhausted (2)
Fever with total absence of thirst (2), cold skin with sticky sweat (2)
Accentuation of the nasolabial furrow (3) with expression of anxiety and pain (2)
Rapid emaciation (2)
Diarrhea in infants during dentition (3), in hot summer (3)

Arsenicum album (2)

Putrid, rotten smelling stool (3)
Bloody (2), small (2), dark (2) stool
Diarrhea worse at night (2), after cold drinks (2)
Simultaneous vomiting and diarrhea (3) from the least intake of food or drink (2)
Great anxiety with prostration (3)

Arundo mauritanica (2)

Diarrhea in infants during dentition (2)
Red sand-like debris (2)
Insomnia (2) and weeps at night (2)

Chamomilla (3)

Diarrhea in infants during dentition (3), child screams, better from being carried or rocked (3)

Diarrhea brought on from anger (2)

Stool smells like rotten eggs (2), with mucus (2), frequent movements (2), acrid and corrosive (2)

Stool looks like cooked spinach (2)

Colicky pain (2), with irritability (3), capriciousness (3), restlessness (3), peevishness (3)

Diarrhea is intolerable to the patient (3)

Hot sweaty face (2)

One cheek is red and the other pale (3)

Croton tiglium (2)

Diarrhea that is greenish (3), explosive (2)

Diarrhea worse in Summer (3), from eating (3), drinking (2), motion (2)

Diarrhea associated with colicky pains (2), followed by great prostration (2)

Constant gurgling in the abdomen (2) as if full of water (2)

Painful vesicular eruption on buttocks (2), diaper rash makes infant cry

Guaiacum (3)

Diarrhea with a bad odor of the whole body (2)

Intestinal fermentation, large amounts of gas

Diarrhea in infants—child appears old (3), exhausted and emaciated (2)

Magnesium carbonicum (2)

Diarrhea associated with colicky pain which makes them double over in pain (2)

Stool is acrid (3), greenish (3), frothy (2), like scum on a pond

Sour odor to the entire body (3)

In nursing infants—milk passes undigested (2)

Mercurius solubilis (3)

Diarrhea is greenish (3), bloody (3), acrid (2) with mucus (3)

Worse in Spring and Fall (2), when days are warm and nights are cold

Bowel movements associated with violent tenesmus (3), during (2) and after passing stool (3)

Profuse foul smelling night sweats (3) which do not ameliorate (3)

Excess salivation (3), intense thirst (3), tongue indented by teeth (3)
Drooling (3)
Fetid odor of all secretions and excretions (3)

Podophyllum (3)

Worse after eating (3), early morning (2), forenoon (2)
Stools: copious (3), fetid (3), yellow (2), watery (2), explosive (3)
Stool "spray paints" the toilet bowl
Passing stool associated with tenesmus (2) and rumbling in the abdomen (2)
Rectal prolapse (2) when severe
Diarrhea in infants during dentition (2), after bathing the child (2)
Traveler's diarrhea

Rheum (3)

Stools are sour smelling (2), pasty (2)
Patient is irritable (2), impatient (3)
Cold sweat on the face (2)
Diarrhea in infants during dentition (2), child cries each time it needs to pass stool (2)
Child's whole body smells sour (3) even after washing (3)

Abdominal Bloating

Carbo vegetabilis (3)

Tremendous bloating (3), especially upper abdomen or pubic area
Better from frequent eructations (3)—may desire carbonated drinks to increase belching (2)
Flatulence (2) worse at night, worse lying
Irritable, especially with family (2), poor memory and concentration (2)
Apathy (3), negative personality (3), makes cutting remarks (3)
Generally cold (3) but may be not want to be covered (3)
May want to be fanned (3), fainting and collapse (3)

China officinalis (3)

Gas, bloating and distention (3), better from eructations or passing flatus (3)
Borborigmus (3), cramping and pain (2), better flexing legs on trunk (2)
Worse after beer, fruit, fat, milk (2); gallbladder disease (3)
May wake during the night with hunger (2), craves sweets (3)
Dislikes fruit (especially cherries), fat, hot food (temperature)

Generals; worse from loss of body fluids (3), periodicity of symptoms (3)
Irritable (3), sensitive (3), dreams or fantasies of heroic deeds (3)

Colchicum autumnale (3)

Enormous distention (3), cannot pass the gas (3), gas is trapped (3)
Especially in the ileocecal region (2)
Nausea (3); in pregnancy (3), nausea increases from smelling food
Gout (3), joint pain worse from any motion (see Bryonia)
Associated with diarrhea (2), may be worse in Autumn

Lycopodium clavatum

Bloating (3), especially right lower quadrant (2), better from eructations or passing flatus
Easy satiety (3), even from a few bites of food, yet may be ravenously hungry
Constipation (1), stools hard at first followed by liquid (2)
Loud borborigmus (3)
Desires warm drinks and sweets
Worse from cold drinks (3) or cold food (2)
May wake during the night with hunger (3), craves sweets (3)
Generally right sided ailments or that start on the right side
Irritability (3), worse in the morning when waking (3), intolerant of contradiction
Worse from 4-8 PM (3)

Raphanus sativus

Sensation of trapped gas, especially in the left upper quadrant (3)
Post-surgical ileus and other bowel obstruction (2)

Constipation

Alumen (2)

No desire whatsoever for many days (2)
Rectal inertia (2)
Stools as hard as rocks (3), like little black balls (3)
Large stools (2)

Alumina (3)

Stools pass with great difficulty (3) and effort (3) even though the stools are soft (3)
Rectal inactivity (3) for up to one or two weeks (2)

No way of passing stool until there is a great accumulation (Allen)
Constipation in the aged
Constipation in babies fed cow's milk
Constipation in sedentary pregnant women
Constipation when traveling (2)
Patient may only be able to have a bowel movement when standing (2)
Insufficient stools like hard little balls (3), dark (2), knotted (2), covered with mucus (2)

Bryonia alba (2)

Large difficult stools (2)
Rectal inactivity (2)
Stools are scanty (2), dry (2), hard (2), as if burnt (3)

Causticum (3)

Difficult stools to pass (3)
Unproductive efforts (3)
Patient may only be able to have a bowel movement when standing (3)
Burning, pressing pain in rectum after stool (2)

Collinsonia (3)

Obstinate constipation (3), associated with painful hemorrhoids (2)
Sensation of the rectum being full of sharp sticks (3)
Large (2), bulky (2), clear (2), hard (2), knotted (2), like little balls (2), black stools (2)
Urge and effort are ineffectual (2)

Lac defloratum (2)

Pain in the rectum makes them cry (3)
Deficient urge for a bowel movement (2)
Dry, hard, large stools (3)
Can go up to 15 days without passing stools
Needs to make great efforts which causes soreness of the anus (2)

Lycopodium clavatum (2)

Dry, hard, knotted, stools in children
Constipation when away from home (2), when traveling
Associated with flatulence (3) gurgling (2) especially in the epigastrium

Nux vomica (3)

Constant (3) but ineffectual urge for stool (3)

Constipation from: excess use of laxatives (3), sedentary habits (3), in the elderly (3) in pregnancy (3), during the menstrual flow (2), while traveling (2)

painful spasmodic constriction of the anus (3)

large, hard, dry stools (2)

Opium (Oreodaphne) (3)*

Constipation from total rectal inactivity (3) without any urge for stool (3)

Constipation from: overuse of drugs (2), sedentary habits (2), in the elderly (2), while traveling (2)

Stools are black, hard, dry balls (3)

Plumbum metallicum (3)

Constipation during pregnancy (3)

Painful bowel movement from anal spasms (3)

Stool is knotted, hard, black little balls (3) like sheep dung (2)

Hemorrhoids

Aesculus hippocastanum (3)*

Purple hemorrhoids (3)

Rectal pain worse from standing (2), walking (3) or sitting (2)

Rectal pain better from kneeling (2)

Associated with pulsating sacroiliac or sacrolumbar pain

The rectum feels full of sharp sticks (3)

Heat (3), heaviness (3) and burning sensation (2)

Dryness (2) and pruritis (2) is felt one hour after passing stool (2) which continues for 2-6 hours

Aloe socotrina (3)

Bluish hemorrhoids like a bunch of grapes (3)

With soreness (2) and burning pain, better from cold applications (3)

Can't tolerate the least contact (3), bleed easily (2)

Intense pruritis and heat (2) at night which prevents sleep

Encopresis (3) from loss of sensation of anal sphincter (3)

Patient does not trust the sphincter (3) when passing flatus or urinating—they can't tell if stool will pass involuntarily (3)

Sensation of a plug (3) or bearing down sensation in the rectum (2)

Collinsonia canadensis (3)

Painful (3), bleeding (3) hemorrhoids with sensation of having the rectum full of sharp sticks (3) or sand

Pain worse during a bowel movement (3) especially if the stool is hard

Sensation of constriction of the rectum

Hamamelis virginiana (2)

Bluish hemorrhoids with soreness from least contact (3)

Pulsating (3) rectal pains associated with soreness in the spine

Passive venous hemorrhage of dark unclotted blood (2) while passing stool (3) hemorrhage followed by prostration (2) disproportionate to the loss of blood

Pulsatilla nigricans (3)

Especially for internal hemorrhoids (2)

Worse at night (2) and when lying (3)

Paroxysmal (2), burning (2), pressing (2) pain after passing stool (2)

Associated with colic, pruritis, passing mucus (even without stool) and bleeding with stool

Pruritis ani

Aesculus hippocastanum (2)

Pruritis ani (1) with burning (2) and chills running up and down the spine (2)

Pruritis associated with hemorrhoids (3)

Main remedy for hemorrhoids

Large (3), purplish (3) hemorrhoids that have only modest amounts of bleeding (2)

Pain and pruritis, worse walking (3) and moving around (3)

Throbbing pain in the sacroiliac region (3)

Agaricus (2)

Burning pruritis ani (2)

Voluptuous itching (2), worse from scratching (2), worse after passing stool

Associated with hemorrhoids

Aloe socotrina (2)

Anal pruritis especially at night and after passing stool

Associated with blue hemorrhoids which protrude from the anus like grapes (2)

Painful, bloody, burning (2) hemorrhoids; better from cold applications

Sense of insecurity of the anal sphincter (3)

Passes stool involuntarily when passing gas in bed at night (3) or while urinating (3)

Cina (3)

Intense voluptuous pruritis ani (2) from parasites, especially in children

Worm infestation causes itching of both anus and nose

Voracious appetite (3), after eating, bruxism during sleep (3)

Bad temper (3), anger and irritability (3), capricious, unstable, crying, does not want to be touched or looked at, asks for something and then throws it away (see Stramonium, Chamomila)

Hard, swollen abdomen

Fluoric acid (2)

Pruritis ani, better cold sitz bath; worse from heat

Associated with protruding hemorrhoids or rectal prolapse (2)

Graphites (3)*

Violent pruritis (2)

Patient rubs the anus until it is raw (2)

Sticky, irritating, oozing appears after rubbing (3) which aggravates the raw swollen anus (2)

Associated with constipation (3) with large stools (3) which are hard to pass (2)

Chapter 12

Hiatal Hernia Syndrome

Clinical Picture
Etiology
Assessment
Visceral Manipulation
Post-manipulation Exercises
Dietary Basics
Functional Breathing and Lifting

Hiatal hernia syndrome is one of the most common functional GI disorders. The recognition and management of this syndrome was greatly advanced by the work of Dr. Ralph Failor, a Naturopathic and Chiropractic physician who practiced in Hillsboro, Oregon in the latter half of the 20th century.

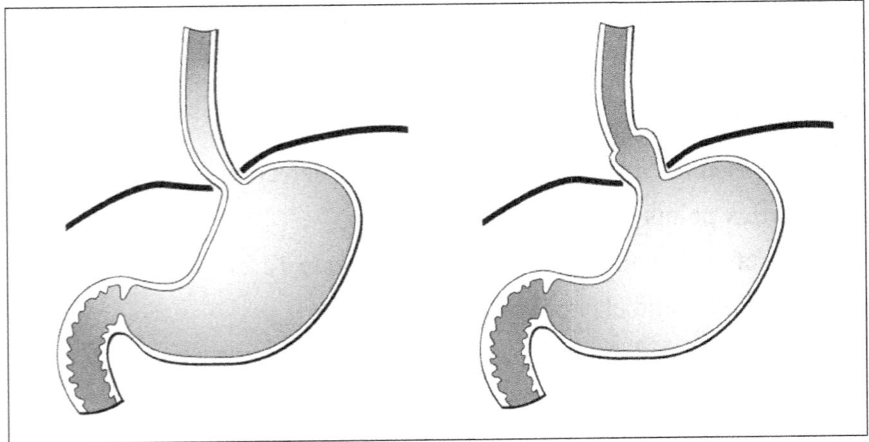

FIGURE 12.1 NORMAL STOMACH AND HIATAL HERNIA

This syndrome is a functional relative to the true hiatal hernia, a gastric pathology in which the proximal stomach is herniated into the mediastinum. Hiatal hernia syndrome is distinguished by the fact that the proximal stomach may only cause upward pressure against the diaphragmatic hiatus and not actually protrude into the chest. Treatment is identical for sliding hiatal hernia and for hiatal hernia syndrome.

Clincial Picture

The possible symptoms are the same for both the true hernia and the syndrome. These include fatigue, mental dullness, easy satiety, shallow thoracic breathing, relatively rapid respiratory rates, globus sensation, dysphagia, chest oppression, reflux, stitching chest pains, regurgitation, aversion to abdominal constriction, flatulence, "spare tire" bulge just below the inferior margin of the ribs, and a tickling non-productive cough.

Etiology

This syndrome may be due to an inherited wide diaphragmatic hiatus or may be acquired from trauma or increased intra-abdominal pressure. Examples of trauma include abdominal surgery, the impact of jumping, horseback riding, abdominal exercise, retching or vomiting, a blow to the abdomen or a "belly flop" dive, falling from a height or merely exertion with breath holding.

An increase in intra-abdominal pressure may also be due to pregnancy or abdominal obesity or any space occupying lesion of the abdomen.

Assessment

Dr. Failor used the following tender points for detection of the syndrome:

- Reflex points
  - Left of xyphoid (HHS point – see Figure 12.2)
  - 4th ICS mid clavicular
  - 4th ICS mid axillary
  - T 10-11 left paravertebral area

I use the hiatal hernia point and ask the patient to rate the tenderness on a 0-4 scale and reassess after treatment.

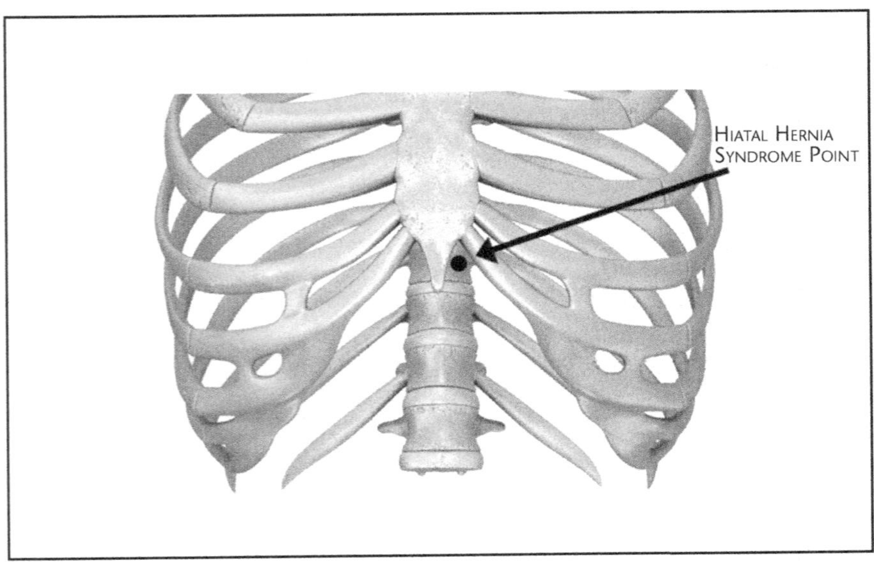

Figure 12.2 Location Of The Hiatal Hernia Syndrome Point

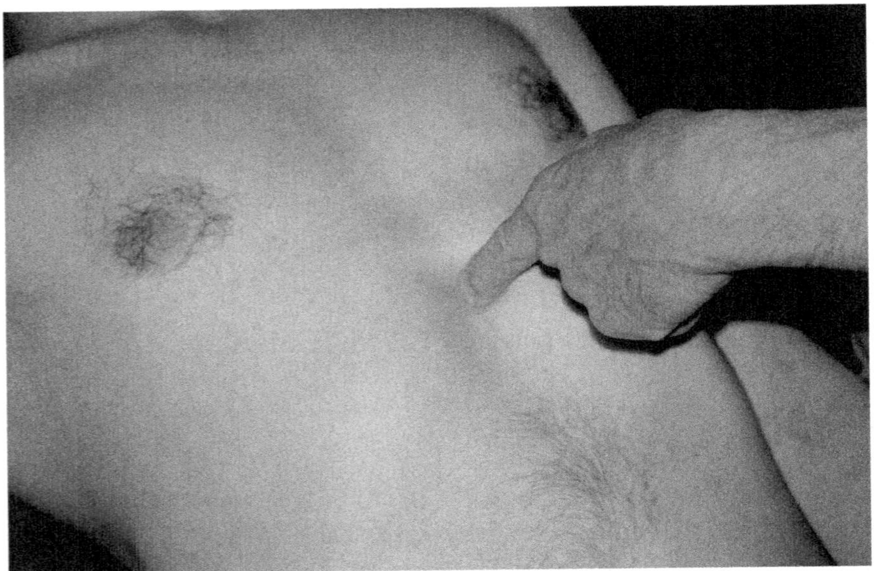

Figure 12.3 Reflex Testing Point For Hiatal Hernia Syndrome

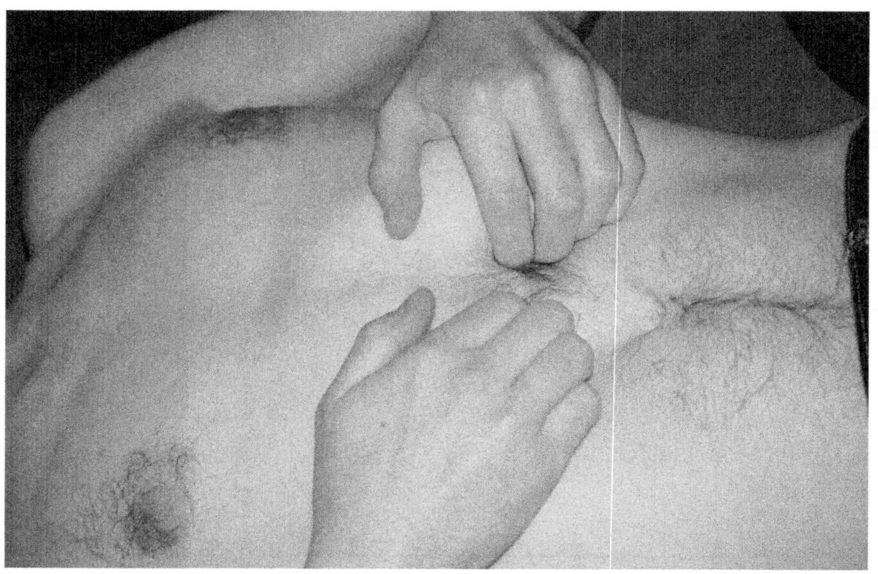

FIGURE 12.4 POSITION OF PATIENT'S HANDS FOR MUSCLE TESTING HIATAL HERNIA SYNDROME

Another method that I have found very useful is an applied kinesiology test. Find any muscle which tests strong. I often use the rectus femoris.

- Retest the strong muscle while having the patient use both hands to press the upper abdomen anteroposterior and cephalad (increases the pressure of the proximal stomach against the diaphragm). If the muscle weakens, this is a positive indicator (Figure 12.4).

Treatment

Treating the syndrome (or an actual sliding hiatal hernia) involves the following:

Visceral Manipulation

Dr. Failor taught us his technique in 1977 and many doctors still use it (for details see *The New Era Chiropractor,* R.M.Failor, D.C, N.D., self-published, 1979.) It is effective, but can be a bit forceful. I trained in structural integration in 1996 and over the last twenty years I've developed a gentler method. I contact the epigastric area just inferior to the costosternal angle. I use a "claw" hand contact and support the contact hand with my other hand (Figure 12.5).

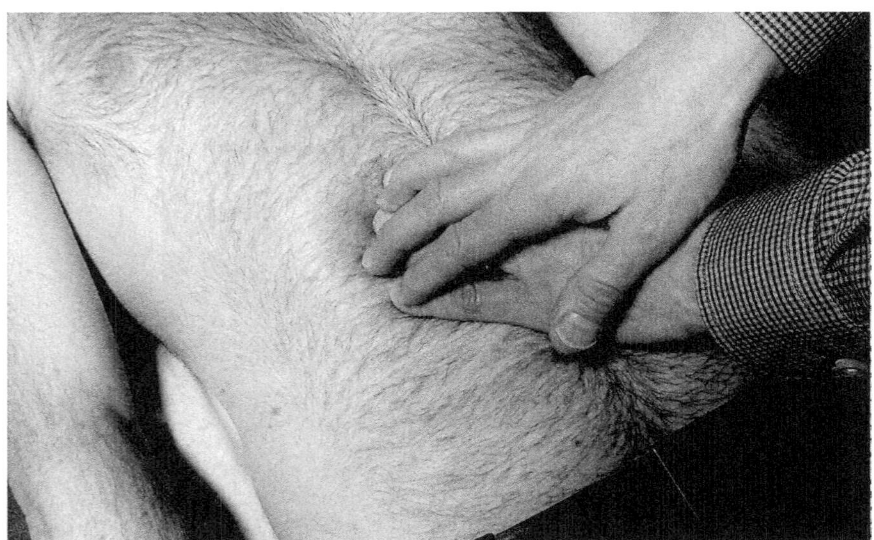

FIGURE 12.5 HAND POSITIONING FOR HIATAL HERNIA SYNDROME CORRECTION

I traction toward the left ASIS and wait for the soft tissue to begin a counter clockwise rotation. I just allow my fingers to follow the movement while continuing to apply the traction. In most cases, the rotation

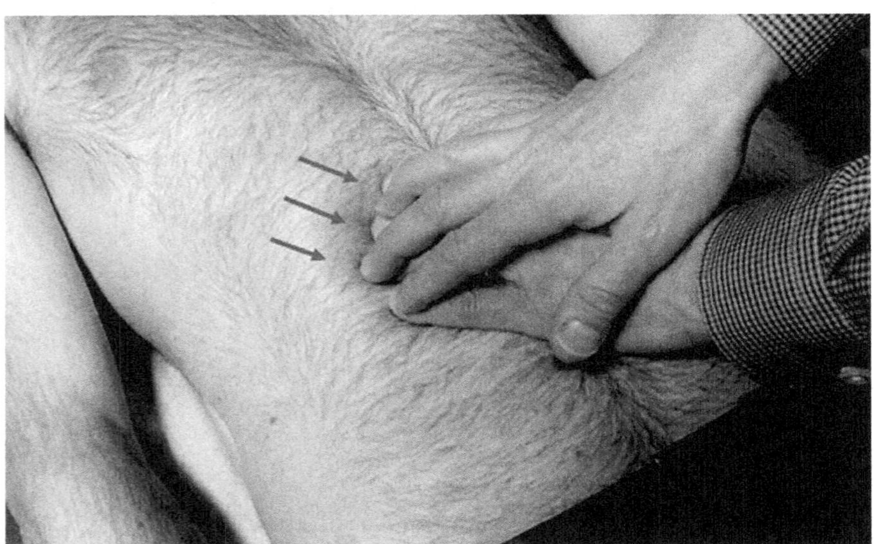

FIGURE 12.5A VISCERAL TECHNIQUE—STEP I: TRACTION TOWARD LEFT ASIS

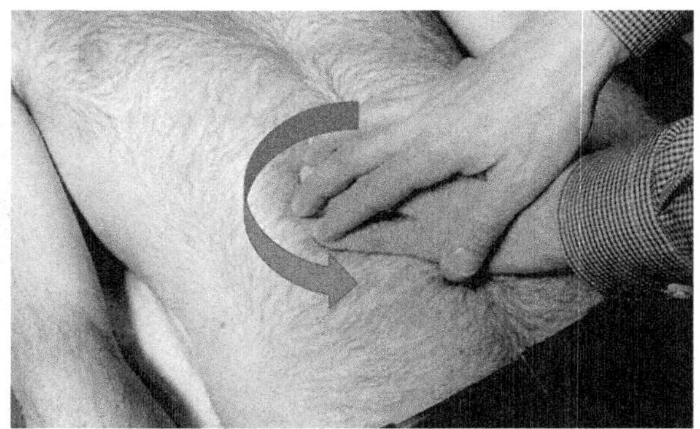

Figure 12.5b Visceral Technique—Step 2: Continue Traction And Follow The Rotation

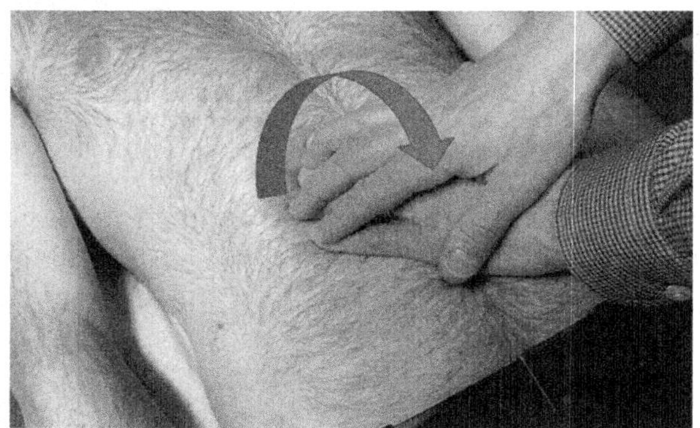

Figure 12.5c Visceral Technique—Step 3: Continue Traction And Follow The Rotation

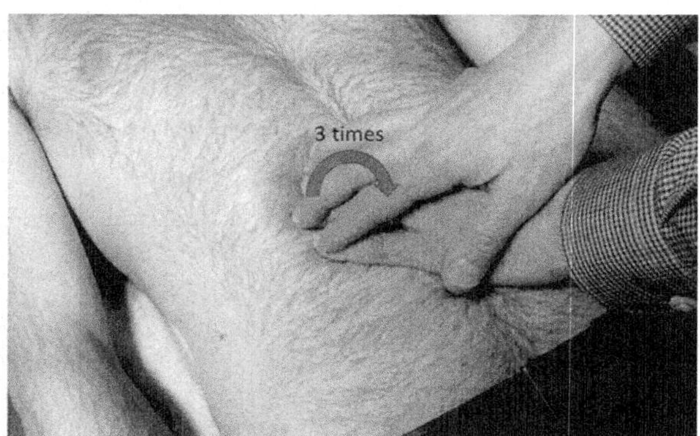

Figure 12.5d Visceral Technique—Step 4: "Ballooning The Stomach"—Perform 3 Clockwise Rotation

will shift to clockwise as I continue the traction. When the rotation is finished (usually 3-4 minutes at the longest) I add three additional clockwise gentle thrusts of my hands. Dr. Failor called this "ballooning the stomach" and felt that it was important in allowing the manipulation to hold. After treatment, recheck the HHS point or kinesiology testing. The change should be immediate.

Any additional techniques that you already use to free the thoracic vertebrae, ribs and diaphragm muscle in general are helpful, should you find these necessary. Figure 12.6 shows a diaphragm release I use. The vector of traction is toward the umbilicus. Hold the traction while having the patient rotate the ribs. I ask them to imagine that each side of the ribcage is a cylinder and that the cylinders can slowly rotate externally and then internally. Have them continue this until the tissue softens or elongates.

Dr. Failor found that T10 and T11 were especially important to assess for fixations or dysarticulations, so I tend to check these carefully. In addition, the occiput is an essential area to check and correct. The osteopathic "cranial base release" is effective or you may use myofascial or other techniques as per your preference.

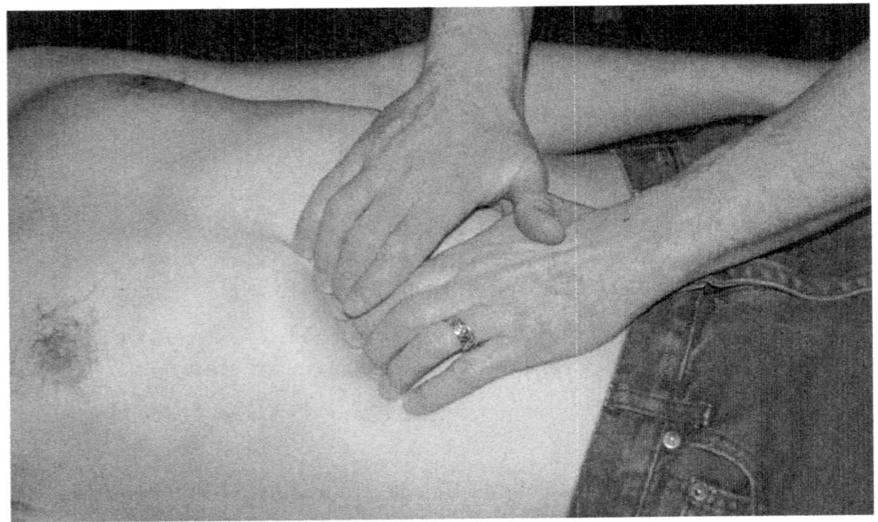

FIGURE 12.6 BASIC MYOFASCIAL RELEASE OF THE DIAPHRAGM

Table 12.1 Hiatal Hernia Syndrome Summary		
Onset	Abdominal surgery Impact of jumping Horseback riding Retching or vomiting Pregnancy	Blow to the abdomen "Belly Flop" dive Falling from a height Exertion with breath holding Abdominal obesity
Symptoms	Fatigue Mental dullness Easy satiety Shallow thoracic breathing Chest oppression Stitching chest pains Relatively rapid respiration	Globus sensation Dysphagia Reflux/regurgitation Aversion to constriction at the waist Flatulence "Spare tire" bulge just below the rib margin Tickling, non-productive cough
Asssessment	Reflex points Left of xyphoid (HHS point) 4th ICS mid clavicular 4th ICS mid axillary T 10-11 left paravertebral	Retest a previously strong lower extremity muscle while having the patient use both hands to press the upper abdomen anteroposterior and cephalad. If the muscle weakens, this is a positive indicator for the syndrome.
Treatment	Stand to the left of the supine patien. Use a left hand "claw" contact. Support the contact hand with your right hand (Figure 12.5). Use continuous traction toward the left ASIS and wait for the soft tissue to begin a counter clockwise rotation. Follow the rotation as it shifts to clockwise—maintaining traction. When the rotation is finished (duration 3-4 minutes) perform three clockwise thrusts (ballooning the stomach). Check the spine with a focus at the occiput and T 10/11.	

Post-manipulation Exercises

Heel drops

The patient drinks (not sipping) 12-16 ounces of warm water on waking, stands, rises onto the toes and then drops onto the heels eleven times in succession. The downward momentum of the water-filled pendulous stomach supports the benefits of the visceral work.

Leg raise (more strenuous)

Lying supine on a flat surface with legs adducted, the patient inhales—and while exhaling very slowly—raises both legs 12-18 inches, slowly abducts and adducts the legs and then lowers them to the resting position. Gradually increase the number of repetitions over time.

Knee raise (less strenuous)

Sitting in a chair, the patient supports the upper body by holding the arms or seat of the chair. Keeping the knees abducted, the patient inhales, then exhales and flexes the legs on the trunk (as far as possible). Gradually increase repetitions over time.

Dietary Basics

These will vary with your patient's individual needs. In general, I find having patients avoid their food sensitivitiesis important. Just as important as "what" they eat is "how" they eat.

- Avoid overeating and large meals
- Take time to sit and chew food until it becomes liquid before swallowing (Flecherizing)
- Avoid stressful discussions or watching television while eating
- If family of origin eating issues are still affecting the patient's eating habits, consider counseling or energetic psychology interventions

Treat hypochlorhydria or achlorhydria if present (see Chapter 13).

Functional Breathing And Lifting

Functional breathing and lifting is crucial. Teach these patients functional lifting and exertion. That is, exertion should be preceded by slow abdominal inhalation and accompanied by exhalation throughout the exertion. This prevents a build-up of intra-abdominal pressure, thus preventing reinjury. This admonition also applies to bearing down with defecation.

Developing your skills and protocols for treatment of hiatal hernia technique will gain you many referrals and the ability to get rapid, lasting results with many cases of functional esophageal, gastric and diaphragmatic syndromes.

Case Example

A thirty-three year old Canadian woman had been an avid ice-hockey player until an injury three years prior. During a match, she and a member of the opposing team collided. The impact was on her left flank and it took her down to the ice with intense abdominal pain. Over time, anxiety, tremendous fatigue and a desire to protect the abdomen developed. She was no longer able to work at her career as a librarian. She had seen a chiropractor about a year prior who had performed a visceral maneuver which had given her a few days of significant relief from her symptoms. Her description of the maneuver seemed to indicate a Failor-like technique.

I used my hiatal hernia visceral technique as well as some general freeing of the diaphragm and ribs (using myofascial release). I instructed her to use the heel drops exercise each morning for at least two weeks following our visit. Dramatic improvement lasted for about three months. We had another visceral session at three months and then again after nine months. At that time she rated her recovery at 90%. At ten year follow-up, she continues improved and is back at work.

Chapter 13

Gastric Secretion And Suppression

Gastric hydrochloric acid secretion is a key factor which initiates protein digestion, triggers duodenal hormones, prepares vitamin B_{12} and folic acid for absorption, prepares minerals for absorption and prevents overgrowth of upper GI flora.

Table 13.1 Major Functions Of Gastric Acid
• Converts pepsinogen to pepsin • Kills some ingested bacteria, fungi and parasites • Aids in digestion of vitamin B_{12} and folic acid • Aids in mineral digestion • Stimulates duodenal CCK and secretin • May modulate leukocyte function

What Is The Effect Of Gastric HCL On GI Hormones?

As the acid bolus exits (gastric emptying) and enters the duodenum it triggers release of cholecystokinin (CCK) and secretin. The secretin effect is thought to be the more potent response in humans.

Table 13.2 Physiologic Effects Of CCK

Stimulates	Inhibits
Gall bladder contraction Mucosal and pancreatic growth Pancreatic enzyme and bicarbonate release Insulin release	Gastric emptying Sphincter of Oddi muscle tone Local GI immunity (transiently) Appetite

Table 13.3 Physiologic Effects Of Secretin

Stimulates	Inhibits
Gallbladder contraction Gallbladder bicarbonate secretion Pancreatic enzyme and bicarbonate release Pancreatic growth Insulin release	Gastric acid secretion Gastrin secretion Gastric emptying Gastric and intestinal motility

Etiology Of Low Stomach Acid Secretion

Helicobacter pylori pangastritis is a common cause of atrophic gastritis and hypochlorhydria.[1] This is due to the effect of VacA, an H. pylori virulence gene. VacA alters apical membrane-cytoskeletal interactions in gastric parietal cells, reducing acid secretion.[2] Atrophic gastritis is one of the most common conditions in the U.S. According to Cotran, "In the Western world, the prevalence of histologic changes indicative of chronic gastritis in the later decades of life is higher than 50%."[3]

Autoimmune gastritis is thought to be present in only 10% of chronic gastritis cases (2-5% of the U.S. population)[81], but occurs in 6-15% of patients with type 1 diabetes and Hashimoto's thyroiditis.[4] The clinical picture of autoimmune gastritis includes mucosal atrophy, autoantibodies against the parietal cell and intrinsic factor, hypo/achlorhydria, iron and B_{12} deficiency anemias, cognitive impairment, peripheral neuropathy and an increased risk of stomach cancer. See Chapter 7 for a case presentation of a sixty-six year-old male with epigastic pain and peripheral paresthesias.

Chronic gastritis is seen in autoimmune adrenal disease (Addison's) as well, but this is an exceedingly rare condition. I test gastric acid levels in all patients with autoimmune disorders. I see functional adrenal maladaption syndromes very often in my practice and these tend to manifest with hypochlorhydria.

Abuse of toxins such as alcohol and tobacco leads to chronic gastritis. It may also manifest following gastric surgery or radiation; from mucosal disease such as Crohn's; uremia and after gastric obstruction. Golan adds that dietary conditions such as devitalized diet, chronic overeating of fat or sugar and salt restricted diets can cause hypochlorhydria.[5]

Clinical Picture Of Hypochlorhydria

Hypochlorhydria may be considered asymptomatic. That is, the patient believes the symptoms to be normal digestive sensations and does not recognize problematic symptoms. Often, symptoms of indigestion or functional dyspepsia develop during or after meals. These may include some combination of gas formation, bloating, belching, a heavy or full sensation in the epigastrium after meals and easy satiety. A chronic iron, vitamin B_{12} or folic acid deficiency (with or without anemia) may be present. H. pylori overgrowth may be detected.

Patients may also fail to respond to medications or nutritional supplements taken in tablet form due to decreased absorption. Signs of mineral deficiency, such as muscle cramps and twitches or soft, brittle or peeling nails may be seen. Diffuse hair loss may be a sign in women. Maxillary telangiectasia and rosacea are associated with hypochlorhydria.[6] Coated tongue and halitosis may also be present. There may be tenderness to digital pressure at the gastric Riddler's point at the left anterior rib margin (see Chapter 6.) Hypochlorhydria should be considered in the prescription and dosage of drugs whose absorption is altered by high gastic pH. Several studies have researched the effect of H. pylori induced hypochlorhydria and absorption of L-dopa, thyroxine, and delavirdine. Eradication of the bacteria increased absorption of L-dopa in Parkinson's disease as much as 54%. TSH levels in treated hypothyroid subjects decreased by 94% after eradication (oral thyroxine absorption improved.) In HIV-positive hypochlorhydric subjects, delavirdine absorption increased by 150% after eradication.[7]

Table 13.4 Signs And Symptoms Of Hypo/Achlorhydria	
Gas	Epigastric heaviness, full feeling after meals
Bloating	Easy satiety
Eructations	Maxillary telangiectasia
Muscle cramps	Diffuse hair loss (females)
Soft or brittle nails	Halitosis
Coated tongue	

With respect to pernicious anemia, vitamin B_{12} deficiency develops insidiously, but progressively. In an article discussing B_{12} deficiency in *Postgraduate Medicine*, Goodman and Salt report:

> ...early manifestations may be generalized weakness or fatigue, indigestion, diarrhea, or depression. Pernicious anemia is considered the classic cause (of B_{12} deficiency), but others include malabsorption because of achlorhydria or other gastric dysfunction, fish tapeworm infection, and strict vegetarianism (veganism.) Iron deficiency often coexists. Because presentation is often atypical, vitamin B_{12} deficiency is a diagnostic consideration whenever neuropsychiatric signs or symptoms are unexplained.[9]

Table 13.5 Conditions Associated With Hypochlorhydria	
Heartburn–non-cardiac chest pain	HIV/AIDS[8]
Allergy	Childhood asthma
Bacterial overgrowth/ stomach & small intestine	Depression
Pernicious anemia	Cholelithiasis
Chronic atrophic gastritis	Rheumatoid arthritis
H. pylori gastritis	Lupus erythematosis
Gastric cancer	Grave's disease
Acne, eczema, urticaria, vitiligo, rosacea	Hashimoto's thyroiditis
Ulcerative colitis	Osteoporosis
Chronic hepatitis	Type 1 diabetes mellitus
	Adrenal maladaption syndromes

B_{12} deficiency is common, with a prevalence of 10-20% in the elderly, but only 5-10% of these are clinically symptomatic (glossitis, peripheral neuropathy, anemia, etc.) Typical findings such as macrocytic anemia may be absent, especially in the elderly,[10] and for this reason I suspect B_{12} or folate deficiency when the mean corpuscular volume (MCV) is 93 fL or higher. These patients are at high risk for cognitive decline.[11] The serum cobalamin assay is a reasonable first line test, but the results must be carefully interpreted, since a normal level does not exclude deficiency. Markers of cobalamin activity, such as serum homocysteine or methylmalonic acid, may be helpful in this situation.

In the atrophic gastritis of H. pylori colonization, the pangastritis-induced hypochlorhydic secretions are not sufficient to cleave cobalamin from proteins. Helicobacter pylori eradication may cure some of these B_{12} deficiencies.[12] Only about half of the patients with neurological signs, and even fewer psychiatric patients respond to treatment with B_{12},[13] so using the early markers (methylmalonic acid) is essential for prevention of cognitive decline. Herschko reporting in *Blood* discusses an autoimmune polyendocrine syndrome with atrophic gastritis beginning in youth as iron deficiency and progressing by a gradual increase in MCV into middle age.[14]

Herrmann and Geisel describe the diagnostic stages of cyanocobalamin deficiency.[15] Vitamin B_{12} deficiency can be divided into four stages. Stages I and II are signaled by a low plasma level of holotranscobalamin II indicating that the plasma and cell stores are depleted. Stage III is seen as homocysteine and methyl malonic acid increase in addition to the low holotranscobalamin II. In stage IV, the typical signs of B_{12} deficiency are seen (macroovalocytes, MCV >98 fL, and signs of anemia).

An adequate serum folate should be >10 nmol/L and red cell folate >340 nmol/L. This is based on a correlation with plasma homocysteine. For serum vitamin B12, the value should be >300 pmol/L based on correlation with homocysteine.[16] In a paper published in the *American Journal of Clinical Nutrition*, doubling the holotranscobalamin concentrations from 50 to 100 pmol/L reduced the rate of cognitive decline by 30% over a ten year study.[17]

Lovat, writing a lead article in *Gut*, explains the toll of aging, polypharmacy and subclinical hormonal imbalance on digestion. Drugs, along with psychological as well as physical disability can affect taste sensation, which lowers appetite. Hypochlorhydria causes protein, mineral and vitamin malabsorption and can lead to small bowel bacterial overgrowth. Subclinical hypothyroidism may lead to GI dysmotility (which improves with physical exercise). He states:

> Evidence is now mounting that thorough investigation of gastrointestinal disturbances in elderly patients coupled with intensive nutritional support can make a very real impact on their outcome. Gastroenterologists should therefore seek out and actively treat gastrointestinal disorders in the elderly and not just ascribe them to old age.[18]

How Does An Alkaline Stomach Cause Symptoms Of Reflux/ Heartburn?

Reflux of duodenal contents into the stomach and esophagus is called duodenogastroesophageal reflux (DGER). Alkaline reflux (containing achlorhydric gastric contents and/or bile) causes esophageal pain and/or esophagitis.[19] Although it occurs in non-surgically treated patients, bile-induced gastritis occurs more commonly after gastric surgery, cholecystectomy, or ampullary sphincteroplasty. If mild, alkaline reflux may be the only result. If severe, this may include chronic epigastric pain exacerbated by meals, bilious vomiting, weight loss, iron deficiency anemia, hypo/achlorhydria, and gastritis. Gastric or esophageal bile staining may be seen on esophagogastroduodenoscopy. These patients do not respond significantly to standard allopathic acid suppressive treatment or promotility agents. Only about 30% of patients with acid reflux have DGER.[20] In a study of 146 patients with reflux symptoms, 32% had bile reflux alone, while another 32% had acid and bile reflux. Only 19% had acid reflux alone. In esophageal pathology, the incidence of DGER increases with the severity of esophageal lesions.[21]

How May A Diagnosis Of Hypochlorhydria Be Formed?

Gastric string test or Heidelberg capsule test (See Chapter 9)

Riddler's gastric acid point (See Chapter 8)

Clinical picture (Table 13.4)

Lab indicators:

- Low serum levels

  Total protein, globulin, ferritin, calcium, magnesium, blood urea nitrogen (BUN)

  B_{12} below <300 pmol/L
- Neutrophilic hypersegmentation index > 10%
- Hair analysis—5 or 6 low minerals (other than Na, K)
- Complete blood count—Mean corpuscular volume above 93.0 fL
- Stool testing

  Persistent/excessive dysbiosis or fungal overgrowth

Treatment Of Hypochlorhydria

1. ***Optimizing the psychophysiology of digestion*** is central in improving parasympathetic tone. This is so important, I am repeating it:
   - Maximize the cephalic phase of digestion by smelling and savoring the food while it is being prepared and eating food that is prepared in an appetizing way.
   - Say grace before meals or employ a minute of slow abdominal breathing or other mindfulness practice.

- Avoid overeating and large meals
- Take time to sit and chew food until it becomes liquid before swallowing (Fletcherizing)
- Avoid stressful discussions, watching television or working at the computer, while eating. With too much distraction, a person may fail to experience the meal—hence overeating and "underdigesting"
- Avoid driving a car while eating
- Sit and relax while eating, rather than eating on the run
- If family of origin eating issues are related to present eating habits, consider counseling or energetic psychology interventions

2. ***Avoid excessive or cold fluid w/ meals***—If the water is used to"wash" the food into the esophagus rather than chewing thoroughly, this may lead to indigestion. Otherwise, sips of cool or room temperature water at a meal (rather than ice water) in between swallowing the bolus of food is generally not a problem. Cold liquids slow transit, while hot liquids enhance motility. These facts apply to the esophagus in patients with esophageal dysmotility.[22] A Japanese study looked at the effect of the female endocrine cycle on cold liquids and transit time. Drinking cold milk accelerated orocecal transit time only during the luteal phase but not the follicular phase of the menstrual cycle.[23]
3. ***Avoid excess fat and sugar at meals***—High fat meals delay gastric emptying (as does hypochlorhydria).
4. ***Employ basic food combining***—Simple meals with fewer ingredients may significantly improve digestion.
5. ***Consider leisurely walks after meals***
6. ***Treat adrenal, thyroid, and autoimmune disease***
7. ***Treat H. pylori if indicated***—H. pylori gastritis is a known cause of hypochlorhydria. Children with iron deficiency anemia due to H. pylori gastritis have normalization of the anemia after antibiotic treatment alone—without iron supplementation.[24] H. pylori should only be treated if there is a clear indication.
8. ***Bitters (ie. Gentian lutea) or vinegar 10-15 minutes prior to meals***

9. ***Betaine HCl (or glutamic acid HCl) with pepsin***—Glutamic acid hydrochloride did not decrease fasting gastric pH in euchlorhydric subjects, but significantly reduced pH in subjects with simulated hypochlorhydria produced by orally administered ranitidine.[25]
10. ***Consider the need to supplement minerals, B_{12}, and folate***
11. ***Treat underlying unresolved stress and improve coping skills***

Case example

A 29 year-old male presented to our clinic with severe digestive problems that began about age 12. His episodic abdominal pain tended to be either right or left sided which came on after eating, so he tended to eat very small amounts of food. There was also intense nausea (7-9/10) which was present on waking and often lasted until mid-afternoon. He did not vomit. He did not eat breakfast because of the nausea. The pain was intense (8/10) and daily. His stools alternated between diarrhea and constipation – small, incomplete, difficult to pass. There was a generalized bloating of the abdomen. Energy was very low (3/10) and he had become quite socially isolated. This man had a successful business that he had to give up three years prior, due to the fatigue and pain.

A Heidelberg test revealed hypochlorhydria. A stool fungal culture grew 3+ Candida albicans. There was no H. pylori colonization. Treatment began with 500,000 units of nystatin powder daily, working up to 2 million units per day over time. He took 1400 mg betaine hydrochloride per meal, based on Heidelberg testing. A probiotic supplying 4 billion Lactobacillus and Bifidobacter organisms was used. His response over 3-6 months was a complete resolution of nausea and abdominal pain.

Proton "Pumpaganda"

A 2008 article in *Digestion* asks "Do we need gastric acid?"[26] My experience is a resounding yes! In Jonathan Wright's book, *Why Stomach Acid is Good For You,* he attempts to re-educate the lay public exposed to decades of proton pumpaganda. Proton pump inhibitors are often symptomatically effective in the management of peptic ulcer disease, Barrett's esophagus, pyrosis, reflux esophagitis, chronic cough[27] and asthma[28] and they are adjunctive treatment for H. pylori along with antibiotics.

These drugs were designed to be used for a period of six to eight weeks in order to allow the healing of peptic ulceration. The common application has become one of lifelong use, since these medications provide symptom relief and protection against the inflammatory, ulcerogenic and dysplastic effects of refluxing acid *only as long as they are administered.*

Proton Pump Inhibitors And Hypochlorhydria

Proton pump inhibitors (PPIs) are an $11 billion a year industry in the US. It is believed that these are significantly overprescribed.[84] There were 95 million prescriptions written for these in 2005. Most are also available OTC.[29]

Table 13.6 PPI Generic/Brand Names	
Omeprazole (Prilosec)	Pantoprazole (Protonix)
Omeprazole and aspirin (Yosprala)	Rabeprazole (Aciphex)
Lansoprazole (Prevacid)	Esomeprazole (Nexium)
Dexlansoprazole (Dexilent)	

PPIs block the H+/K+ ATPase enzyme system on parietal cells. This action increases pepsinogen and gastrin and lowers pepsin and HCl.[30]

Proton Pump Inhibitors And Bacterial Overgrowth

Gastric alkalinity increases the level of nitrate rendering bacteria and increases carcinogenic nitrosamines in gastric juice. A pH > 3.8 allows gastric bacterial overgrowth. Thirty-five percent of patients on omeprazole had overgrowth compared to ten percent of controls.[29]

Omeprazole also causes small intestinal bacterial overgrowth[30] (see Chapter 6). A study performed by the Pfizer corporation revealed that lansoprazole use increases the incidence of commensal overgrowth leading to Clostridium difficile associated diarrhea (CDAD).[31] An article by Metz reiterates the link between hypochlorhydria and PPIs and recommends the lowest effective dose be used when patients enter a hospital. "Clostridium difficile colitis, an epidemic of major importance among hospitalized individuals, is potentially facilitated by the fourth mechanism (hypochlorhydria) in PPI users."[32] PPIs are commonly prescribed to prevent acute gastritis and stress ulcers in patients admitted to intensive care units. A group at Seton Hall University showed that if the analysis is limited to first-time use during a hospital stay, PPIs are strongly associated with CDAD. They concluded that "these data suggest that the widespread prescription of PPIs for stress ulcer prophylaxis in acute care facilities may contribute to the increased incidence of CDAD."[33]

Nosocomial systemic Candida fungal infections have a mortality rate as high as forty-eight percent. Risk factors are hypochlorhydria, parenteral nutrition, surgery, and placement of central venous catheters.[34]

Hydrochloric acid may aid in the prevention of murine prion infection.[35] Mice given ranitidine (an H_2 receptor antagonist) contracted scrapie—analogous to Creutzfeldt-Jakob disease at a significantly lower dose than mice with adequate gastric acid.

Proton Pump Inhibitors, Hypergastrinemia And Neoplasia

Hypergastrinemia has several implications which increase the risk of gastric polyps and may have relevance to gastric and colon cancer. An article by Waldum in 2000 states:

> A decrease in acidity always causes an increase in plasma gastrin. The trophic effect of gastrin leads to hyperplasia and neoplasia of the enterochromaffin-like (ECL)* cell. ECL cell derived tumours in man were previously regarded as rare, and also as rather benign. It is now clear that the ECL cell gives rise to a significant proportion of gastric carcinomas. Moreover, ECL cell carcinoids secondary to hypergastrinaemia may develop into highly malignant tumours.[36]

There are reports indicating development of ECL cell carcinoids after long-term treatment with proton pump inhibitors. Moreover, the ECL cell may give rise to colonic cancer [37] and gastric carcinomas of diffuse type, which have increased during the last few decades. Gastric cancers occurred significantly more often in lanzoprazole-treated rats with duodenogastric reflux (50%) compared with controls (27%).[38]

---

*ECL (enterochromaffin-like cell) is synonymous with EEC (enteroendocrine cell).

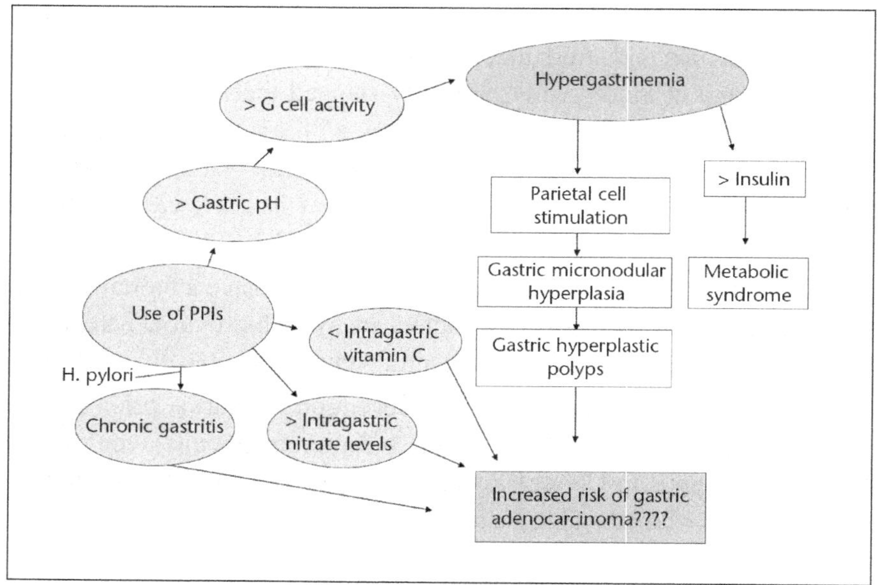

FIGURE 13.1 PPIs, H. PYLORI AND GASTRIC MUCOSAL HYPERPLASIA

Gastric hyperplastic polyps are usually multiple, <1cm, and sessile and occur after a mean of 32.5 months on PPIs. Most carcinoids develop in patients with long lasting hypergastrinemia and are of ECL origin. It is estimated that, in humans, it takes at least ten years to induce ECL cell carcinoids.[39] H. pylori overgrowth profoundly decreases intragastric vitamin C levels.[40] Vitamin C has an important role in reducing gastric nitrosamine formation.[41,42] It is also well proven that H. pylori overgrowth can cause hypochlorhydria.[43] High intragastric pH markedly raises intragastric nitrite levels, profoundly lowers gastric juice ascorbic acid and allows colonization by nitrosating bacteria and formation of n-nitroso compounds.

Freeman, writing in the *World Journal of Gastroenterology* says:

> [An] epidemic of fundic gland polyposis will be defined. Studies are needed to determine if further follow-up of patients on long-term therapy with proton pump inhibitors and fundic gland polyps is warranted. In spite of an early record of safety with long-term use, there remain concerns regarding the potential risk of cancer with

long-term exposure, not only in those with familial adenomatous polyposis, but also in those (otherwise) genetically predisposed to cancer.[44]

The stomach is capable of absorbing alcohol or converting it to acetaldehyde, which is a known carcinogen in the digestive tract and heart of humans. Ethanol conversion to acetaldehyde is enhanced by the bacterial overgrowth caused by lansoprazole induced hypochlorhydria.[45]

Reg protein is expressed in gastric fundic ECL cells. It is stimulated by gastrin, H. pylori overgrowth and certain cytokines (CINC-2β). Its effect is to increase proliferation of gastric mucosal cells. Reg protein is produced in many gastric cancers, especially the more advanced and poorly differentiated types. The hypergastrinemia induced by PPIs may increase proliferation of these gastric cancer cells.[46]

A British study investigated the effect of PPI induced hypergastrinemia on human colonic adenoma when grown in mice. They found that the use of omeprazole and lansoprazole increased the weight of human adenoma grafts by 43-70%.[47] A review of the risk of long-tern PPI use found a non-significant increase in colon cancer with higher dosage ranges and increasing duration of use.[48]

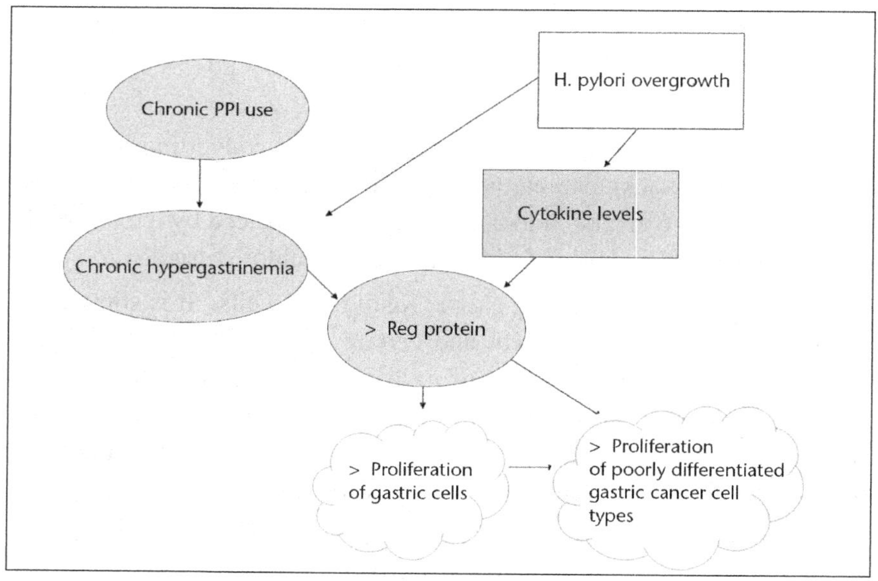

FIGURE 13.2 PROTON PUMP INHIBITORS, H. PYLORI, REG PROTEIN AND GASTRIC CANCER

Excessive G cell production of gastrin is an adaptive response as the system tries to upregulate the parietal cell. Research published in 2006 in the *Journal of Rheumatology* reported that TSH levels are significantly altered in patients treated with PPIs.[49] Other hormones are affected by PPIs as well (Table 13.7).

TABLE 13.7 ENZYME, ACID AND HORMONAL EFFECTS FROM CHRONIC USE OF PPIs

Increases	**Decreases**
Pepsinogen Gastrin Calcitonin[50] Parathyroid hormone (in chickens)[51] Cortisol (rabeprazole and lansoprazole)[52] TSH (in treated hypothyroidism due to poor absorption of oral thyroxine)[53]	Pepsin Hydrochloric acid

Proton Pump Inhibitors And Pathological Fracture

Hydrochloric acid is needed for functional protein and calcium absorption. Not surprisingly there is a significant increase in the risk of hip fracture in women over age 50 on long term acid suppression therapy. When these women take PPIs for more than a year they have a 44% increased risk of hip fractures. In addition, long term high dose use increases hip fracture by 245%.[54] No increase in fracture risk was found for H2 receptor antagonists (cimetadine, etc.) Roux, et al, found a three-fold increase in vertebral fractures in post-menopausal women taking omeprazole.[55] A Canadian study of 15,792 subjects with osteoporotic fractures linked significant risk with at least seven years of PPI use.[56] In a review, Yang points out that inhibition of the osteoclastic proton pumps may actually reduce bone resorption, while potent acid suppression decreases intestinal calcium absorption. In addition, PPI-induced hypergastrinemia may speed bone resorption due to parathyroid hyperplasia.[57]

Proton Pump Inhibitors And Pneumonia

Reduction of gastric acid secretion may lead to bacterial and viral colonization of the stomach and small intestine. These organisms may originate in the oral cavity and gastroenteric overgrowth is normally prevented by proteolysis. I hypothesize that fluid reflux may then introduce these organisms to the respiratory tract or the organisms may be inhaled as an aerosol. Leheij reported that the use of PPIs is associated with a 1.89 risk ratio for community acquired pneumonia while H2 receptor antagonists carry a 1.63 risk ratio.[58] Several studies specified an even higher risk (odds ratio of 5.0) in the first 30 days of initiating the acid blockade.[59,60]

Proton Pump Inhibitors And Myocardial Infarction

Research is active on this topic. PPIs may be an independent risk factor for heart attacks. The number needed to harm is over 4000, so the risk is relatively low.[83]

Table 13.8 Other Common Side Effects Of PPIs	
CNS	Headache, dizziness, asthenia
GI	Diarrhea, constipation, abdominal pain, nausea and/or vomiting
Miscellaneous	URI, rash, alopecia, cough, back pain,myositis, polymyositis, rhabdomyolysis[61]

Rare cases of interstitial nephritis and cutaneous vasculitis have occurred as a reaction to pantoprazole (Protonix).[62] Peripheral edema is a side effect of PPIs in women.[63] One of my patients developed fulmanent hepatic failure when started on a PPI course when she was hospitalized for pancreatitis. The drug reactions were recognized and her liver function normalized several days after cessation of the drug.

Proton Pump Inhibitors And Drug Interactions

The FDA advises patients taking PPIs to warn their physician or pharmacist if they are also taking diazepam, warfarin, antifungals, digoxin, tacrolimus, or atazanavir. Co-administration of PPIs and warfarin, clarithromycin, or corticosteroids increases the risk of medical complications.[64] All PPIs except for rabeprazole are metabolized by the P450 system enzyme CYP 2C19. The bioavailability of omeprazole and esomeprazole increases after the first week of dosage due to a progressive reduction in their hepatic clearance. In other words, these drugs impair the activity of CYP 2C19.[67] Melatonin appears to reduce some of the negative effects of ranitidine and omeprazole.[66]

Table 13.9 Proton Pump Inhibitor—Drug Interactions	
Decreased levels Related to phase I CYP 2C19 competition	Diazepam Warfarin Antifungals Digoxin Tacrolimus Atazanavir
Increased levels Related to decreased renal clearance[67]	Methotrexate

Proton Pump Inhibitors And Laboratory Testing

Table 13.10 Effects Of Lansoprazole On Lab Values		
Increases	Transaminases Globulin LDH Creatinine	Glucocorticoids Alkaline phosphatase Bilirubin Eosinophils
Increases or decreases	Electrolytes Total cholesterol	

Table 13.11 Effects Of Rabeprazole On Lab Values	
Increases	Glucose Albumin Total cholesterol Transaminases PSA CPK
Increases or decreases	RBCs WBCs Platelets

Proton Pump Inhibitors And Cognition

Increased brain burden of β-amyloid is seen in subjects taking PPIs. Significant impairment in attention, executive function and visual memory has been found in those taking all the major forms of PPIs.[85]

Proton Pump Inhibitors And Nutrient Absorption

Long term PPI use may cause deficiencies of calcium, iron, vitamin B_{12} and zinc.

Calcium

Gastric acid is needed for proper absorption of dietary calcium.[68] O'Conell writes:

> In vitro calcium carbonate disintegration and dissolution is pH dependant, as pH increases, disintegration and dissolution slows, decreasing from 96% at a pH of 1.0 to 23% at a pH of 6.1. Proton pump inhibitors effectively reduce gastric acid production and increase gastric pH to an average of 5.5 with 19% of the day spent above a pH of 6.0.[69]

Dietary supplementation with lactic acid or lactic acid dairy products improves calcium absorption in hypochlorhyric rats.[70] Compared to placebo, omeprazole decreased calcium absorption by 41% in a seven day trial. A study at Tufts University found no decrease in calcium absorption in subjects exposed to a *single dose of omeprazole* even though it induced transient hypochlorhydria.[71]

Iron

Long term use of PPIs increases the risk of iron malabsorption. This is especially important in patients who are iron deficient prior to commencing acid suppression.[72] Treatment of H. pylori overgrowth has cured several cases of chronic iron deficiency anemia in children and adults.[73,74] Perhaps this is due to correction of the hypochlorhydria induced by many cases of H. pylori overgrowth.

Magnesium

PPIs are associated with magnesium deficiency and the risk of magnesium deficiency-associated cardiac issues. [82]

Vitamin B_{12}

Case reports of B_{12} in patients taking long term PPIs indicate a gradual decrease in serum levels.[75,76] Some studies find no significant decline. Research using more accurate markers than serum cyanocobalamin such as methyl-malonic acid, holotranscobalamine II, homocysteine or neutrophilic segmentation index may be more definitive and should be pursued.

Zinc

Omeprazole decreases intestinal zinc absorption.[77] A Jordanian study found that zinc, copper and cobalt form complexes with omeprazole.[78]

Proton Pump Inhibitors And Rebound Hypersecretion

Significant rebound acid hypersecretion lasts from 8 to 26 weeks after long-term proton pump inhibition is discontinued.[79,80]

Clearly, the naturopathic approach to digestive wellness with a focus on improving function is the ideal approach. Optimizing the tone of the lower esophageal sphincter as well as the tone of the parasympathetic nervous system, and normalizing gastric and pancreatic secretion with resultant reduction or obliteration of reflux symptoms, is the ideal treatment for GERD. I agree with the following quote from the *Digestive and Liver Disease Journal*:

> The relatively common use of acid inhibitors in uncomplicated GERD or in the prevention of NSAID and steroid gastropathy is often unsubstantiated and should be limited to very specific situations.

1 Lahner E, Annibale B, Delle Fave G. Systematic Review: Heliocobacter Pylori Infection and Impaired Drug Absorption. *Aliment Pharmacol Ther.* 2008 Nov 26. [Epub ahead of print]

2 Wang F, Xia P, Wu F, et al Helicobacter pylori VacA disrupts apical membrane-cytoskeletal interactions in gastric parietal cells. *J Biol Chem.* 2008 Sep 26;283(39):26714-25. Epub 2008 Jul 14.

3 Robbins , Cotran, Pathologic Basis of disease Page

4 De Block, CE *J. Clin Endocrinol Metab.* 2008 Feb;93(2):363-71.

5 Golan, R, *Optimal Wellness*, Ballantine Books, NY, New York, 1995.

6 Daković Z, Vesić S, Vuković J, Milenković S, Janković-Terzić K, Dukić S, Pavlović MD. Ocular rosacea and treatment of symptomatic Helicobacter pylori infection: a case series. *Acta Dermatovenerol Alp Panonica Adriat.* 2007 Jun;16(2):83-6.

7 Lahner E, Annibale B, Delle Fave G Systematic Review: Heliocobacter Pylori Infection and Impaired Drug Absorption. *Aliment Pharmacol Ther.* 2008 Nov 26. [Epub ahead of print]

8 Herzlich, B C : Schiano, T D : Moussa, Z : Zimbalist, E : Panagopoulos, G : Ast, A : Nawabi, I. Decreased intrinsic factor secretion in AIDS: relation to parietal cell acid secretory capacity and vitamin B12 malabsorption. *Am J Gastroenterol.* 1992 Dec; 87(12): 1781-8.

9 Goodman KI, Salt WB 2nd. Vitamin B12 deficiency. Important new concepts in recognition. *Postgrad Med.* 1990 Sep 1;88(3):147-50, 153-8.

10 Lechner K, Födinger M, Grisold W, Püspök A, Sillaber C.Vitamin B12 deficiency. New data on an old theme. *Wien Klin Wochenschr.* 2005 Sept;117(17:579-91.

11 Koike T, Kuzuya M, Kanda S, Okada K, Izawa S, Enoki H, Iguchi A. Raised homocysteine and low folate and vitamin B-12 concentrations predict cognitive decline in community-dwelling older Japanese adults. *Clin Nutr.* 2008 Dec;27(6):865-71.

12 Dali-Youcef N, Andrès E An update on cobalamin deficiency in adults. *QJM.* 2008 Nov 5. [Epub ahead of print]

13 Lechner K et al Vitamin B12 deficiency, New data on an old theme. Wien Klin Wochenschr. 2005 Sep;117(17):579-91.

14 Hershko C, Ronson A, Souroujon M, Maschler I, Heyd J, Patz J. Variable hematologic presentation of autoimmune gastritis: age-related progression from iron deficiency to cobalamin depletion. Blood. 2006 Feb 15;107(4):1673-9.

15 Herrmann W, Geisel J. Vegetarian lifestyle and monitoring of vitamin B-12 status Clin Chim Acta. 2002 Dec;326(1-2):47-59.

16 Selhub J, Jacques PF, Dallal G, Choumenkovitch S, Rogers G. The use of blood concentrations of vitamins and their respective functional indicators to define folate and vitamin B12 status. *Food Nutr Bull.* 2008 Jun;29(2 Suppl):S67-73.

17 Clarke R, Birks J, Nexo E, Ueland PM, Schneede J, Scott J, Molloy A, Evans JG. Low vitamin B-12 status and risk of cognitive decline in older adults *Am J Clin Nutr.* 2007 Nov;86(5):1384-91.

18 Lovat LB. Age related changes in gut physiology and nutritional status. *Gut.* 1996 Mar;38(3):306-9.

19 Nath BJ, Warshaw AL. Alkaline reflux gastritis and esophagitis. *Annu Rev Med.* 1984;35:383-96.

20 Fein M, Fuchs KH, Freys SM, Maroske J, Tigges H, Thiede A. Is duodeno-gastroesophageal relux just a bystander of acid reflux? *Zentralbl Chir* 2002 Dec;1279120: 1068-72.

21 Kunsch S, Linhart T, Fensterer H, Adler G, Gress TM, Ellenrieder V. [Prevalence of a pathological DGER (duodeno-gastric-oesophageal reflux) in patients with clinical symptoms of reflux disease] *Z Gastroenterol* 2008 May;46(5):409-14.

22 Triadafilopoulos G, Tsang HP, Segall GM. Hot water swallows improve symptoms and accelerate esophageal clearance in esophageal motility disorders. *J Clin Gastroenterol.* 1998 Jun;26(4):239-44.

23 Kagaya M, Iwata N, Toda Y, Mitsui T, Nakae Y, Kondo T. Cold milk accelerates oro-cecal transit time during the luteal phase but not the follicular phase in women. *Nagoya J Med Sci.* 1999 May;62(1-2):57-62.

24 Cardamone M, Alex G, Harari MD, Moss WP, Oliver MR Severe iron-deficiency anaemia in adolescents: consider Helicobacter pylori infection. *J Paediatr Child Health.* 2008 Nov;44(11):647-50.

25 Knapp MJ, Berardi RR, Dressman JB, Rider JM, Carver PL. Modification of gastric pH with oral glutamic acid hydrochloride. *Clin Pharm.* 1991 Nov;10(11):866-9.

26 Pohl D, Fox M, Fried M, Göke B, Prinz C, Mönnikes H, Rogler G, Dauer M, Keller J, Lippl F, Schiefke I, Seidler U, Allescher HD. Do we need gastric acid? *Digestion.* 2008;77(3-4):184-97.

27 Yu L, Qiu Z, Lü H, Wei W, Shi C. Clinical benefit of sequential three-step empirical therapy in the management of chronic cough. *Respirology.* 2008 May;13(3):353-8.

28 Littner MR, Leung FW, Ballard ED 2nd, Huang B, Samra NK Effects of 24 weeks of lansoprazole therapy on asthma symptoms, exacerbations, quality of life, and pulmonary function in adult asthmatic patients with acid reflux symptoms. *Chest.* 2005 Sep;128(3):1128-35.

29 Theisen J, Nehra D, Citron D, Johansson J, Hagen JA, Crookes PF, DeMeester SR, Bremner CG, DeMeester TR, Peters JH. Suppression of gastric acid secretion in patients with gastroesophageal reflux disease results in gastric bacterial overgrowth and deconjugation of bile acids. *J Gastrointest Surg.* 2000 Jan-Feb;4(1):50-4.

30 Paiva SA, Sepe TE, Booth SL, Camilo ME, O'Brien ME, Davidson KW, Sadowski JA, Russell RM, Interaction between vitamin K nutriture and bacterial overgrowth in hypochlorhydria induced by omeprazole. *Am J Clin Nutr.* 1998 Sep;68(3):699-704.

31 Hauben M, Horn S, Reich L, Younus M. Association between gastric acid suppressants and Clostridium difficile colitis and community-acquired pneumonia: analysis using pharmacovigilance tools. *Int J Infect Dis.* 2007 Sep;11(5):417-22.

32 Metz DC, Clostridium difficile colitis: wash your hands before stopping the proton pump inhibitor. *Am J Gastroenterol.* 2008 Sep;103(9):2314-6.

33 Jayatilaka S, Shakov R, Eddi R, Bakaj G, Baddoura WJ, DeBari VA. Clostridium difficile infection in an urban medical center: five-year analysis of infection rates among adult admissions and association with the use of proton pump inhibitors. *Ann Clin Lab Sci.* 2007 Summer;37(3):241-7.

34 Costa-de-Oliveira S, Pina-Vaz C, Mendonça D, Gonçalves Rodrigues A. A first Portuguese epidemiological survey of fungaemia in a university hospital. *Eur J Clin Microbiol Infect Dis.* 2008 May;27(5):365-74.

35 Martinsen TC, Taylor DM, Johnsen R, Waldum HL. Gastric Acidity Protects Mice Against Prion Infection? *Scand J Gastroenterol.* 2002 May;35(2):497-500.

36 Waldum HL, Brenna E. Personal review: is profound acid inhibition safe? Aliment Pharmacol Ther. 2000 Jan;14(1):15-22.

37 Watson SA, Morris TM, McWilliams DF, Harris J, Evans S, Smith A, Clarke PA.

Potential role of endocrine gastrin in the colonic adenoma carcinoma sequence. *Br J Cancer.* 2002 Aug 27;87(5):567-73.

38 Viste A, Øvrebø K, Maartmann-Moe H, Waldum, H. Lanzoprazole promotes gastric carcinogenesis in rats with duodenogastric reflux *Gastric Cancer*. 2004;7(1):31-5.

39 Choudhry U, Boyce HW Jr, Coppola D. Proton pump inhibitor-associated gastric polyps: a retrospective analysis of their frequency, and endoscopic, histologic, and ultrastructural characteristics. *Am J Clin Pathol.* 1998 Nov;110(5):615-21

40 McColl KE, el-Omar EM, Gillen D. Alterations in gastric physiology in Helicobacter pylori infection: causes of different diseases or all epiphenomena? *Ital J Gastroenterol Hepatol.* 1997 Oct;29(5):459

41 Combet E, Paterson S, Iijima K, Winter J, Mullen W, Crozier A, Preston T, McColl KE. Fat transforms ascorbic acid from inhibiting to promoting acid-catalysed N-nitrosation. *Gut.* 2007 Dec;56(12):1678-84. Epub 2007 Sep

42 Porubin D, Hecht SS, Li ZZ, Gonta M, Stepanov I. Endogenous formation of N'-nitrosonornicotine in F344 rats in the presence of some antioxidants and grape seed extract. *J Agric Food Chem.* 2007 Aug 22;55(17):7199-204

43 Wang F, Xia P, Wu F, Wang D, Wang W, Ward T, Liu Y, Aikhionbare F, Guo Z, Powell M, Liu B, Bi F, Shaw A, Zhu Z, Elmoselhi A, Fan D, Cover TL, Ding X, Yao X. Helicobacter pylori VacA disrupts apical membrane-cytoskeletal interactions in gastric parietal cells. *J Biol Chem.* 2008 Sep 26;283(39):26714-25.

44 Robertson DJ, Larsson H, Friis S, Pedersen L, Baron JA, Sorensen HT. Proton pump inhibitor use and risk of colorectal cancer: a population-based, case-control study. *Gatroenterol.* 2007 Sep;133(3):755-60.

45 Väkeväinen S, Tillonen J, Blom M, Jousimies-Somer, Salaspuro M. Acetaldehyde and other ADH-related characteristics of aerobic bacteria isolated by hypochlorhydric human stomach *Alcohol Clin Exp Res* 2001 Mar; 25(3): 421-6.

46 Kinoshita Y, Ishihara S, Kadowaki Y, Fukui H, Chiba T. Reg protein is a unique growth factor of gastric mucosal cells. *J Gastroenterol.* 2004 Jun;39(6):507-13.

47 Watson SA, Morris TM, McWilliams DF, Harris J, Evans S, Smith A, Clarke PA. Potential role of endocrine gastrin in the colonic adenoma carcinoma sequence. *Br J Cancer.* 2002 Aug 27;87(5):567-73.

48 Yang, YX, Hennessy S, Propert K, Hwang WT, Sedarat A, Lewis JD. Chronic proton pump inhibitor therapy and the risk of colorectal cancer. *Gastroenterol.* 2007 Sep;133(3):748-54.

49 Sachmechi I, Reich DM, Aninyei M, Wibowo F, Gupta G, Kim PJ. Effect of proton pump inhibitors on serum thyroid-stimulating hormone level in euthyroid patients treated with levothyroxine for hypothyroidism. Endocr Pract. 2007 Jul-Aug;13(4):345-9.

50 Erdogan MF, Gursoy A, Kulaksizoglu M. Long-term effects of elevated gastrin levels on calcitonin secretion. *J Endocrinol Invest.* 2006 Oct;29(9):771-5.

51 Gagnemo-Persson R, Samuelsson A, Hâkanson R, Persson P. Chicken parathyroid hormone gene expression in response to gastrin, omeprazole, ergocalciferol, and restricted food intake. *Calcif Tissue Int.* 1997 Sep;61(3):210-5.

52 Katagiri F, Inoue S, Sato Y, Itoh H, Takeyama M.Comparison of the effects of proton pump inhibitors on human plasma adrenocorticotropic hormone and *Biomed Pharmacother.* 2006 Apr;60(3):109-12.

53 Lahner E, Annibale B, Delle Fave G. Systematic Review: Heliocobacter Pylori Infection and Impaired Drug Absorption. *Aliment Pharmacol Ther.* 2008 Nov 26. [Epub ahead of print]

54 Yu-Xiao Yang, MD, MSCE; James D. Lewis, MD, MSCE; Solomon Epstein, MD; David C. Metz, MD Long-term Proton Pump Inhibitor Therapy and Risk of Hip Fracture *JAMA*. 2006;296:2947-2953.

55 Roux C, Briot K, Gossec L, Kolta S, Blenk T, Felsenberg D, Reid DM, Eastell R, Glüer CC. Increase in Vertebral Fracture Risk in Postmenopausal Women Using Omeprazole. *Calcif Tissue Int*. 2008 Nov 21. [Epub ahead of print]

56 Targownik LE, Lix LM, Metge CJ, Prior HJ, Leung S, Leslie WD. Use of proton pump inhibitors and risk of osteoporosis-related fractures. CMAJ. 2008 Aug 12;179(4): 319-26.

57 Yang YX, Proton pump inhibitor therapy and osteoporosis. *Curr Drug Saf.* 2008 Sep;3(3):204-9.

58 Laheij RJ, Sturkenboom MC, Hassing RJ, Dieleman J, Stricker BH, Jansen JB Risk of community-acquired pneumonia and use of gastric acid-suppressive drugs. *JAMA*. 2004 Oct 27;292(16):1955-60.

59 Sarkar M, Hennessy S, Yang YX. Proton-pump inhibitor use and the risk for community-acquired pneumonia. *Ann Intern Med*. 2008 Sep 16;149(6):391-8.

60 Gulmez SE, Holm A, Frederiksen H, Jensen TG, Pedersen C, Hallas J. Use of proton pump inhibitors and the risk of community-acquired pneumonia: a population-based case-control study. *Arch Intern Med.* 2007 May 14;167(9):950-5.

61 Clark DW, Strandell J. Myopathy including polymyositis: a likely class adverse effect of proton pump inhibitors? *Eur J Clin Pharmacol.* 2006 Jun;62(6):473-9. Epub 2006 Apr 22.

62 Jacobs-Kosmin D, Derk CT, Sandorfi N. Pantoprazole and perinuclear antineutrophil cytoplasmic antibody-associated vasculitis. *J Rheumatol*. 2006 Mar;33(3):629-32.

63 Brunner G, Athmann C, Boldt JH. Reversible peripheral edema in female patients taking proton pump inhibitors for peptic acid diseases. *Dig Dis Sci*. 2001 May;46(5): 993-6.

64 McCarthy DM, McLaughlin TP, Griffis DL, Yazdani C. Impact of cotherapy with some proton pump inhibitors on medical claims among HMO patients already using other common drugs also cleared by cytochrome P450. *Am J Ther*. 2003 Sep-Oct;10(5):330-40.

65 *Horn J. Review* article: relationship between the metabolism and efficacy of proton pump inhibitors—focus on rabeprazole. *Aliment Pharmacol Ther.* 2004 Nov;20 Suppl 6:11-9.

66 Reiter RJ, Tan DX, Sainz RM, Mayo JC, Lopez-Burillo S. Melatonin: reducing the toxicity and increasing the efficacy of drugs. *J Pharm Pharmacol.* 2002 Oct;54(10):1299-321.

67 Beorlegui B, Aldaz A, Ortega A, Aquerreta I, Sierrasesúmega L, Giráldez J Potential interaction between methotrexate and omeprazole. *Ann Pharmacother*. 2000 Sep;34(9):1024-7.

68 Graziani G, Badalamenti S, Como G, Gallieni M, Finazzi S, Angelini C, Brancaccio D, Ponticelli C. Calcium and phosphate plasma levels in dialysis patients after dietary Ca-P overload. Role of gastric acid secretion. *Nephron.* 2002 Jul;91(3):474-9.

69 O'Connell MB, Madden DM, Murray AM, Heaney RP, Kerzner LJ. Effects of proton pump inhibitors on calcium carbonate absorption in women: a randomized crossover trial. *Am J Med.* 2005 Jul;118(7):778-81.

70 Chonan O, Takahashi R, Yasui H, Watanuki M. Effect of L-lactic acid on calcium absorption in rats fed omeprazole. *J Nutr Sci Vitaminol* (Tokyo). 1998 Jun;44(3): 473-81.

71 Serfaty-Lacrosniere C, Wood RJ, Voytko D, Saltzman JR, Pedrosa M, Sepe TE, Russell RR. Hypochlorhydria from short-term omeprazole treatment does not inhibit intestinal absorption of calcium, phosphorus, magnesium or zinc from food in humans. *J Am Coll Nutr.* 1995 Aug;14(4):364

72 Sharma VR, Brannon MA. Carloss EA. Effect of omeprazole on oral iron replacement in patients with iron deficiency anemia. *South Med J.* 2004 Sep;97(9):887-9.

73 Ashorn M, Ruuska T, Mäkipernaa A. Helicobacter pylori and iron deficiency anaemia in children. *Scand J Gastroenterol.* 2001 Jul;36(7):701-5.

74 Sugiyama T, Tsuchida M, Yokota K, Shimodan M, Asaka M. Improvement of long-standing iron-deficiency anemia in adults after eradication of Helicobacter pylori infection. *Intern Med.* 2002 Jun;41(6):491-4.

75 Ruscin JM, Page RL 2nd, Valuck RJ Vitamin B(12) deficiency associated with histamine(2)-receptor antagonists and a proton-pump inhibitor. *Ann Pharmacother.* 2002 May;36(5):812-6.

76 Termanini B, Gibril F, Sutliff VE, Yu F, Venzon DJ, Jensen RT. Effect of long-term gastric acid suppressive therapy on serum vitamin B12 levels in patients with Zollinger-Ellison syndrome. *Am J Med.* 1998 May;104(5):422-30.

77 Ozutemiz AO, Aydin HH, Isler M, Celik HA, Batur Y. Effect of omeprazole on plasma zinc levels after oral zinc administration. *Indian J Gastroenterol.* 2002 Nov-Dec;21(6):216-8.

78 Hamdan II. In vitro study of the interaction between omeprazole and the metal ions Zn(II), Cu(II), and Co(II). *Pharmazie.* 2001 Nov;56(11):877-81.

79 Fossmark R, Johnsen G, Johanessen E, Waldum HL. Rebound acid hypersecretion after long-term inhibition of gastric acid secretion. *Aliment Pharmacol Ther.* 2005 Jan 15;21(2):149-54.

80 Waldum HL, Arnestad JS, Brenna E, Eide I, Syversen U, Sandvik AK. Marked increase in gastric acid secretory capacity after omeprazole treatment. *Gut.* 1996 Nov;39(5):649-53.

81 Coati I et al, Autoimmune gastritis: Pathologist's viewpoint. *World J Gastroenterol.* 2015 Nov 14;21(42):12179-89.

82 Cheungpasitporn W et al, Proton pump inhibitors linked to hypomagnesemia: a systematic review and meta-analysis of observational studies. *Ren Fail.* 2015 Aug;37(7):1237-41

83 Shih CJ et al, Proton pump inhibitor use represents an independent risk factor for myocardial infarction. *Int J Cardio.* 2014 Nov 15;177(1):292-7.

84 Heidelbaugh JJ et al, Overutilization of proton-pump inhibitors: what the clinician needs to know. *Therap Adv Gastroenterol.* 2012 Jul; 5(4): 219–232.

85. Akter S et al, Cognitive impact after short-term exposure to different proton pump inhibitors: assessment using CANTAB software. *Alzheimers Res Ther.* 2015 Dec 27;7:79.

Chapter 14
Pancreatic Exocrine Insufficiency

Etiology of Pancreatic Dysfunction

Celiac Disease, Cow's Milk Enteropathy, and Pancreatic Insufficiency

Bone Mineral Density and the Pancreas

Other Factors

Diagnosis—Stool Chymotrypsin and Elastase

Treatment Options in Pancreatic Insufficiency

- *Failor's Pancreactic Technique*
- *Pancreatic Enzyme Replacement*
- *Organotherapy*
- *Antioxidant Nutrition*

Etiology Of Pancreatic Dysfunction

Pancreatic insufficiency (fecal elastase <200ug/g) occurs in up to 40% of diabetics. It is also common in persons who are obese, have hyperlipidemia or insulin resistance.[1,2] Tobacco use is an independent risk factor for pancreatic insufficiency.[20] Some cases of pancreatic insufficiency may be caused by a hormonal deficiency secondary to H. pylori colonization.[3] An article in *Medical Hypothesis* discusses impaired secretin release and reduced numbers of duodenal S cells as a result of H. pylori overgrowth and the gastric metaplasia it causes in the duodenum. Without adequate secretin, reduced bicarbonate levels from hepatic, pancreatic, biliary and submucosal glands increase the risk of peptic ulceration. Loss of secretin may also reduce pancreatic exocrine secretion.[4] The study used a cutoff of 200ug/g, for fecal elastase, which indicates moderate insufficiency. Note that H. pylori may be part of the commensal gastrobiota.[21] Carefully consider the risks versus benefits before treating patients who do not have recurrent peptic ulcer disease or other classic H. pylori related diseases. Chronic viral hepatitis B or C can cause pancreatic insufficiency. A Russian study found enzyme deficiency in 18% of viral hepatitis patients.[5]

Celiac Disease, Cow's Milk Enteropathy, And Pancreatic Insufficiency

It is estimated that greater than 20% of patients with celiac disease have pancreatic insufficiency.[6] Celiac patients maintained on a gluten-free diet who continue to have chronic diarrhea have a five-fold greater incidence of low fecal elastase than celiac patients who are free from digestive complaints on a gluten-free diet.[7] The pathophysiology is thought to be related to villous atrophy with loss of S cells and I cells. Protein malnutrition probably leads to pancreatic acinar atrophy and deficient precursors of enzyme synthesis.[8] A study of children with villous atrophy secondary to celiac disease found that stool chymotrypsin levels returned to normal after following a gluten-free diet for twelve months.[9] The dietary protocol restored CCK production and pancreatic secretion to normal, as it regenerated the intestinal mucosa.[10] A similar trend was seen with fecal elastase levels in patients suffering from cow's milk protein enteropathy before and after six months on a milk-free diet. Residual pancreatic exocrine dysfunction should be considered in gluten or casein sensitive patients who fail to respond to a gluten or casein-free diets.

TABLE 14.1 POSSIBLE UNDERLYING ETIOLOGIES FOR PANCREATIC INSUFFICIENCY
Small intestinal bacterial overgrowth
Tobacco, alcohol or other causes of chronic pancreatitis
Pancreatic adenocarcinoma
Biliary stasis (including pancreatic and ampullary neoplasms)
Hypochlorhydria—induces low pancreatic output due to decreased secretin release
Diabetes mellitus
Gluten or casein intolerance
Adrenal maladaption
Hepatitis B or C
Cystic fibrosis

Imaging of the pancreas may be important in diagnosing underlying causes of pancreatic insufficiency in cases of chronic pancreatitis. Remember that chronic pancreatitis can lead to pancreatic adenocarcinoma.

Steroid Hormones And The Pancreas

There is a fascinating and little-appreciated relationship between the pancreas and steroid hormones. Pancreatic tissue synthesizes estrogen, progesterone and testosterone, responds to steroid hormones and expresses steroid receptor molecules. Estradiol induces exocrine enzyme production but not secretion in mice.[11] A short term effect of glucocorticoids is up-regulation of pancreatic enzyme secretion but chronic exogenous administration of cortisol may lead to pancreatic exocrine dysfunction.[12]

With respect to the endocrine pancreas, glucagon producing α-islet cells activate glucocorticoids which elevate blood glucose.[13] Insulin synthesis and release are modulated by steroids such as cortisol.[14]

Table 14.2 Steroid Effects On The Exocrine And Endocrine Pancreas

Estrogen	Increases amylase and trypsin production but not secretion by regulation of the CCK receptor density (murine)
Cortisol	Up-regulates pancreatic T3 receptors, thereby up-regulating exocrine secretions (murine) Prolonged exogenous cortisol inhibits secretion (esp. amylase)
Testosterone	Promotes pancreatic growth (murine)

Bone Mineral Density And The Pancreas

Malabsorption in pancreatic exocrine insufficiency (PEI) decreases bone mineral density. Fat soluble vitamin deficiencies are thought to be part of the mechanism for osteopenia. A Swedish study examined the effect of PEI on bone density in males with chronic pancreatitis. Bone pain and a history of fracture were common in these men, 56% of whom tested positive for PEI. Supplementation with pancreatic enzymes was significantly associated with higher bone mineral density.[23] In another study, decreased levels of fecal elastase were also correlated with altered vitamin D, calcium and parathyroid hormone values in men and women with osteoporotic fractures.[24]

Other Factors

Either an excessively acidic intestinal pH or bacterial overgrowth may prevent adequate fat digestion, therefore these problems should be considered when a patient fails to respond to treatment for pancreatic insufficiency.[15]

A controlled study of patients with pancreatic insufficiency secondary to chronic pancreatitis found rapid gastric emptying and a decrease in gallbladder ejection fraction. Administration of pancreatic enzymes with meals normalized gastric emptying but not gallbladder function.[16]

Hyperchlorhydria or decreased bicarbonate production may increase the acidity of the duodenum which inactivates pancreatic enzymes. Note that this is not an enzymatic pancreatic insufficiency, but will create the same symptoms.

Diagnosis—Stool Chymotrypsin And Elastase

Fecal chymotrypsin and pancreatic elastase are markers of total pancreatic exocrine output and are screening tests for pancreatic insufficiency. A patient who is supplementing most forms of plant pancreatic enzymes or pancreatin with meals will have a falsely elevated chymotrypsin level, but an accurate elastase level. Pancreatic enzyme supplements do not contain elastase which is unique to the human pancreas, but most do contain chymotrypsin. A patient should discontinue these enzyme supplements prior to the stool chymotrypsin test. An acute diarrhea with a more liquid stool consistency may lead to a falsely low elastase level (positive test).[22]

TABLE 14.3 CHYMOTRYPSIN LEVELS AND PANCREATIC EXOCRINE OUTPUT
*Very low output = <4
*Low output = 4-9
Adequate output = >9
**Falsely low levels may occur with stool transit time >96 hours*

TABLE 14.4 PANCREATIC ELASTASE AND PANCREATIC EXOCRINE OUTPUT
Severe pancreatic insufficiency = <100 ug/g
Moderate pancreatic insufficiency = 100-200 ug/g
Indeterminate pancreatic output = 200-400 ug/g
Ideal pancreatic exocrine function = >400 ug/g
Note: Falsely low levels of elastase may occur with excessively liquid stool due to dilution of the sample.

PEI is described as occurring after 90% of the acini have been lost.25 I would suggest considering treatment for patients with elastase levels between 200-400 ug/g rather than waiting for 90% destruction of the gland before intervening.

Treatment Options In Pancreatic Insufficiency

Treat gastroparesis (see Chapter 7)

Treat hypochlorhydria (see Chapter 13)

Treat insulin resistance if present (see Chapter 7)

Stimulate the Chapman's pancreatic reflex—in the right or left 7th intercostal space.

Pancreatic Enzyme Replacement (or stimulation with organotherapy)

Failor's Pancreas Technique

Teach the patient to use Failor's Pacreas Technique. This simple visceral maneuver was taught by Ralph Failor, DC, ND. With the patient seated or supine, begin by stabilizing the skin with the left hand at the left mid-axillary line at the level of the umbilicus (see Figure 14.1). Take a tissue pull from right to left with a finger of the other hand (See figure 14.2) and let it recoil from left to right (see figure 14.3). Move the stabilizing fingers a few inches to the right and repeat the procedure, continuing across to the right mid-axillary line. Have the patient do this before each meal.

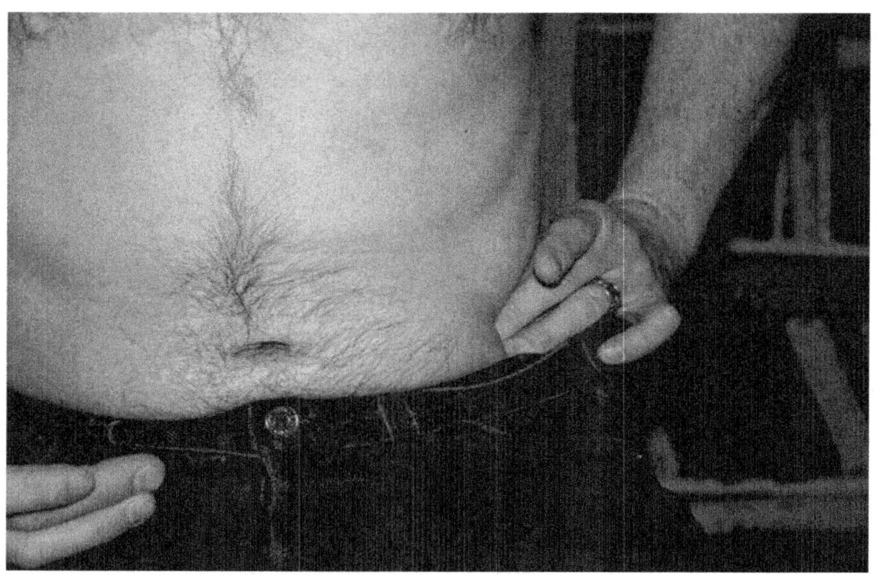

FIGURE 14.1 FAILOR'S PANCREATIC TECHNIQUE—
STABILIZE THE SKIN WITH THE LEFT HAND

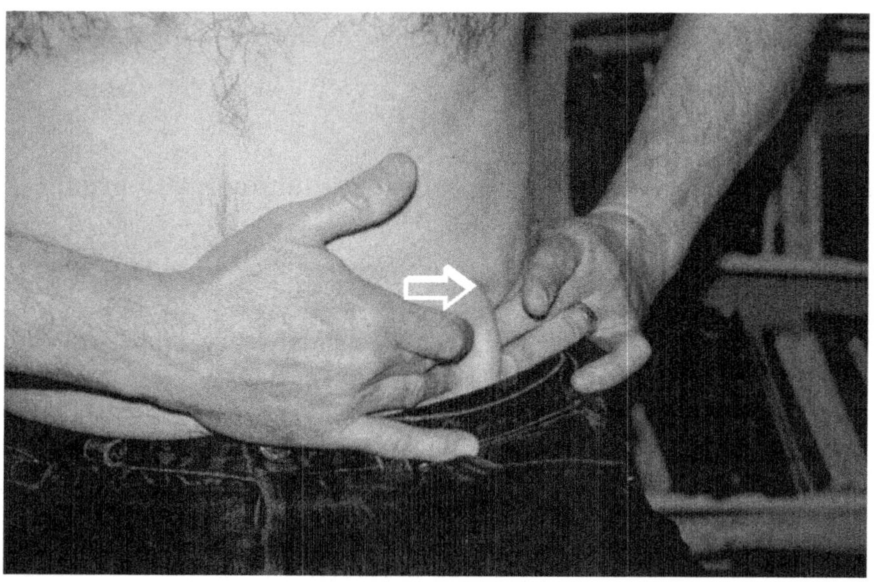

FIGURE 14.2 FAILOR'S PANCREATIC TECHNIQUE—
TISSUE PULL FROM RIGHT TO LEFT WITH THE FINGERS OF THE RIGHT HAND

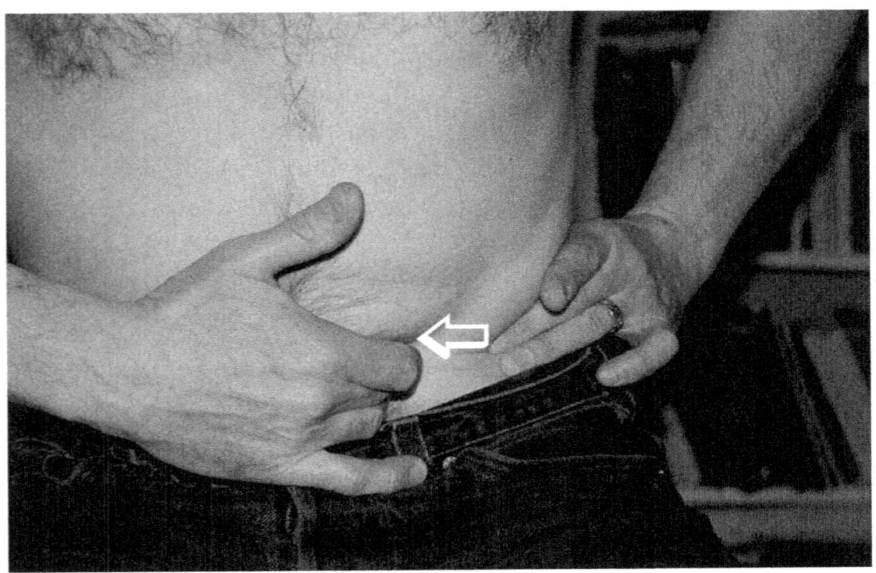

FIGURE 14.3 FAILOR'S PANCREATIC TECHNIQUE—LET THE TISSUE RECOIL FROM LEFT TO RIGHT

Pancreatic Enzyme Replacement

Two main approaches are available. There are several units of measurement for pancreatic enzymes. Pancreatin is derived from porcine pancreas and is active at an alkaline pH. It is taken with or after meals. *Remington's Science and Practice of Pharmacy* defines pancreatin as containing no less than 2 U of lipase, 25 U of amylase and 25 U of protease. Higher potencies are noted by multiples such as 4X or 8X. Pancrealipase is defined as containing not less than 24 U of lipase, 100 U of amylase and 100 U of protease. These are taken after meals because their activity begins in the duodenum.

Plant enzymes are derived from Aspergillus niger, so they are fungal enzymes, but the term "fungal" is often considered undesirable by consumers. Various formulations may also contain lactase, cellulase, sucrase and maltase. These are active at a pH range of 2-12 and taken before meals to take advantage of their gastric action.

Papain, derived from Carica papaya, and bromelain, derived from Ananas comosus, are also excellent sources of plant proteases.

My approach to enzyme replacement for pancreatic insufficiency is to have the patient perform serial trials of various blends of plant enzymes at increasing doses before meals. If significant improvement in symptoms is not experienced, I ask them to try various blends of pancreatin after meals in increasing dosage. Finding the right formula and dosage for each patient can make the difference between success and failure. Do not let the patient give up on pancreatic replacement therapy after trying one or two products. If the diagnosis is definitive, significant improvement can be achieved by matching the patient with the right blend of enzymes.

TABLE 14.5 COMPARISON OF PORCINE AND PLANT ENZYMES

Enzyme	Source	pH range	Digestion begins	When taken
Pancreatin	Porcine	6.8 – 8.0	In the duodenum	pc
Plant enzymes	Aspergillus	2-12	In the stomach	ac

Organotherapy

Homeopathically prepared pancreas (pancreatinum) or vagus nerve (nervinum vagum) may be used to stimulate exocrine pancreatic function.

Antioxidant Nutrition

Patients with moderate to severe chronic pancreatitis were found to have significantly lower mean selenium levels than controls.[18] Those with alcoholism induced chronic pancreatitis had significantly reduced levels of vitamin E, vitamin A, selenium, and plasma glutathione peroxidase compared to controls with similar dietary intakes of these nutrients.[19]

1 Vsterhus, M et al, *Diabetes Care.* 2008 Feb;31(2):306-10.
2 Hardt PD et al, *Dig Dis Sci.* 2003 Sep;48(9):1688-92.
3 Love JW. Peptic ulceration may be a hormonal deficiency disease. *Med Hypotheses.* 2008;70(6):1103-7.
4 Wasielica-Berger J et al, Exocrine pancreatic function in biliary tract pathology treated with the endoscopic methods. *Adv Med Sci.* 2007;52:222-7
5 Shamychkova AA, Nikushkin EV, The activity of gastrointestinal enzymes in chronic viral hepatitis B and C. *Klin Lab Diagn.* 2006 Mar;(3):16-8.
6 Carroccio A et al, Exocrine pancreatic function in children with coeliac disease before and after a gluten free diet. *Gut.* 1991 Jul;32(7):796-9.
7 Leeds JS et al, Is exocrine pancreatic insufficiency in adult coeliac disease a cause of persisting symptoms? *Aliment Pharmacol Ther.* 2007 Feb 1;25(3):265-71.
8 Freeman HJ, Kim YS,, Seisenger MH. Protein digestion and absorption in man. Normal mechanisms and protein-energy malnutrition. *Am J Med.* 1979 Dec;67(6): 1030-6.
9 Freeman HJ. Pancreatic endocrine and exocrine changes in celiac disease.*World J Gastroenterol.* 2007 Dec 21;13(47):6344-6.
10 Nousia-Arvanitakis S et al, Subclinical exocrine pancreatic dysfunction resulting from decreased cholecystokinin secretion in the presence of intestinal villous atrophy. *J Pediatr Gastroenterol Nutr.* 2006 Sep;43(3):307-12.
11 Hilgendorf I et al, Estradiol has a direct impact on the exocrine pancreas as demonstrated by enzyme and vigilin expression. *Pancreatology.* 2001;1(1):24-9.
12 de Dios I, Manso MA, Calvo JJ Alterations of pancreatic juice amylase by glucocorticoid levels in the rat. *Biochem Med Metab Biol.* 1988 Aug;40(1):76-85.
13 Swali A et al, 11beta-Hydroxysteroid dehydrogenase type 1 regulates insulin and glucagon secretion in pancreatic islets. *Diabetologia.* 2008 Nov;51(11):2003-11.
14 Morales-Miranda A, Robles-Díaz G, Díaz-Sánchez V. Steroid hormones and pancreas: a new paradigm] *Rev Invest Clin.* 2007 Mar-Apr;59(2):124-9.
15 Domínguez-Muñoz JE et al, Pancreatic enzyme therapy for pancreatic exocrine insufficiency. *Curr Gastroenterol Rep.* 2007 Apr;9(2):116-22.
16 Mizushima T et al, Pancreatic enzyme supplement improves dysmotility in chronic pancreatitis patients. *J Gastroenterol Hepatol.* 2004 Sep;19(9):1005-9.
17 Kampa nis, P et al *Ann Clin Biochem.* 2008 Nov 13. [Epub ahead of print]
18 Vaona B, Stanzial AM, Talamini G, Bovo P, Corrocher R, Cavallini G, Serum selenium concentrations in chronic pancreatitis and controls. *Dig Liver Dis.* 2005 Jul;37(7):522-5
19 Van Gossum A, Closset P, Noel E, Cremer M, Neve J. Deficiency in antioxidant factors in patients with alcohol-related chronic pancreatitis. *Dig Dis Sci.* 1996 Jun;41(6):1225-31.
20 Raphael KL et al, Pancreatic Insufficiency Secondary to Tobacco Exposure: A Controlled Cross-Sectional Evaluation. *Pancreas.* 2017 Feb;46(2):237-243.
21 Whalen MB, Massidda O. Helicobacter pylori: enemy, commensal or, sometimes, friend? *J Infect Dev Ctries*, 2015 Jul 4;9(6):674-8.
22 Campbell JA et al, Should we Investigate Gastroenterology Patients for Pancreatic Exocrine Insufficiency? A Dual Centre UK Study. *J Gastrointestin Liver Dis.* 2016 Sep;25(3):303-9.

23 Haas S et al, Altered bone metabolism and bone density in patients with chronic pancreatitis and pancreatic exocrine insufficiency. *JOP*. 2015 Jan 31;16(1):58-62.
24 Mann ST et al, Fecal elastase 1 and vitamin D3 in patients with osteoporotic bone fractures. *Eur J Med Res*. 2008 Feb 25;13(2):68-72

Chapter 15

Ileocecal Valve Syndrome (ICVS)

Anatomy And Physiology Of The Valve

The ileocecal valve (ICV) is located in the last several centimeters of the ileum. This area contracts to slow chyme from entering the cecum and prevents reflux of colonic contents into the terminal ileum. It is a thickening of the circular muscle layer with an architecture of anastomosing cords.[1] A study of seven fresh ICV specimens revealed the gross structure to be an intussusception of terminal ileum into the cecum.[2] Both the muscular and mucosal layers of the terminal ileum fold into the cecal wall.

As is true for all GI sphincters, the resting state is tonic. Relaxation occurs during the gastroileac reflex. Cecal distention or irritation increases the tone of this region, hence the tendency for acute appendicitis to cause constipation. This cecoileal excitatory reflex helps to prevent cecoileal reflux.[3] Similar to the lower esophageal longitudinal muscles and lower esophageal sphincter's action on esophageal reflux of gastric contents, the distal ileum muscles contract and the ICV transiently relaxes to clear reflux of colonic contents from the small intestine. This function of preventing reflux of large bowel flora is thought to be important for decreasing the risk of small intestinal bacterial overgrowth (see Chapter 6).[4] Short chain fatty acids in the distal ileum—when sensed by endocrine cells or vagal afferents—trigger this clearance mechanism.[5] Ehlers-Danlos Syndrome —Joint Hypermobility Type is associated with an increased incidence of a hypotonic ('open") ICV.

The ileocecal region is essential to immune control. In neoplasia, lymphoid infiltration of the terminal ileum may lead to an altered mucin secretion and protect against invasive and metastatic processes in the proximal colon.[6] Bazar and Lee at San Mateo Medical Center wrote the following explanation of this region's role in immune surveillance:

> Neural systems are the traditional model of intelligence. Their complex interconnected network of wired neurons acquires, processes, and responds to environmental cues. We propose that the immune system is a parallel system of intelligence in which the gut, including the appendix, plays a prominent role in data acquisition. The immune system is essentially a virtual unwired network of interacting cells that acquires, processes, and responds to environmental data. The data is typically acquired by antigen-presenting cells (APCs) that gather antigenic information from the environment. The APCs chemically digest large antigens and deconstruct them into smaller data packets for sampling by other cells. The gut performs the same function on a larger scale. Morsels of environmental content that enter the gut are sequentially deconstructed by physical and chemical digestion. In addition to providing nutrients, the componentized contents offer environmental data to APCs in mucosa-associated lymphoid tissues (MALT) that relay the sampled information to the immune intelligence network. In this framework, positioning of the appendix immediately after the ileocecal valve is strategic: it is ideally positioned to sample environmental data in its maximally deconstructed state after small bowel digestion. For single-celled organisms, digestion of the environment has been the primary way to sample the surroundings. Prior to the emergence of complex sensory systems such as the eye, even multi-cellular organisms may have relied heavily on digestion to acquire environmental information. While the relative value of immune intelligence has diminished since the emergence of neural intelligence, organisms still

use information from both systems in integrated fashion to respond appropriately to ecologic opportunities and challenges.[7]

This view of the ICV and terminal ileum fits in well with the function of the vermiform appendix as a "safe house" for commensal bacteria. In the event of purging of the intestinal tract in response to a pathogen, re-inoculation of the gut takes place from the appendiceal flora.[8]

The Ileocecal Valve Syndrome

Dysfunctional motility or tonicity of the ileocecal valve leads to the ileocecal valve syndrome (ICVS). The valve may be hypertonic—"spastic" or "closed", or hypotonic—"open"—which may predispose to small intestine bacterial overgrowth.

According to Francis and Walther, clues that should put this syndrome in your differential diagnosis are acute onset of pain, inflammation or swelling anywhere in the body which has not been preceded by a traumatic event.

Etiology Of ICVS

Inciting causes may include dehydration, pregnancy (progesterone relaxes smooth muscle), intestinal dysbiosis, parasites anywhere in the body, unresolved emotions/sympathetic dominance, food intolerances and irritant foods. Francis uses the mnemonic DAPEs representing D–diet, A–allergy, P–parasites, E–emotions. Systemic symptoms are theorized to be due to fluid retention as an adaptive response to toxicity.[9] I believe that systemic symptoms may also stem from small intestinal bacterial overgrowth secondary to cecoileal reflux.

Clinical Picture Of ICVS

Local symptoms include right or left upper quadrant pain, right lower quadrant pain, nausea, diarrhea or constipation. Referred pain may be right shoulder "bursitis", carpal tunnel syndrome, low back pain, headache or non-cardiac chest pain.

Systemic symptoms include a viral-like syndrome with general achiness, stiff neck, arthritis, tinnitus, dizziness—especially mid-afternoon—syncope, near syncope, dependent edema, halitosis, facial pallor, and dark circles under the eyes.

Table 15.1 "Open" And "Closed" Forms Of ICVS (After Francis And Walther)	
Open	**Closed**
Associated with the iliacus muscle Associated with C5 and L1 spinal levels Diarrhea is most common Chlorophyll, digestive enzymes or adrenal gland supplements may be needed Patient likely to have relative hypoadrenia	Associated with the quadriceps muscle group Associated with C3 and L3 spinal levels Constipation is most common Calcium, vitamin D, HCl or choline supplements may be required Patient is likely to have relative hyperadrenia Symptoms aggravated if patient "sleeps in" Pains improve after rising with activity Pains improve after a bowel movement

Indicators Of ICVS

Muscle Testing For An "Open" Ileocecal Valve

Test the iliacus muscle with the patient supine. Have the foot externally rotated and elevate the patient's leg 6-8 inches above the table. Stabilize

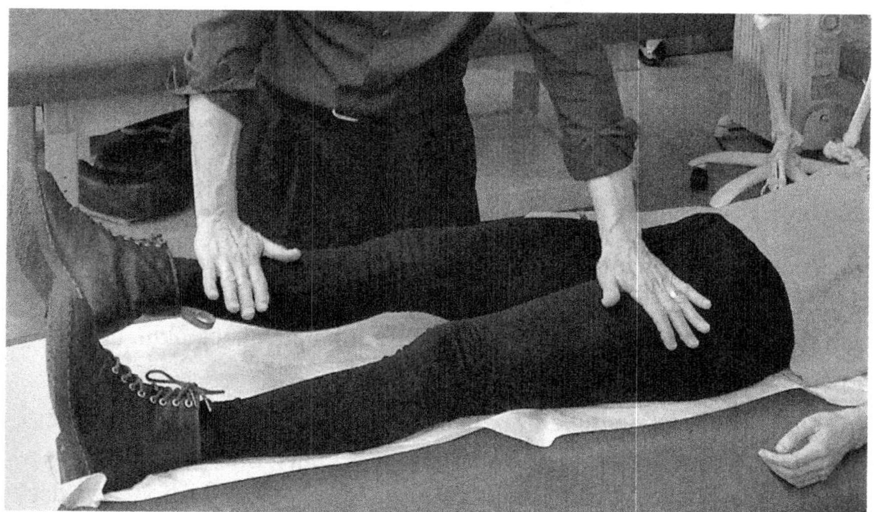

Figure 15.1 Iliacus Test For An "Open" Valve

the contralateral hip just inferior to the ASIS. The physician presses down toward the table with a contact just above the medial malleolus while the patient resists (attempts to keep the leg from being moved.) Note: The patient must keep the knee extended during the test. Also, consider that the iliacus is a small muscle and the physician is pushing at the end of a long lever, so push gradually and with moderate force so as not to overpower the muscle. A solid locking of the muscle is a negative test. This test should be performed bilaterally. If either test reveals a weak muscle it indicates a possible "open" ileocecal valve.

Muscle Testing For A "Closed" Ileocecal Valve

To test the quadriceps as a group, again the patient is in a supine position, but for this test the patient has both knees flexed and the feet flat on the

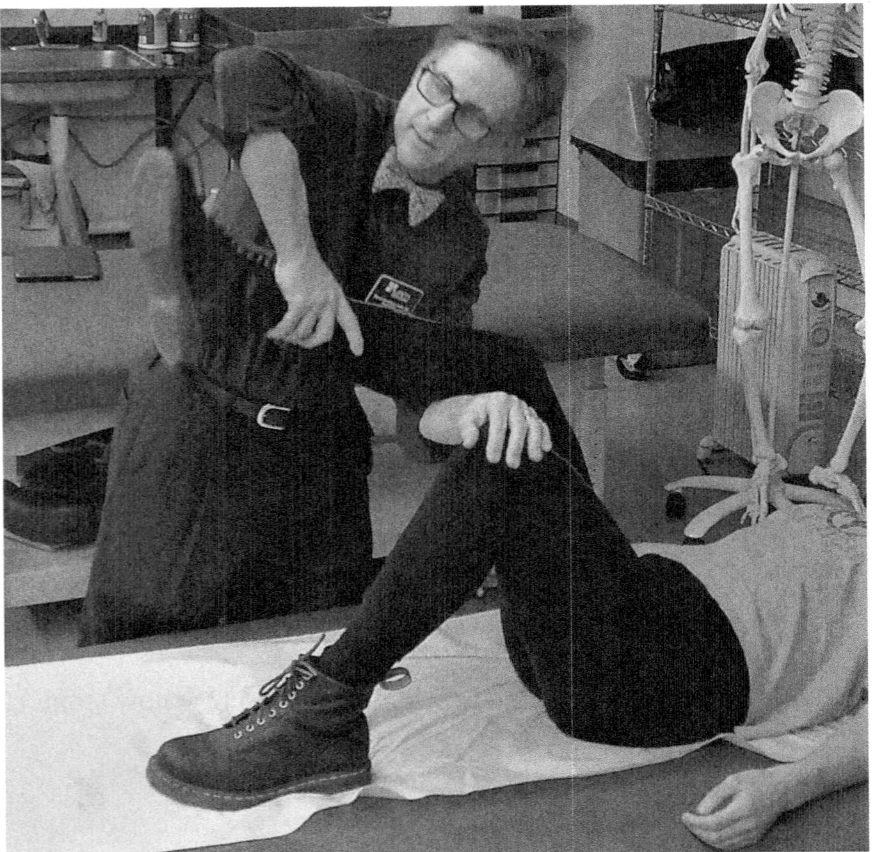

Figure 15.2 Quadriceps Test For A "Closed" Valve

table. To test the right leg the doctor reaches under the right knee and puts the palm of her left hand on the patient's left patella. Extending the right knee greater than 90 degrees, instruct the patient to resist your force as you push the right leg—contact just above the ankle—down in an arc toward the patient's buttocks. The quadriceps should be tested with full pressure, keeping the physician's shoulder directly above the line of force. This test should be performed bilaterally. If either test reveals a weak muscle it indicates a possible "closed" ileocecal valve.

Confirming The Testing When A Weak Iliacus Or Quadriceps Is Found

1) Instruct the patient to make a loose fist with the right hand. Place the patient's right hand over the RLQ (McBurney's point) and the patient's open left palm on top of the positioned right hand.

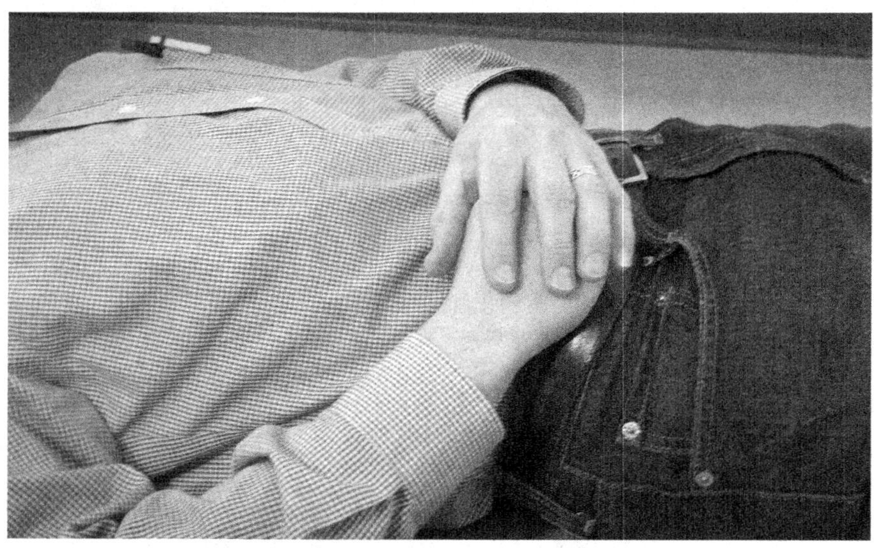

FIGURE 15.3 PATIENT'S HAND POSITION FOR ICVS CONFIRMATION

2) Retest the previously weak muscle. If the muscle is now stronger, you have confirmed ICVS.

Treatment Of ICVS

Visceral manipulation

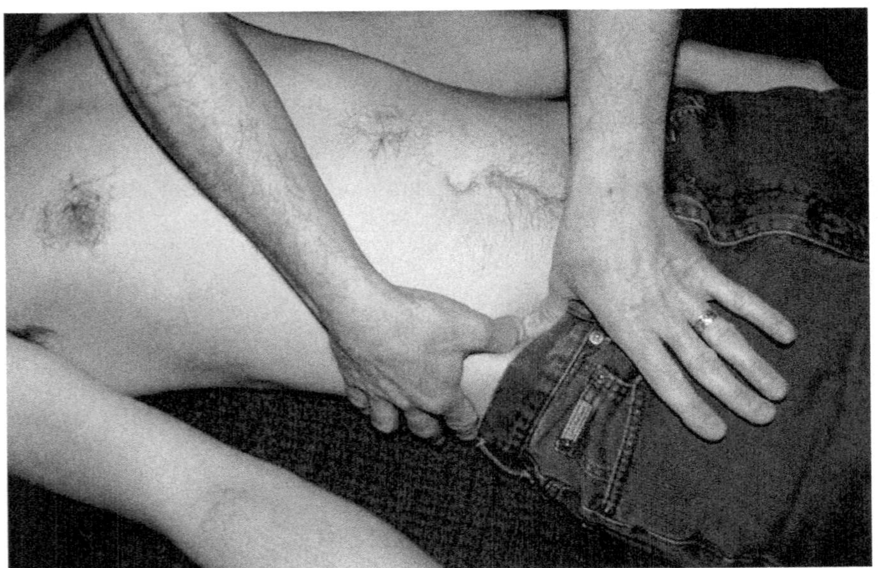

FIGURE 15.4 VISCERAL MANEUVER FOR ICVS

Using the pads of your thumbs or other digits, roll the tissue immediately superior to the inguinal ligament in an anterior to posterior and superior arc, searching for trigger points from the iliac crest to the pubic symphysis. "Pin" the tissue in that position and hold it while the patient elongates his leg through the heel (extended knee, dorsiflexed foot) and instruct him to slowly rotate the knee internally and then externally. The range of motion that increases the patient's tenderness beneath your fingers is the most efficient movement to release the trigger point. It may take one or two minutes for the tenderness to decrease at each point you treat. Clear all tender points along the iliac-pubic ramus.

Note: This region may be very tender to palpation. When acute, appendicitis, Crohn's disease, salpingitis, ovarian cyst, and ectopic pregnancy are in the differential. If organic disease is present, the tenderness/pain will not abate and symptoms may increase with this technique. This is a red flag that pathology must be ruled out.

Spinal Manipulative Therapy

C3-5 and L1-3 are spinal segments often needing attention in patients with ICVS. Use your typical thorough spinal exam with special attention to fixations or dysarticulations at these levels.

Diet

Temporary guidelines to consider during the acute stage of symptoms include avoidance of:

- High fiber and irritant foods: popcorn, chips, pretzels, nuts, seeds, whole grains
- Raw fruits and vegetables
- Strong spices such as chili, black and cayenne pepper
- Methyl xanthines such as coffee, black tea and chocolate
- Alcohol

Nutritional Supplements To Be Considered

- Liquid chlorophyll—1 tablespoon TID ("open" ICV)
- Betaine hydrochloride with pepsin (see Chapter 13)
- Pancreatic enzymes or alternate therapy (see Chapter 14)
- Calcium—400-800 mg in divided doses ("closed" ICV)
- Choline—200-400 mg per day
- Adrenal support

1 Faussone-Pellegrini MS, Pantalone D, Cortesini C. Morphological evidence for a cecocolonic junction in man and its functional implications. *Acta Anat (Basel).* 1993;146(1):22-30.

2 Awapittaya B et al, New concept of ileocecal junction: Intussusception of the terminal ileum into the cecum. World J Gastroenterol 2007; 13(20): 2855-2857.

3 Shafik A et al, Assessment of the function of the ileocecal junction with evidence of ileocecal reflexes. *Med Sci Monit.* 2002 Sep;8(9):CR629-35AA.

4 Quigley EM, Phillips SF. The Ileocecal (ileocolonic) sphincter. *Z Gastroenterol.* 1983 Feb;21(2):47-55.

5 Malbert, CH *Neurogastroenterol Motil.* 2005 Jun;17 Suppl 1:41-9.

6 Honma K. Mucin histochemical analysis of the ileocecal valve and lymphoid tissues of the terminal ileum: role against tumour invasion. *Asian J Surg.* 2002 Jul;25(3): 220-5.

7 Bazar KA, Lee PY, Joon Yun A. An "eye" in the gut: The appendix as a senitinel sensory organ of the immune intelligence network. *Med Hypotheses.* 2004;63(4):752-8

8 Randal Bollinger R et al, Biofilms in the large bowel suggest an apparent function of the human vermiform appendix. *J Theor Biol.* 2007 Dec 21;249(4):826-31.

9 Walther, D (2000). *Applied Kinesiology*. Pueblo, Colorado. Systems DC.

Index

A

B

C

D

E

H

I

K

L

M

N

O

P

T

U

V

W

Y

Z

About The Author

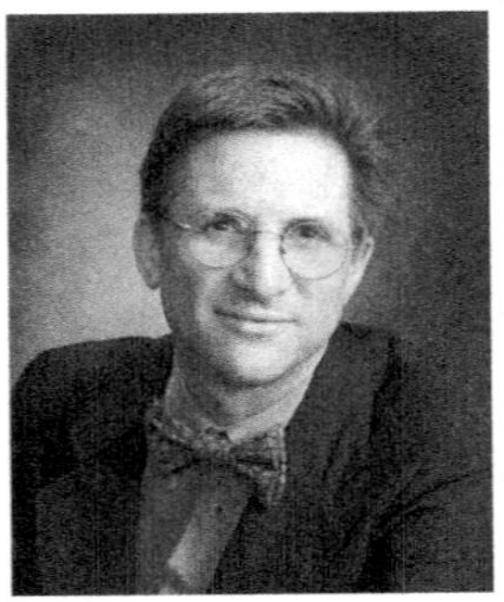

Dr. Steven Sandberg-Lewis has been a practicing naturopathic physician for nearly 40 years in the Pacific Northwest region of the USA and a professor at the National University of Natural Medicine (NUNM) in Portland, Oregon since 1985. In 2010 he co-founded the SIBO Center at NUNM which is one of only four centers in the USA for Small Intestine Bacterial Overgrowth diagnosis, treatment, education and research.

Within gastroenterology he has special interest and expertise in inflammatory bowel disease (including microscopic colitis), irritable bowel syndrome (including post-infectious IBS), Small Intestine Bacterial Overgrowth (SIBO), hiatal hernia, gastroesophageal and bile reflux (GERD), biliary dyskinesia, and chronic states of nausea and vomiting.

Dr. Sandberg-Lewis receives referrals of patients with digestive diseases who desire naturopathic treatment options; and often these are conditions that have defied diagnosis or effective resolution by other physicians. He understands the diseases of the gastrointestinal tract, but also can assess function and often find successful treatments to regain a balance in the digestive system.

In addition to supervising clinical rotations at the NUNM Health Center, as a full-time faculty member, Dr. Sandberg-Lewis teaches gastroenterology, advanced gastroenterology and GI physical medicine practicum at NUNM. He also maintains a part-time practice at 8 Hearts Health and Wellness in Portland, Oregon. He lectures frequently at functional medicine seminars, presents webinars and is frequently interviewed on issues of digestive health and disease. He is the author or co-author of several *Townsend Letter* award winning articles (Hiatal Hernia Syndrome, Dysbiosis Has a New Name, Small Intestine Bacterial Overgrowth: Common but Overlooked Cause of IBS) and the author of the medical textbook *Functional Gastroenterology: Assessing and Addressing the Causes of Functional Digestive Disorders*. In 2014 he was named one of the "Top Docs" in Portland monthly magazines yearly healthcare issue and in 2015 was inducted into the OANP/NUNM Hall of Fame.

Dr. Sandberg-Lewis lives in Portland with his wife, Kayle. His interests include mandolin, guitar and voice; cross country skiing; writing and lecturing.

CPSIA information can be obtained
at www.ICGtesting.com
Printed in the USA
FSOW03n1557020817
37153FS

9 780692 864661